FAT-SOLUBLE VITAMIN ASSAYS IN FOOD ANALYSIS

A Comprehensive Review

FAT-SOLUBLE VITAMIN ASSAYS IN FOOD ANALYSIS

A Comprehensive Review

G. F. M. Ball

Scientific Services Division, J Sainsbury plc, London, UK

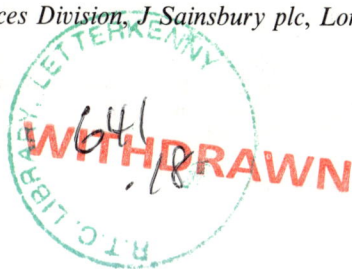

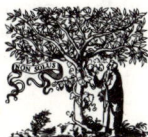

ELSEVIER APPLIED SCIENCE
LONDON and NEW YORK

ELSEVIER SCIENCE PUBLISHERS LTD
Crown House, Linton Road, Barking, Essex IG11 8JU, England

Sole Distributor in the USA and Canada
ELSEVIER SCIENCE PUBLISHING CO., INC.
52 Vanderbilt Avenue, New York, NY 10017, USA

WITH 30 TABLES AND 122 ILLUSTRATIONS

© 1988 ELSEVIER SCIENCE PUBLISHERS LTD

British Library Cataloguing in Publication Data

Ball, G. F. M.
  Fat-soluble vitamin assays in food analysis.
  1. Food. Fat-soluble vitamins. Analysis
  I. Title
  641.1′8

Library of Congress Cataloging in Publication Data

Ball, G. F. M.
  Fat-soluble vitamin assays in food analysis.

  Bibliography: p.
  1. Vitamins, Fat-soluble. 2. Food—Vitamin content.
  3. Food—Composition. I. Title.
  TX553.V5B35 1988   641.1′8   88-16541

ISBN 1-85166-239-1

Printed in Great Britain by Galliard (Printers) Ltd, Great Yarmouth

Foreword

The estimation of vitamin content presents special problems. Almost always, in natural products, several vitamers, each able to act as the vitamin, may be present. All the functions of Vitamin A, for instance, may be met not only by the parent alcohol, retinol, but also by numerous related compounds, which vary very much in quantitative activity, stability and other properties. The Vitamin A active compounds include the related retinaldehyde, and numerous esters typified by the acetate and palmitate, as well as various isomers and homologues. The estimation of vitamin activity is often complicated by the presence of provitamins. Many carotenoids for instance, may, depending on their chemical structures, be converted into retinol in the body and so act as provitamin A. The efficacy of this conversion is related not only to the structure of the carotenoid itself, but also to the extent to which it is released from the plant cells of the ingested food. The biological value of the vitamers may also depend on other factors. The absorption of retinol, and hence its bioactivity, is for instance, much greater from aqueous dispersions than from oily solutions.

Over the last fifty years there have been major advances in many fields of analytical chemistry, but in none more so than in vitamin assays. Tests which once took weeks are now easily completed within the working day. Preliminary isolations have developed from simple extractions and phase separations to swift and powerful chromatographic methods. Measurement techniques have changed from laborious bioassays through rapid microbiological, titrimetric, colorimetric and spectrophotometric procedures, while mass spectrometry awaits routine application.

Previous difficulties may be judged by the Vitamin D bioassay which for over three decades, from the 1930s to the 1960s, was the only procedure capable of estimating Vitamin D in foods as opposed to concentrated

v

pharmaceutical preparations. The test involved dosing groups of specially bred animals (rats or chicks)—in all about 50 animals—over a period of two weeks, with subsequent evaluation of bone healing by visual assessment of X-ray photographs or silver stained bones. This assay was the first to which statistical evaluation and calculation of fiducial limits was applied. Though one of the more precise of the bioassays, the fiducial limits were seldom less than $\pm 30\%$ even when the vitamin D potency was within the anticipated range. The statistical evaluations, which are now carried out instantly by computer, then required painstaking calculations with the aid of log tables!

The assessment of vitamin activity for Vitamin A, Vitamin D, Vitamin E and Vitamin K in foods and concentrates is even now seldom a simple matter. The separate estimation of several vitamers, provitamins and previtamins may be essential, often with the application of officially recognised conversion factors derived from the results of nutritional investigations.

This comprehensive review is opportune because of the presently increasing public interest in nutrition and the consequent demand for more informative food labelling. The critical evaluation and comparison of the numerous published methods will be of great assistance to all concerned with food analyses and their interpretation. The manuscript has also given great pleasure to one who, in the past, spent long hours in laborious, but fascinating tasks which could now be completed in but a fraction of the time then needed.

W. F. J. CUTHBERTSON, OBE

Preface

The object of this book is to provide a comprehensive survey of physico-chemical methods for determining the fat-soluble vitamins in foods and feedstuffs.

I have tried to bear in mind the requirements of the analytical chemist, food scientist and research worker who is concerned with vitamin assays in foods or feeds. I hope to supply such readers with the present state of knowledge of the subject, and to enable the analyst to select or develop a suitable assay technique.

As to the scope of the book, chapter two (which follows the introduction) sets out to acquaint the reader with a brief account of the chemical, physical, and biological properties of vitamins A, D, E and K. These fat-soluble vitamins are notoriously prone to decomposition when exposed to oxygen, heat and light, hence factors affecting their stability are given special attention. The biological properties of the vitamins illustrate that they are physiological substances which are essential in maintaining normal health. A detailed discussion of bioassays is beyond the scope of this book, since bioassays are of limited use, and most laboratories do not maintain the personnel or facilities for their evaluation.

In the subsequent chapters, I have attempted to explain the basic principles of the various techniques encountered in vitamin assays and, by reference to representative published methods, to illustrate and discuss the applications of these techniques. Thus the first step in a vitamin assay is to extract the vitamin from the bulk of the food or feed matrix, and to obtain a vitamin-rich fraction. Purification of the vitamin-rich fraction may then be necessary before quantification of the vitamin(s) can be performed.

Purification procedures rely largely upon some form of chromatography, whilst the quantification procedures discussed range from older, well-established techniques, such as colorimetry and spectrophotometry, to sophisticated modern techniques, particularly high-performance liquid chromatography.

I have described the older purification and quantification procedures because they dominate many of the official fat-soluble vitamin assay methods to the present day, and because most of the vitamin data in food compositional tables have been obtained using such procedures. Therefore, techniques such as gravity-flow column chromatography and thin-layer chromatography, used in conjunction with colorimetry or spectrophotometry, may be required for certain analyses, and are of necessity where laboratory resources are restricted.

The emphasis of the book is, inevitably, upon the application of high-performance liquid chromatography to the determination of fat-soluble vitamins in foods and feeds, since this technique has emerged as the method of choice for the foreseeable future.

I would like to acknowledge the support of Dr Roy Spencer, Director of Scientific Services, J Sainsbury plc, throughout the construction of this book.

For the preparation of the manuscript, I am indebted to Mrs Ruth Harrisson, proprietor of Action Desk.

I am grateful to Mr Martin Clemance of BDH Ltd for providing the ultraviolet absorption spectra of the vitamins, and to Dr Steve Upstone of Perkin Elmer Ltd for the spectra of other lipids. The fluorescence spectra of vitamins A and E were kindly provided by Dr Mark Upton of Perkin Elmer Ltd.

Dr Stuart Jones, Director of Laserchrom Analytical Ltd, injected enthusiastic advice, and the Vitamin and Chemical Division of Roche Products Ltd contributed useful additional material.

G. F. M. Ball

Contents

Chapter 1

Introduction

Definitions of vitamins, provitamins and vitamers

Vitamins are organic micro-nutrients that occur naturally in foods, and that are essential in maintaining normal health. Lack of a vitamin produces a specific deficiency syndrome, and supplying it prevents and cures this deficiency. Vitamins may be conveniently divided into two distinct groups based upon their solubility characteristics. The fat-soluble vitamins (A, D, E and K) dissolve readily in fat and in non-polar organic solvents, whilst the water-soluble vitamins (B-complex and C) dissolve readily in aqueous solutions. The fat-soluble vitamins form the subject of this literature review.

Many definitions of vitamins state that they cannot be produced in the body and must, therefore, be supplied in the diet. This definition is valid for vitamins A and E, but is not strictly true for vitamins D and K, which can also be obtained from non-dietary sources. Vitamin D can be formed in the skin upon adequate exposure to sunlight, whilst vitamin K is normally produced in sufficient amounts by intestinal bacteria.

Vitamin A is implicated in the physiology of vision as a part of the visual pigment, rhodopsin; the vitamin is also essential in maintaining normal cell growth and differentiation in epithelial tissues and in bone. Vitamin D is a precursor of a hormone involved in the regulation of calcium and phosphorus metabolism; vitamin E acts as an antioxidant in stabilizing unsaturated lipids in biological membranes; and vitamin K is involved in the synthesis of blood clotting factors.

Provitamins are vitamin precursors, i.e. naturally occurring substances which are not themselves vitamins, but which can be converted by normal body metabolism into vitamins. Provitamin A carotenoids refer to those carotenoids (e.g. α-, β-, γ-carotene and β-cryptoxanthin) that exhibit

1

vitamin A activity due to their conversion in the intestine or liver to retinol via retinaldehyde. Provitamin D_3 refers to 7-dehydrocholesterol which occurs in the animal's skin and its secretions and which, under the influence of ultraviolet light, is converted to an intermediate compound, previtamin D_3, and thence, under the influence of body heat, to cholecalciferol (vitamin D_3). The corresponding plant provitamin, ergosterol, gives rise to ergocalciferol (vitamin D_2) by a similar process.

For each of the fat-soluble vitamins, vitamin activity is attributed to a number of structurally related compounds known as vitamers. The vitamers display, in most cases, similar biological properties for a given parent vitamin but, because of subtle chemical differences, exhibit varying degrees of potency. The vitamers of vitamin A comprise retinol (vitamin A_1), 3-dehydroretinol (vitamin A_2), retinaldehyde and the various *cis-trans* isomers of these compounds. Ergocalciferol and cholecalciferol, together with their respective previtamin isomers, are vitamers of vitamin D.

The most active vitamin E vitamer, α-tocopherol, is accompanied in plant sources by the various tocopherol and tocotrienol vitamers of lower vitamin E activity. Vitamin K vitamers occur as phylloquinone (vitamin K_1) and the various analogues of menaquinone (vitamin K_2).

Why fortify foods with vitamins?
Reasons for fortifying foods with fat-soluble vitamins are presented below:

(i)   Revitaminization; to replace vitamins removed or destroyed during food processing. For instance, the removal of cream from milk takes almost all of the natural vitamins A and D with it. Therefore, skimmed milk may be fortified to the same vitamin levels as fluid whole milk.

(ii)   Standardization; to compensate for natural fluctuations in vitamin content. For instance, milk and butter are subject to seasonal variations in the vitamin A and D contents. Some dairy products are fortified with vitamins A and D in order to maintain constant vitamin levels.

(iii)   Enrichment; addition of vitamins over and above the initial natural levels to make a product more marketable by being fortified (e.g. breakfast cereals).

(iv)   Vitaminization; addition of vitamins to foods which represent ideal carriers for a particular vitamin, but which do not necessarily contain that vitamin naturally. For instance, margarine is fortified with vitamins A and D to render it nutritionally equivalent to butter.

(v) To perform specific processing functions. For instance, β-carotene (the principal source of dietary vitamin A) is added to products such as pasta, margarine, cakes and processed cheeses to impart colour. Vitamin E can be used as an antioxidant to stabilize pure oils and fats, including margarines.

Vitamins A, D, E and K, and certain provitamin A carotenoids (e.g. β-carotene), can be economically synthesized on an industrial scale. The use of synthetic vitamins is now the predominant practice in human and animal nutrition, as well as in pharmaceutical products. The synthetic forms have a high degree of purity, and, unlike vitamin-rich natural materials, are able to meet the critical requirements of modern processing industries. The instability of the pure vitamins towards oxygen, heat, light and adverse pH is overcome by the synthesis of stable ester derivatives or the preparation of formulations containing antioxidants and/or protective coatings such as gelatin.

Fat-soluble vitamins are nowadays added to margarine, milk products, breakfast cereals, infant formula foods and dietetic foods. Although it is not possible experimentally to determine the precise vitamin requirements of man, certain quantities of each vitamin have been shown to be necessary for the maintenance of good health. Recommended Dietary Allowances (RDA) have been derived after assessment of human epidemiological and experimental animal studies. In the United Kingdom and in the United States, figures for RDAs have been published by the Department of Health and Social Security (DHSS) and the National Research Council (NRC), respectively. Other international bodies such as the Food and Agricultural Organization (FAO) of the United Nations have compiled similar recommendations. The Ministry of Agriculture, Fisheries and Food (MAFF) in the United Kingdom proposed in 1985 that the nutrient levels stated on food labels should be expressed in terms of the RDA for each nutrient. Thus the addition of vitamins to a certain food is designed to provide a specific proportion of the RDA.

Why analyse foods for vitamins?
Vitamin determinations in foods are carried out for many purposes.

(i) For legal purposes in connection with nutritional labelling.
(ii) To provide quality assurance for fortified products.

(iii) In food technology it is desirable to know the fate of vitamins during processing, and to study the effects of different types of packaging and storage.

(iv) To assess the effects of geographical, environmental and seasonal conditions.

(v) In nutritional surveys, the vitamin contents of meals at the point of consumption has to be measured.

(vi) The vitamin content of foods has to be determined for establishing food compositional tables.

(vii) Detection of adulteration of certain foods. For instance, knowledge of the distribution of the various tocopherols and tocotrienols that comprise vitamin E in vegetable oils can be utilized for identification and purification assessment.

The role of vitamins in animal nutrition
The intensification of animal production systems is associated with a restriction of a free choice of feed and the increased use of manufactured feeds, a lower feed consumption per unit of production, stress, and the increased susceptibility to infections. Dietary supplementation with vitamins is necessary to overcome the potential risk of vitamin deficiency under such conditions.

Fat-soluble vitamin supplements currently used are (Anon., 1976):

(i) In cattle feeds (for rearing, milk production and fattening) and in milk replacers for calves: A, D_3, E.

(ii) In pig feeds and in milk replacers for piglets: A, D_3, E, K.

(iii) In poultry feeds: A, D_3, E, K.

Bioassays versus physico-chemical assays
It must be appreciated that the term 'vitamin' is a physiological one, rather than a chemical one. Bioassays, using experimental animals, provide a measure of vitamin activity in terms of a particular physiological response, and take into account the combined response of the various vitamers, provitamins, and biologically active metabolites of the vitamin in question. Bioassays also take into account the complexities of absorption, inactivation, metabolism and storage within the particular species of animal tested. Physico-chemical assays permit the quantification of the substances that are responsible for the biological activity but, in many cases, they do not provide values for total vitamin activity. Modern physico-chemical assays, such as high-performance liquid chromatography, permit the distinction between the naturally occurring and the

supplemental forms of vitamins A and E. Thus the analyst is able to report the weight of a given vitamin in its various forms within a food product.

Ideally, all forms of a given vitamin should be assayed separately by chemical means, and the result for each vitamer should be multiplied by its biological activity. Unfortunately, this procedure is not always feasible since the separate determination of each vitamer on a routine basis is not practicable and, in any case, the biological activity in man of many vitamers is not known. A further problem is the varying degree of utilization or bioavailability of the vitamin from different foods. For instance, β-carotene in raw carrots has only a low vitamin A activity, whereas the same compound in oily solution is almost completely transformed to vitamin A. The incomplete utilization of the β-carotene of vegetable origin may be due to the binding of this provitamin to certain parts of the plant cell, and a consequent incomplete liberation of vitamin A in the intestine. This missing information is of concern when the results of chemical assays are used to estimate the nutritional value of food, but is of little concern where the results are used in quality assurance to check fortification levels, or to satisfy legal requirements in connection with nutritional labelling.

Expression of dietary values for the fat-soluble vitamins
In the early days of vitamin assays, when bioassays were the only methods for estimating the vitamin contents of foods, the vitamin activity of a food sample was expressed in International Units (IU), and was determined by comparing the activity in the bioassay with the activity of an official international standard. These standards were single preparations of a compound, either isolated from natural sources or synthesized in the laboratory, and were maintained and distributed by an international agency. The more recent international standards for vitamin A were crystalline β-carotene (provitamin A) and retinyl acetate (preformed vitamin A). For vitamin D the international standard was crystalline cholecalciferol (vitamin D_3) prepared from irradiated 7-dehydrocholesterol. The international standard for vitamin E was a synthetic ester, racemic α-tocopheryl acetate (Bieri & McKenna, 1981). Nowadays, the bioassays are performed using highly pure reference standards, the original international standards being no longer in existence.

A committee of the FAO and the World Health Organization (WHO) in 1965 proposed that the vitamin A value of foods should no longer be expressed in IU. Instead, the value should be designated as the amount of retinol plus the equivalent amount of retinol that can be obtained from the provitamin A carotenoids. The total would be termed the 'retinol equivalent' and would be expressed in micrograms. Bieri & McKenna (1981) pointed out that the term 'retinol equivalent' is a dietary concept for estimating the vitamin A activity in foods, and is not an equivalency in the usual chemical sense. The term, therefore, applies specifically to retinol or the provitamin A carotenoids; retinoic acid, for example, cannot be expressed as a retinol equivalent. Thompson (1986) warned that the retinol equivalent, whilst being appropriate for human nutrition, is not always applicable in animal nutrition.

In 1970, another joint FAO/WHO report recommended that the intake of vitamin D be expressed as μg of cholecalciferol rather than as IU.

In the 1980 edition of the Recommended Dietary Allowances the designation of vitamin E activity has been changed from IU to an expression of equivalents, similar to that used for vitamin A. In this notation, all vitamin E activity is expressed relative to the naturally occurring, most active form of the vitamin, d-α-tocopherol. The total vitamin E activity in a food should be given as mg of d-α-tocopherol equivalent, and would represent the sum of the weight of d-α-tocopherol plus the weights of other vitamers (tocopherols or tocotrienols) after correction to their equivalency as d-α-tocopherol (Bieri & McKenna, 1981).

Chapter 2

Chemical and Biological Nature of the Fat-Soluble Vitamins

2.1 VITAMIN A

Discovery. In 1915 McCollum and Davis isolated 'growth factor A' from animal fats or fish oils, which proved to be essential for the normal development of experimental animals. Vitamin A deficiency was later shown to be responsible for xerophthalmia (non-specific lesions of the eye), and in 1935 Wald established the role of vitamin A in the biochemistry of vision. The provitamin A activity of the plant pigment, β-carotene, was demonstrated by Moore in 1930.

2.1.1 Chemical Structure

Vitamin A-active compounds fall into two basic groups: preformed vitamin A (retinoids) and provitamin A carotenoids.

Preformed vitamin A

The chemical structures of the main vitamin A-active retinoids are shown in Fig. 1. The commonest and most biologically active form of vitamin A is all-*trans*-retinol (vitamin A_1), which comprises a β-ionone ring attached at C-6 to a side chain composed of two unsaturated isoprene units. The four double bonds in the polyene side chain theoretically permit sixteen *cis-trans* isomers of reduced biological activity, but only three of these geometric isomers are free from steric hindrance, and are the 'preferred' structures found in nature. The commonest of the unhindered *cis-trans* isomers is 13-*cis*-retinol; the other two are 9-*cis*- and 9,13-di-*cis*-retinol.

In nature, most of the retinol forms esters with long-chain fatty acids, particularly palmitic acid. Retinyl acetate and retinyl palmitate can be synthesized chemically, and are used commercially to supplement the vitamin A content of foodstuffs.

7

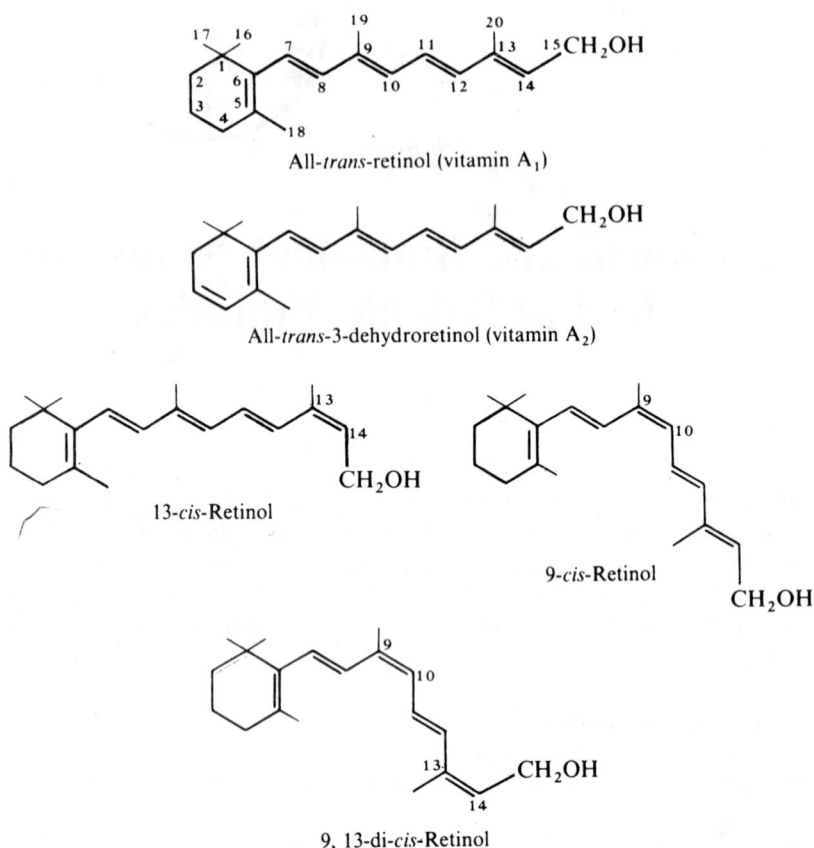

Fig. 1. Chemical structures of the main vitamin A-active retinoids.

3-Dehydroretinol (vitamin A_2) is the main form of vitamin A in the liver and flesh of freshwater fish and has about 40% of the biological activity of all-*trans*-retinol (Sivell *et al.*, 1984).

Provitamin A carotenoids
All vitamin A in nature originates from carotenoids, which are yellow to red pigments responsible for the colour of many vegetables and fruits. Animals are unable to biosynthesize carotenoids, but assimilate them through their diet as a source of vitamin A. Of the five hundred or so naturally occurring carotenoids, about sixty possess vitamin A activity in

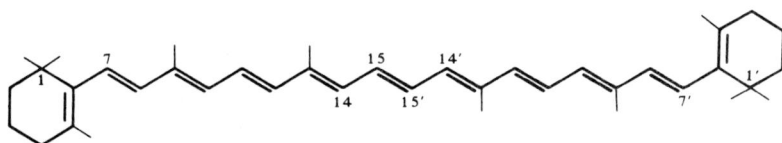

Fig. 2. Chemical structure of β-carotene.

varying degrees, but only five or six of these are commonly found in food (Simpson, 1983). The terms carotenes and xanthophylls designate carotenoid hydrocarbons and oxygenated carotenoids, respectively.

The most common and most active of the provitamin A carotenoids is β-carotene (Fig. 2), which is the main pigment of the carrot root, and is present in all green plant tissues. The biological value of dietary β-carotene varies widely depending upon the efficiency of absorption, but has been taken, on average, as one-sixth of that of all-*trans*-retinol (Bieri & McKenna, 1981). All provitamin A carotenoids are structurally related to one of three carotenes, α-, β- or γ- carotenes, which are derived biosynthetically from a straight-chain carotenoid, lycopene (Fig. 3). β-Carotene is composed of two molecules of retinol joined tail to tail, thus the compound possesses maximal provitamin A activity. The other two active carotenes (α- and γ-) contain one β-ionone ring, hence theoretically contribute 50% of the activity of β-carotene. α-Carotene, which usually accompanies β-carotene, but in smaller amounts, possesses an inactive α-ionone ring; γ-carotene, which is less ubiquitous, possesses only the β-ionone ring.

Other provitamin A carotenoids, which also theoretically possess about 50% of the activity of β-carotene, and which are fairly common in foods, are β-cryptoxanthin, β-carotene-5, 6-epoxide, β-apo-8'-carotenal and β-apo-8'-carotenoic acid ethyl ester (Fig. 4); the substituted rings of the first two mentioned compounds are inactive (Simpson, 1983).

Most naturally occurring carotenoids possess a *trans* configuration for all conjugated double bonds; a few *cis* isomers also exist which possess lower vitamin A activity than the all-*trans* forms.

2.1.2 Natural Occurrence

All sources of vitamin A are derived ultimately from provitamin A carotenoids, which are present in higher plants, and in lower forms of animal and plant life. Humans obtain preformed vitamin A exclusively from animal sources; provitamin A is obtained from plant and certain animal sources.

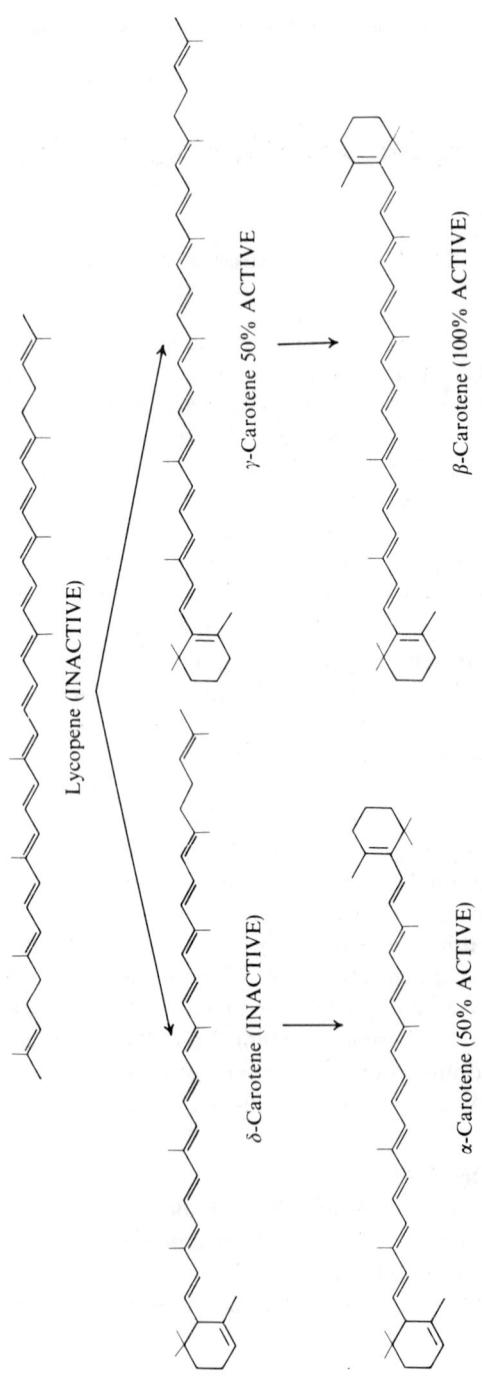

Fig. 3. Part of the biosynthetic pathway of carotenes.

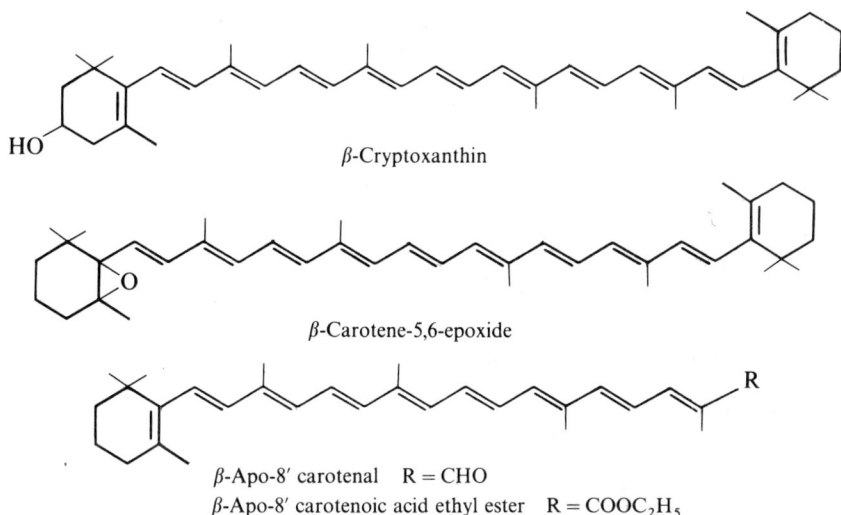

β-Cryptoxanthin

β-Carotene-5,6-epoxide

β-Apo-8′ carotenal   R = CHO
β-Apo-8′ carotenoic acid ethyl ester   R = COOC$_2$H$_5$

Fig. 4.   Chemical structures of some provitamin A carotenoids that occur in foods.

Preformed vitamin A
Animals store vitamin A in the liver, and fish liver oils, particularly halibut liver oil, are especially rich in the vitamin (see Table 1). Vitamin A exists in the liver chiefly as retinyl palmitate, although some unesterified retinol is also present (Holasová & Blattná, 1976).

The distribution of preformed vitamin A in selected foods is given in Table 1. The liver of meat animals is a rich source of the vitamin, and the heart and kidney contain lesser amounts. Whole milk, butter, cheese and eggs provide useful amounts of vitamin A. The edible portion of fatty fish contains moderate amounts of vitamin A, but white fish, apart from the haddock, contain only trace amounts. In most of the above foods the vitamin A occurs mainly as mixed esters of retinol. However, in eggs the unesterified alcohol represents the major form of the vitamin, with retinaldehyde and retinyl esters constituting lesser amounts (Parrish, 1977). *Cis* isomers of vitamin A occur in foods to varying extents, with fish liver oils and eggs containing as much as 35% and 20%, respectively, of their total retinol in this form (Sivell *et al.*, 1984).

Provitamin A carotenoids
Approximately half of the human dietary vitamin A intake is derived from red, yellow and green fruits and vegetables containing α-, β- and γ-carotenes (Hsieh & Karel, 1983). The distribution of vitamin A activity

Table 1
Distribution of preformed vitamin A in foods (typical values)

Food	Vitamin A (μg retinol equivalent per 100 g edible portion)
Animal products	
Liver (sheep and ox)	15 000
Beef, mutton and pork	0–4
Dairy products	
Butter	830
Margarine (fortified with vitamin A)	900
Eggs (fresh, whole)	140
Milk (fresh, whole)	40
Cheese (whole, fatty type)	320
Fatty fish and their oils	
Halibut liver oil	900 000
Cod liver oil	18 000
Herring and mackerel	50
Sardine	Trace

From Passmore, R. & Eastwood, M. A. (1986). *Davidson and Passmore Human Nutrition and Dietetics*, 8th edn. By permission of Churchill Livingstone.

attributable to the provitamin A carotenoids in vegetables and fruits is given in Table 2.

In most vegetables and in many fruits (the major exception being citrus fruits) the majority (85–97%) of all provitamin A activity is due to the *trans* forms of α- and β- carotene, the latter being predominant (Sweeney & Marsh, 1971). The predominant carotenoid in citrus fruits (Stewart, 1977) and in yellow maize (Green, 1970) is β-cryptoxanthin. γ-Carotene constitutes only a small percentage by weight of the total provitamin A content. Provitamin A carotenoids are also found in shellfish and crustaceae. Dairy products and egg yolk contain carotenes derived from the animal's diet (Roels, 1967).

The richest source of provitamin A is red palm oil. Vegetables are also rich sources, with the carrot predominant. Fruits vary, but generally contain lower amounts of activity compared with vegetables. Negligible sources of provitamin A carotenoids include cereals (except yellow maize), vegetable oils, potatoes (but not sweet potatoes), jams and syrups.

With regard to animal nutrition, fresh green pasture herbage is an

Table 2
Distribution of provitamin A carotenoids in foods (typical values)

Food	Vitamin A (μg retinol equivalent[a] per 100 g edible portion)
Red palm oil	30 000
Carrots	2 000
Leafy vegetables	685
Tomatoes	100
Apricots (fresh)	250
Bananas	30
Sweet potatoes (white)	50
Sweet potatoes (red and yellow)	670
Orange juice	8

From Passmore, R. & Eastwood, M. A. (1986). *Davidson and Passmore Human Nutrition and Dietetics*, 8th edn. By permission of Churchill Livingstone.
[a] The number of retinol equivalents is obtained by dividing the β-carotene content (μg) by a factor of 6.

exceptionally rich source of carotene, and supplies about one hundred times the requirement of a grazing cow when eaten in normal quantities. The green tops of mangold, fodder beet, sugar beet, turnip and swede also constitute excellent sources of carotene (McDonald *et al.*, 1972). Root crops (beets), pulses and brewers' grains contain almost no carotene, whilst oilseed cakes and cereals (except yellow maize) are totally devoid of carotene. Regardless of the conservation method used (hay or silage) carotene undergoes a slow degradation in storage. The loss is of the order of 50% in the first six months, but it may be higher (Meissonnier, 1983).

2.1.3 Physico-chemical Properties
Description
Retinol: yellow crystalline powder. Retinyl acetate: pale yellow crystalline powder. Retinyl palmitate: yellow oil, or crystalline mass. β-Carotene: reddish-brown to deep violet crystalline powder. β-Apo-8'-carotenal: deep violet crystalline powder. β-Apo-8'-carotenoic acid ethyl ester: rust red crystalline powder.

Solubility
Vitamin A is insoluble in water; soluble in alcohol; and readily soluble in diethyl ether, petroleum spirit, chloroform, acetone, and fats and oils.

β-Carotene is insoluble in water; very sparingly soluble in alcohol, fats and oils; sparingly soluble in ether and acetone; and slightly soluble in chloroform and benzene (Anon., 1976).

Stability
Vitamin A in the unesterified form is readily oxidized by atmospheric oxygen to yield the 5,6-epoxide among the oxidation products. The acetate and palmitate esters of vitamin A are somewhat more stable towards oxidation than the free alcohol.

Vitamin A is extremely sensitive towards acids, which can cause rearrangements of the double bonds and dehydration, eventually followed by the addition of the solvent and *cis-trans* isomerization (Schwieter & Isler, 1967). Isomerization to the lower potency *cis* isomers occurs during storage at a pH of 4·5 or lower (De Ritter, 1977).

Vitamin A is relatively stable towards alkali, and its stereochemistry is not affected by reducing agents.

Cis-trans isomerization is directly promoted by light containing wavelengths of less than 500 nm. In the photo-isomerization of vitamin A, the relative amounts of the different *cis-trans* isomers formed are dependent on the wavelength and on the solvent used. When a standard ethanolic solution of all-*trans*-retinol in clear glassware (2·76 µg/ml) is exposed to ordinary laboratory light for 12 h there is 14% degradation, and 22% of the remaining vitamin is in the form of the 13-*cis* isomer (Egberg *et al.*, 1977). Landers & Olson (1986) demonstrated that solutions of all-*trans*-retinyl palmitate in chloroform or dichloromethane undergo isomerization fairly rapidly when exposed to white light, i.e. a mixture of indirect sunlight and white fluorescent light. The final mixture, after 23 h irradiation, contains approximately equal amounts of 9-*cis*- and all-*trans*-retinyl palmitate. In hexane solution, retinyl palmitate undergoes only slight isomerization under white light. No significant isomerization of all-*trans*-retinyl palmitate occurs under gold fluorescent light (wavelengths > 500 nm) in chloroform, dichloromethane or hexane solutions, even after exposure for 23 h. The effects of light upon solutions of all-*trans*-retinol are essentially identical to those obtained with the palmitate ester. The photo-isomerization of chlorinated solutions of all-*trans*-retinyl palmitate, previously reported to take place under gold fluorescent light (Mulry *et al.*, 1983), is considered to be due to inadequate exclusion of sunlight, or of white fluorescent light, during the experiment. Thompson *et al.* (1971) reported that irradiation promotes the conversion of retinyl esters to the highly fluorescent retro ethers, the conversion rate being greater in the presence of chlorinated solvents. The stabilized vitamin A preparations supplied to the food industry are not prone to isomerization, and remain in the all-*trans* form after storage for several years (Parrish, 1977).

In general, the carotenoids are destroyed or altered by acids and free halogens, particularly in the presence of light and high temperature, to form mixtures of *cis-trans* isomers from the all-*trans* structure. The carotenoids are easily oxidized in the presence of oxygen or oxidizing agents (catalysed by fluorescent light and lipoxygenase), commonly with the co-oxidation of unsaturated fatty acids. The initial site of attack is the 5, 6 double bond or in-chain double bonds, leading to epoxide formation and chain cleavage (De Ritter & Purcell, 1981; Simpson, 1983).

In foods the retinyl esters and carotenoids are dissolved in the fat matrix, where they are protected from the oxidizing action of atmospheric oxygen by vitamin E and other antioxidants. The antioxidant intercepts the oxygen before it can react with the vitamin; the antioxidant itself is oxidized in the process. On final depletion of the antioxidant, the retinyl esters and carotenoids become vulnerable to oxidation. Under these circumstances unsaturated fats also begin to oxidize and turn rancid, with the production of highly active peroxides. The peroxides produced during oxidative rancidity attack, and finally destroy, the vitamin A and carotenoids. Thus factors that accelerate oxidative rancidity, such as access of air, heat, light, traces of certain metals (notably copper and, to a lesser extent, iron), and storage time will also result in the destruction of the vitamin A compounds (Kläui *et al.*, 1970).

Food processing causes loss of vitamin A activity, largely because of heat-catalysed *trans* to *cis* conversion of retinol and the carotenoids (Lambert *et al.*, 1985). For example, processing of vegetables by cooking or canning lowers the vitamin A values of green vegetables by 15–20%, and values of yellow vegetables by 30–35% (Sweeney & Marsh, 1971). Severe loss of carotene occurs during the dehydration of unblanched vegetables, but blanching exerts a protective effect (Cain, 1975).

In margarine, the various naturally occurring vitamin A isomers and provitamin A carotenoids that may have been present in the original crude oils are removed during the refining process. Thus the only vitamin A that is present in the final margarine is the all-*trans*-retinyl palmitate or acetate that is added during margarine production (Aitzetmüller *et al.*, 1979).

Vitamin A is more stable in whole milk products than in low-fat or skimmed milk products, presumably because of natural antioxidants present in milk fat (Coulter & Thomas, 1968). Vitamin A added to low-fat milk is destroyed more rapidly by light than is naturally present vitamin A.

A certain portion of the native vitamin A is lost rapidly on light exposure, with the remaining portion being resistant to further destruction (de Man, 1981). Ultra-high-temperature (UHT) milk sterilization by direct steam injection and evaporative cooling removes virtually all of the oxygen from the milk; indirect heating and evaporative cooling leaves about one-third of the initial oxygen content; and indirect heat followed by cooling in a heat exchanger causes no change in oxygen content. None of these three treatments caused any significant loss of vitamin A in UHT milk either during processing, or during subsequent storage in aluminium foil-lined cartons at room temperature for up to ninety days (Ford et al., 1969). The stability of vitamin A in direct UHT-treated milk, and also in pasteurized milk, was confirmed by Le Maguer & Jackson (1983). However, Woollard & Fairweather (1985) reported that both natural (retinyl palmitate) and supplemental (retinyl acetate) vitamin A in UHT milk sterilized by indirect heating underwent rapid degradation. In two trials the total loss of vitamin A was 21% and 25% after three weeks' storage; the loss increased to 33% and 45% after fifteen weeks' storage after which there was no further loss up to forty weeks. The cause of the vitamin A degradation was attributed to residual oxygen in the milk.

The loss of vitamin A is confined to the all-*trans* isomers of the natural retinyl palmitate and the supplemental retinyl acetate. *Cis* isomers, which are essentially absent in untreated milk before UHT treatment, but which appear after processing, maintain their concentrations until the onset of proteolysis and gelation (Woollard & Indyk, 1986). Vitamin A isomerization and degradation in dried-milk powder occur in a similar fashion to liquid milk (Woollard & Indyk, 1986).

When animal feeds are pelleted, destruction of vitamin A may occur under the processing conditions of moisture and high temperature, unless sufficient antioxidant is present.

When green herbage is dried in the field, much of the carotene (up to 90%) is destroyed by oxidation. The loss of carotene is reduced to as little as 18% if rapid drying of the crop by tripoding or barn drying is employed. In the case of artificially dried grass, the loss of carotene during drying rarely exceeds 10%, but as much as 50% may be lost during seven months of storage under ordinary conditions (McDonald et al., 1972).

Ultraviolet absorption
All-*trans*-retinol exhibits ultraviolet (UV) absorption with a specific extinction coefficient ($E_{1cm}^{1\%}$) in ethanol (Indyk, 1982) or isopropanol (Strohecker & Henning, 1966) of 1830 at an absorption maximum (λ_{max}) of

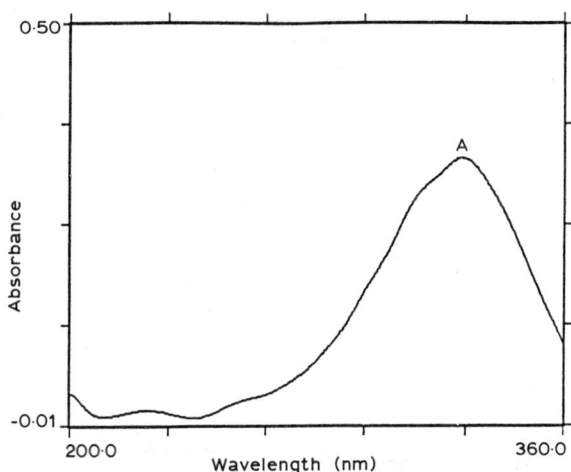

Fig. 5. UV absorption spectrum of retinyl palmitate in isopropanol (λ_{max} of peak A = 326·5 nm).

325 nm. The absorbance of 13-*cis*-retinol is about 92% of that of the all-*trans* isomer (Lawn *et al.*, 1983). The $E_{1cm}^{1\%}$ values of retinyl acetate and retinyl palmitate in isopropanol at λ_{max} 326 nm have been quoted at 1530 and 960 respectively (Olson, 1984). The absorption spectrum of retinyl palmitate in isopropanol is shown in Fig. 5.

Fluorescence
Retinol and retinyl esters exhibit strong native fluorescence with excitation and emission maxima at wavelengths of 325–330 nm and 470–490 nm, respectively (Hubbard *et al.*, 1971). The excitation and emission spectra of retinyl acetate are shown in Fig. 6.

2.1.4 Biological Activity in Man
Functional metabolism
In the body, dietary β-carotene is converted to retinol by enzymic action, whereby molecular oxygen reacts across the central C-15, 15′ double bond to form a peroxide. The peroxide rapidly cleaves to yield two, or in the case of other dietary provitamins, one molecule of retinaldehyde. A small amount of the retinaldehyde is irreversibly oxidized to retinoic acid, but the majority is reduced enzymatically to retinol. This conversion occurs in the intestinal wall and liver of many species, but the liver is believed to be the only organ capable of this conversion in humans (Cremin & Power, 1985).

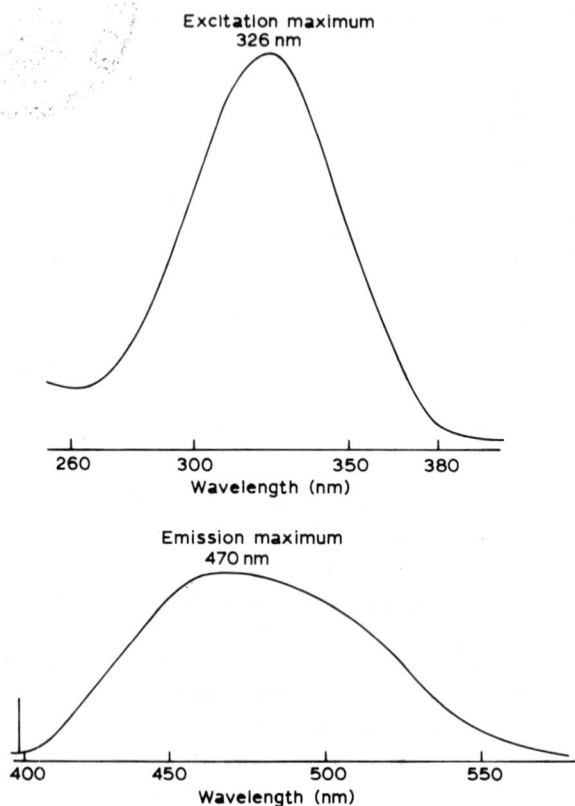

Fig. 6.   Fluorescence excitation and emission spectra of retinyl acetate obtained by stop-flow scanning after passage through a silica HPLC column eluted with hexane containing 0·03% isopropanol.

An alternative pathway for the conversion of β-carotene to retin-aldehyde involves the stepwise degradation of the provitamin at one end of the molecule to form apocarotenoids, e.g. β-apo-8′-carotenal (Schwieter & Isler, 1967). β-Carotene is stored in the body only to a very small extent.

Dietary retinol, which has been formed by another animal from a carotenoid, or synthesized commercially, is usually in the esterified form. During absorption the esters are completely hydrolysed in the small intestine to the free retinol, which is then transferred across the mucosal cell membrane. Inside the mucosal cells, the retinol is re-esterified with long-chain fatty acids, mainly palmitic, followed by stearic and oleic. The retinyl esters are transported to the lymph, and thence into the blood. Retinyl

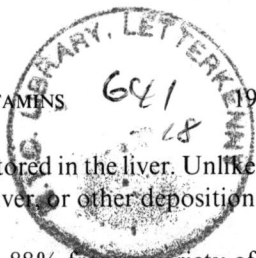

esters in excess of the body's immediate needs are stored in the liver. Unlike retinol, β-carotene cannot be mobilized from the liver or other deposition sites, when required (Lambert *et al.*, 1985).

Human carotene absorption varies from 1% to 88% from a variety of yellow and green vegetables. The FAO/WHO committee decided in 1965 that 33% availability from diet was the best approximation that could be made for practical purposes. Thus, the β-carotene in a food would be only one-third absorbed and this, in turn, would be only one-half converted to retinol, giving a factor of one-sixth for the overall utilization. Since dietary retinol is assumed to be 100% utilized, 1 μg of food β-carotene becomes equivalent to 0·167 μg of retinol. For the other provitamins that theoretically yield only one-half as much retinol as does β-carotene, the factor is one-twelfth (Bieri & McKenna, 1981).

Physiological role

An adequate intake of dietary vitamin A is essential in the chemistry of vision, and for the normal development of the epithelium and of bone. There is also evidence that vitamin A is implicated in antibody production (Omaye, 1984).

An early sign of vitamin A deficiency is night blindness, which is caused by an insufficient amount of visual purple in the retina. Visual purple (rhodopsin) is an addition product of retinaldehyde and the protein opsin, and is essential for normal night vision. Night blindness refers to the lengthening of the time required for the eyesight to adapt from light conditions to dark conditions.

Another sign of vitamin A deficiency is where the epithelial cells of the skin and mucous membranes lining the respiratory, gastrointestinal and urinogenital tracts cease to differentiate, and lose their secretory function. The undifferentiated cells are flattened and multiply at an increased rate, so that the cells pile up on one another and the surface becomes keratinized. This condition promotes dry skin and loss of hair sheen; the symptom of loss of appetite may be due to keratinization of the taste buds. The lack of protective mucus in the affected mucosae leads to an increased susceptibility to infections. Xerophthalmia refers to keratinization of the conjunctiva (the mucous membrane covering the eye) which later spreads to the cornea causing ulceration. The ultimate condition is keratomalacia (softening of the cornea) which, if not treated, leads to permanent blindness. Xerophthalmia, in man, is confined mainly to very young children and has been stated to be the most serious vitamin deficiency disease in the world today (Passmore & Eastwood, 1986).

The clinical effects of vitamin A deficiency in adults are usually seen only in people whose diet has been deficient for a long time in both dairy produce and vegetables. Induced vitamin A deficiency experiments in human volunteers resulted in night blindness and some follicular keratosis (blockage of the sebaceous glands by horny plugs), but there was no xerophthalmia (Passmore & Eastwood, 1986). The most serious manifestations of deficiency are seen in very young children and, in these cases, the deficiency rarely occurs in isolation. A reduced protein intake, for example, dramatically diminishes the intestinal conversion of carotenoids to retinol. Furthermore, carotenoids are poorly absorbed when the diet is low in fat (McLaren, 1967a).

Vitamin A has been regarded as a possible anticarcinogenic agent in view of its properties in re-establishing normal differentiation of malignant epithelial tissues cultured in vitro, and in preventing the development of cancer in response to proven carcinogens in rodents (Hicks, 1983). Moreover, epidemiological investigations have revealed an inverse association between dietary β-carotene and incidence of human cancer (Peto et al., 1981). Naturally occurring retinoids are toxic at high doses, and thus are of limited usefulness for the chemo-prevention of cancer. Synthetic retinoid analogues that have diminished toxicity are under investigation (Pitt, 1985).

The storage of vitamin A in the liver is highly efficient, and an excess intake of the vitamin can produce symptoms of toxicity. Normally, hypervitaminosis A results from the indiscriminate use of pharmaceutical supplements, and not from the consumption of usual diets. The only naturally occurring products that contain sufficient vitamin A to induce toxicity in man are the livers of animals at the top of long food chains, such as large marine fish and carnivores (e.g. bear and dog). Small amounts of vitamin A within the range of the RDA stabilize the cell membrane by providing a cross-link between the membrane lipid and protein. In hypervitaminosis A the membrane is exposed to unbound vitamin A, which disrupts the integrity of the membrane. A daily intake of 100 000 IU of vitamin A for several months has generally been associated with chronic toxicity in adults, with symptoms of anorexia, headache, blurred vision, muscle soreness after exercise, hair loss, bleeding lips, cracking and peeling skin, and nose bleed. These symptoms are relieved promptly when vitamin A dosing is discontinued. Prolonged high vitamin A consumption may eventually result in cirrhosis of the liver. Chronic hypervitaminosis A can also produce teratological effects (malformations) in the foetus. Ingestion of acute high doses of vitamin A (2–5 million IU) produces symptoms of severe headache, dizziness, abdominal pain, nausea and diarrhoea (Miller & Hayes, 1982; Omaye, 1984).

Biopotency

The International Unit of vitamin A is the activity of:

0·300 μg of all-*trans*-retinol
0·344 μg of all-*trans*-retinyl acetate
0·55 μg of all-*trans*-retinyl palmitate
0·6 μg of all-*trans*-β-carotene or 1·2 μg of other provitamin A carotenoids.

The vitamin A value of foods is nowadays more commonly expressed as retinol equivalents (RE).

1 RE = 1 μg of all-*trans*-retinol
= 6 μg of all-*trans*-β-carotene
= 12 μg of other provitamin A carotenoids
= 3·33 IU activity from retinol
= 10 IU vitamin A activity from β-carotene.

For products containing β-carotene and other provitamin A carotenoids (Simpson *et al.*, 1985):

$$\text{Total RE} = \frac{\mu g \ \beta\text{-carotene}}{6} + \frac{\mu g \ \text{other provitamins A}}{12}$$

By both growth and liver storage bioassays 13-*cis*-retinol possesses 75% of the activity of the all-*trans* isomer; 9-*cis*- and 9,13-di-*cis*-retinol possess, respectively, 21% and 24% relative activities (Ames, 1966). Dietary retinaldehyde possesses about 90% of the biological activity of all-*trans*-retinol (Sivell *et al.*, 1984). Retinoic acid cannot be converted *in vivo* to retinaldehyde or retinol, and is thus unable to maintain vision or normal reproductive performance in male and female animals. However, the acid has been shown to support the growth of vitamin A-depleted rats (Ganguly & Murthy, 1967).

Requirement

In 1965, a Joint FAO/WHO Expert Group set a recommended intake of 750 μg of retinol per day for the maintenance of health in nearly all people: requirements during infancy and childhood were related to growth rate (McLaren 1967*b*; Department of Health and Social Security, 1979).

2.1.5 Biological Activity in Animals

Vitamin A deficiency in animals produces a diversity of adverse changes that affect the eyes, skin, nervous system, bones, mucous membranes, and reproductive systems (Anon., 1976). Specific signs of deficiency depend upon the animal species and upon the nutritional conditions. Many of the signs are attributable to the lack of differentiation of mucus-secreting cells in the membranes lining the eyes, respiratory tract, alimentary tract, and urinogenital tract. The membranes become keratinized and dried out, thus losing their function and, in this condition, they are very susceptible to infection. Reproductive changes include atrophy of the testes and male accessory sex glands, and of the ovaries. Other deficiency signs are attributable to disturbed bone growth, impaired food utilization, and lack of antibody formation. Night blindness, which can be diagnosed by special tests, is an early sign of vitamin A deficiency in all animals. An earlier sign of vitamin A deficiency is a raised cerebrospinal fluid pressure.

Typical vitamin A deficiency signs in domestic animals have been described (McDonald et al., 1972; Thompson, 1975; Anon., 1976). In adult cattle a mild deficiency of vitamin A is associated with roughened hair and scaly skin. Prolonged deficiency affects the eyes, leading eventually to xerophthalmia. In breeding animals a deficiency may lead to infertility, and in pregnant animals to abortion or stillbirths. The lowered conception rate in cows is due to the reduced synthesis of sex hormones, and cornification of the vaginal epithelium causing irregular oestrus. Defects in the development of the foetus are attributable to necrosis of the placenta. Bulls continue to produce viable spermatozoa even when blindness through xerophthalmia has developed; continued vitamin A deprivation leads to degeneration of the seminiferous tubules with a consequent reduction in semen volume and sperm count, and an increased proportion of abnormal spermatozoa. The lack of protective mucus in the alimentary and respiratory tracts leads to scours and pneumonia, resulting usually in death. Less severe signs of vitamin A deficiency in calves are loss of appetite and poor growth.

It has been postulated that, besides acting as a vitamin A precursor, β-carotene plays a specific role in the synthesis of progesterone in cattle, and thus is necessary for maintaining regular oestrous cycles (Anon., 1976).

In practice, severe deficiency signs are unlikely to occur in adult cattle, except after prolonged deprivation of vitamin A. Grazing animals generally obtain more than adequate amounts of provitamin A carotenoids from pasture grass, and normally build up liver reserves of vitamin A. If cattle are fed on silage or well-preserved hay during the winter months, deficiencies are unlikely to occur.

Vitamin A deficiency is not common in sheep because of adequate dietary sources of provitamin A carotenoids on pasture.

In pigs, a deficiency in vitamin A may cause eye disorders such as xerophthalmia and blindness. Compression of the brain, due to abnormal bone growth and nerve degeneration, gives rise to nervous disorders such as uncoordinated movements and convulsions. A deficiency in pregnant animals may result in the production of blind, deformed litters. In less severe cases, appetite is impaired and growth retarded.

Poultry differ markedly in their carotenoid metabolism in that they preferentially absorb from their diet, and transfer to tissues, the xanthophylls, and only traces of carotenes (Thompson, 1975). The mortality rate is usually high in vitamin A-deficient poultry. Early signs of deficiency include retarded growth, weakness, ruffled plumage, and a staggering gait. The keratinization of secretory epithelia in the intestine leads to parasitic infestations. The impaired production of antibodies reduces the bird's resistance to infections such as coccidiosis. In mature birds suffering from severe vitamin A deficiency egg production and hatchability are reduced.

2.1.6 Supplementation of Foods and Animal Feeds
Foods
Fat-based foods, particularly margarine and shortenings, are enriched by direct addition of standardized and stabilized solutions of retinyl acetate or retinyl palmitate in oil; the fortification of margarine is under legislation in the United Kingdom. Nowadays, most food manufacturers use retinyl palmitate, which has been shown to exhibit the greatest stability of the retinyl esters toward oxidation, in the fortification process (Widicus & Kirk, 1979). Dry preparations of synthetic retinyl esters are used in dried food products such as milk powder, infant foods and dietetic foods. These preparations provide good stability, high purity and potency, and agreeable flavour characteristics.

Synthetic preparations of provitamin A carotenoids such as β-carotene, β-apo-8'-carotenal and β-apo-8'-carotenoic acid ethyl ester are used primarily as colouring agents for food to impart, standardize or enhance natural colour. Micropulverized dispersions of carotenoids are used in colouring fat-based foods such as margarine, butter, shortenings, cheese and French dressings. Water-dispersible forms of carotenoids have been developed for the colouring of water-based foods such as orange-type beverages, cake mixes, puddings, dried and canned soups. Carotenoids added to juices and carbonated beverages show adequate stability due to the antioxidant property of ascorbic acid (Schwieter & Isler, 1967; Kläui *et al.*, 1970).

Animal feeds
Cattle which are kept indoors are fed on rations which include conserved

fodders (hay or silage), cereal grains (oats, barley, white maize, wheat), oilseed cakes, and roots (beets). These products are either poor sources, or are totally devoid, of provitamin A, hence need to be supplemented with vitamin A. Yellow maize, which contains β-cryptoxanthin, is an important source of provitamin A in the United States, but it tends to colour the carcass fat which, in the United Kingdom, is not considered desirable (McDonald *et al.*, 1972). Dried grass made from young herbage is a valuable source of carotene, and can be made into cubes or pellets. However, dried grass is relatively expensive to produce and generally can only be given in limited quantity to cattle during the winter.

High-yielding dairy cows should be given supplemental vitamin A even during the grazing period, especially in periods of drought. Young cattle during the growing or fattening period should receive daily supplements of vitamin A (Meissonnier, 1983).

Synthetic retinyl esters in stabilized form are added to the feed ration, either by using a vitamin/mineral premix or a protein concentrate with added vitamins and minerals. The oily forms of retinyl esters are unsuitable for processing in dry preparations such as animal feeds. For such purposes, gelatin-coated dry powder preparations have been developed in which the vitamin is dispersed as extremely finely divided droplets (Anon., 1976). A daily supplement of β-carotene is also needed to satisfy the specific requirement for reproduction in cattle.

Supplements of vitamin A must be given to pigs fed on compounded diets.

Poultry feed concentrates need to be supplemented with vitamin A or provitamin A xanthophylls since such feeds are usually low or lacking in these nutrients. The addition of fish liver oil or synthetic vitamin A satisfies the bird's nutritional requirements, whilst the synthetic β-apo-8'-carotenal or β-apo-8'-carotenoic acid ethyl ester are used as pigments to impart a satisfactory colour to the egg yolk (Thompson, 1975).

2.1.7 Bioassays

The most commonly used biological methods for measuring vitamin A activity are rat growth-response tests, liver-storage tests in rats and chicks, and the rat vaginal cornification test (Olson, 1965; Green, 1970).

2.2 VITAMIN D

Discovery. Sir Edward Mellanby in 1921 was the first to show clearly that rickets is a nutritional disease, and that cod liver oil contains a factor that prevents it. In 1922 McCollum and co-workers treated cod liver oil by bubbling oxygen through it. This destroyed the antixerophthalmic properties but left the antirachitic properties, thus indicating the presence of two factors: factor A (or vitamin A) and the antirachitic factor, which they later termed 'fat-soluble' vitamin D. Zucker and co-workers in 1922 found that vitamin D was present in the unsaponifiable fraction of cod liver oil, and suggested that it was closely related to cholesterol.

The beneficial effect of sunlight in curing rickets in children had been recognized in the early 1800s. In 1924, Steenbock and Black discovered that rat rations irradiated with UV light had the same beneficial effects as when rachitic rats were irradiated. Soon afterward, Hess and Weinstock independently reported the increased vitamin D activity of foods exposed to UV light. In 1925, several independent workers demonstrated that it is the sterols in foods that are activated. Ergosterol was identified as the precursor of ergocalciferol (vitamin D_2) in 1927, and 7-dehydrocholesterol as the precursor of cholecalciferol (vitamin D_3) in 1934 (Navia, 1971).

2.2.1 Biogenesis and Chemical Structure

In vertebrates, cholecalciferol can be produced by the action of sunlight on the provitamin D_3 sterol, 7-dehydrocholesterol, in the skin. The provitamin is synthesized in the sebaceous glands, then secreted onto the skin surface, and re-absorbed into the various layers of the epidermis (Lawson, 1985). The ultraviolet light can readily penetrate the skin to the level of the epidermis, and the vitamin D_3 thus formed eventually reaches the bloodstream. In animals and birds, oily secretions are irradiated on the surface of the fur or feathers, and the vitamin D can be ingested by licking the fur or preening the feathers. In cases of insufficient exposure to sunlight, man has become dependent on dietary sources of vitamin D.

In plants, fungi and invertebrates, the chief provitamin D sterol is ergosterol which, under UV irradiation, gives rise to ergocalciferol. Other plant sterols possess provitamin D activity, but their resultant vitamins (D_5, D_6 and D_7) are of low biological activity (Navia, 1971).

In structural terms, vitamins D_2 and D_3 differ only in the C-17 side chain, in which D_2 possesses a double bond and an additional methyl group (Fig. 7). Vitamin D occurs naturally as the 5,6-*cis*-form; *trans*-vitamin D has no significant antirachitic activity. In this review 'vitamin D' refers to vitamins D_2 and D_3.

The biogenesis of vitamin D is represented in Fig. 8. The provitamin D sterols are irradiated to form intermediate previtamin D compounds, which, aided by the warmth of the body, are converted slowly to their respective vitamins. The biogenic process involves the opening of the sterol

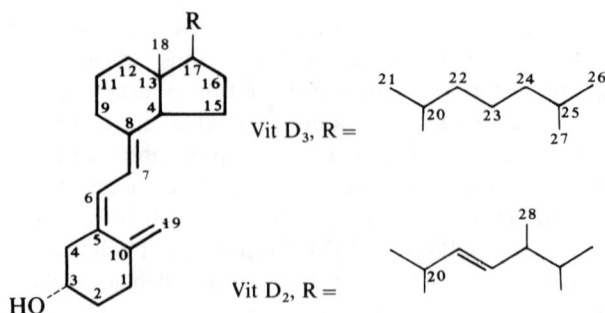

Fig. 7. Chemical structures of cholecalciferol (vitamin D_3) and ergocalciferol (vitamin D_2).

B ring and double bond rearrangement. The previtamin D exhibits approximately one-half of the antirachitic activity of vitamin D when administered to experimental animals. Reported activities are 34, 40 and 56%, for previtamin D_2 in the rat, and 35% for previtamin D_3 in the chick relative to vitamins D_2 and D_3, respectively (Keverling Buisman *et al.*, 1968). Previtamin D itself is considered to be inactive, and the biological activity shown by this isomer is attributable to its in-vivo conversion to vitamin D (Mulder *et al.*, 1971). The previtamin D can, upon further irradiation with UV light, proceed to lumisterol or to tachysterol, both of which are biologically inactive.

2.2.2 Natural Occurrence

Only a very few foods provide vitamin D. The richest natural sources of vitamin D_3 are fish liver oils, especially halibut liver oil. Smaller amounts of the vitamin are found in the edible portion of fatty fish, mammalian liver, eggs and dairy products (see Table 3). The concentration of vitamin D_3 in milk shows a seasonal variation, which is related to the amount of sunlight available to convert 7-dehydrocholesterol in the animal's skin to cholecalciferol. Vitamin D_2 also occurs in milk, but in smaller concentrations than vitamin D_3. Unlike vitamin D_3, ergocalciferol is derived by UV irradiation of ergosterol in sun dried green forage (hay); ergosterol cannot be converted by the animal into vitamin D_2 (Cremin & Power, 1985). Cereals, vegetables and fruit contain no vitamin D, whilst meat, poultry and white fish contribute insignificant amounts.

Of the provitamins D, ergosterol occurs in plants, and is the main sterol of many fungi. Ergosterol is obtained in high yield from bakers' yeast for the commercial preparation of vitamin D_2. 7-Dehydrocholesterol occurs

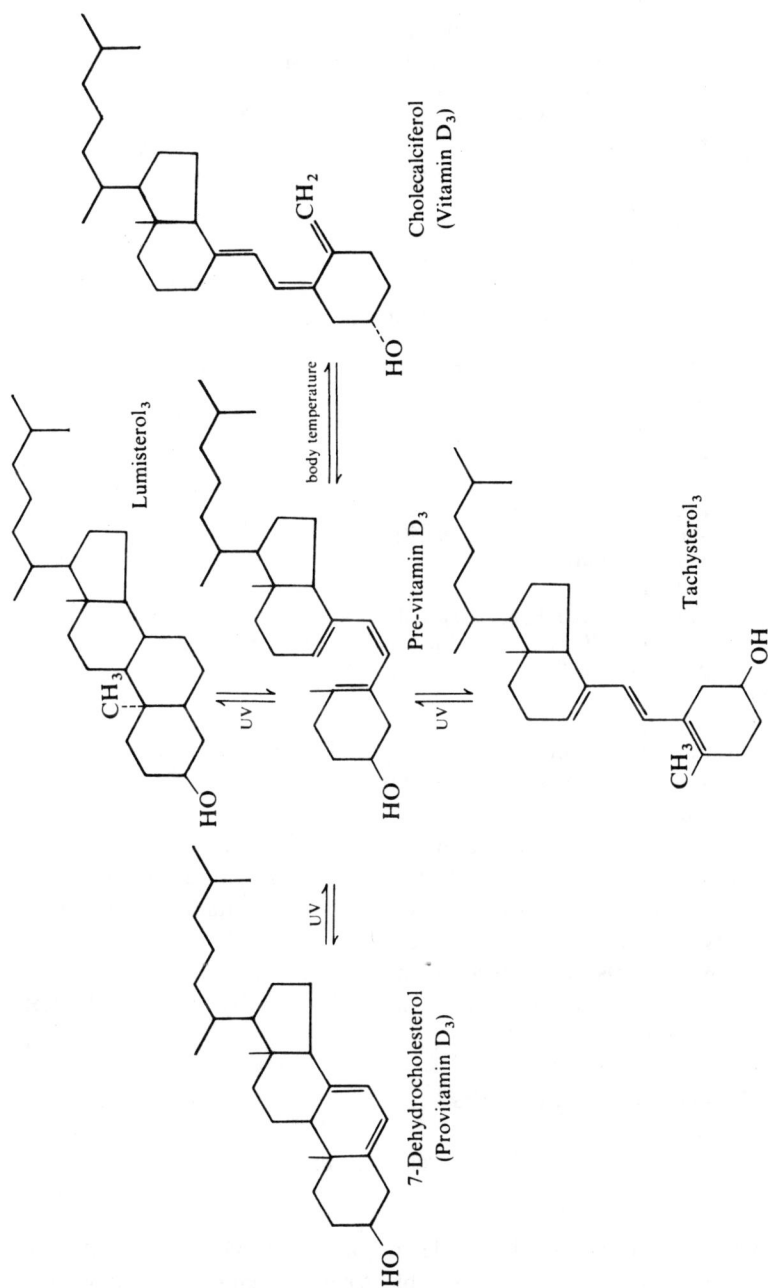

Fig. 8. The biogenesis of vitamin D_3 (from DeLuca, 1978).

Table 3
Distribution of vitamin D in foods (Mean values)

Food	Vitamin D (μg per $100\,g$)
Animal products	
Liver	0·75
Dairy products	
Butter	0·75
Margarine (fortified with vitamin D)	8·8
Eggs	1·75
Milk (unfortified, summer)	0·03
Cream (double)	0·25
Cheese (Cheddar)	0·25
Fatty fish and their oils	
Cod liver oil	210
Herrings and kippers	22
Sardines and pilchards (canned)	8
Tuna (canned)	6

From Passmore, R. & Eastwood, M. A. (1986). *Davidson and Passmore Human Nutrition and Dietetics*, 8th edn. By permission of Churchill Livingstone.

with cholesterol in many animals, especially the lower forms, but is produced commercially from cholesterol for conversion to vitamin D_3 (Green, 1970).

With regard to animal nutrition, young grass at the usual harvesting stage is almost devoid of vitamin D, but hay contains variable amounts of vitamin D_2 produced from irradiated ergosterol. The vitamin D content of dried grass is very low, since the drying process does not allow the irradiation of sterols to take place. Concentrated animal feedstuffs such as cereals, oilseed cakes, root crops and industrial by-products do not contain vitamin D.

2.2.3 Physico-chemical Properties
Description
Vitamins D_2 and D_3 are white to yellowish crystalline powders.

Solubility
Vitamins D_2 and D_3 are insoluble in water; soluble in 95% ethanol, acetone, fats and oils; and readily soluble in benzene, chloroform and ether.

Stability

Grady & Thakker (1980) studied the effects of temperature (25 and 40°C) and relative humidity (RH) (dry air at 45% RH and very moist air at 85% RH) on the stability of vitamin D_2 and D_3 powders in the absence of light. After twenty-one days, vitamin D_2 samples stored in dry air at 25°C had only about 66% ergocalciferol remaining, whilst samples stored under very moist air had >95% remaining. Vitamin D_3 was more stable, and had >99% remaining under both sets of conditions. Both compounds were less stable at the higher temperature. After seven days, samples of vitamin D_2 stored at 40°C and 85% RH had 87% remaining; those stored at 40°C and 45% RH had only 20% remaining. Conversely, samples of vitamin D_3 stored for seven days at 40°C and 85% RH had 15% of the cholecalciferol remaining; those stored at 40°C and 45% RH had about 65% remaining.

In oily solutions at 0°C the biological activity of vitamin D drops by about 50% within three to five years, whilst in emulsions this drop takes place within three weeks (Krampitz, 1980). Vitamin D is also unstable towards acids. Under conditions of even mild acidity, the vitamin D molecule isomerizes to form the 5,6-*trans* isomer and the isotachysterol isomer (DeLuca, 1978) (Fig. 9). Vitamin D is stable towards alkali (Kutsky, 1973).

In solution, vitamin D exhibits reversible thermal isomerization to previtamin D, forming an equilibrium mixture. In the solid state, vitamin D does not isomerize. Equations and calculations have been described to determine the ratio of previtamin D to vitamin D as a function of the temperature and the reaction time (Keverling Buisman *et al.*, 1968). The previtamin D/vitamin D ratios and the equilibrium times attained at different temperatures are given in Table 4. At 100°C, equilibrium is

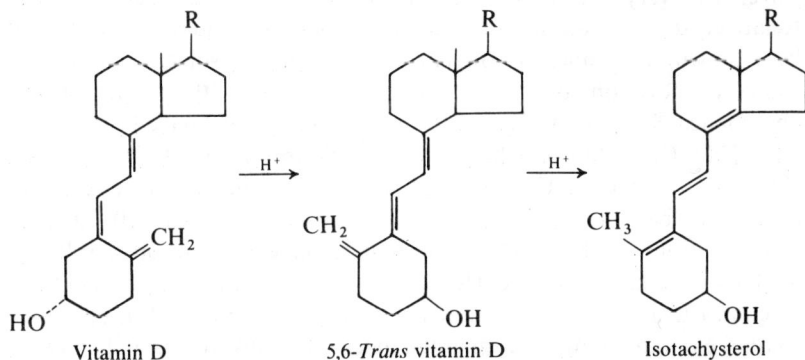

Fig. 9. Isomerization of vitamin D under acid conditions (from DeLuca, 1978).

Table 4

The previtamin D/vitamin D equilibrium (Mulder *et al.*, 1971)

Temperature (°C)	% previtamin D	% vitamin D	Equilibrium time[a]
−20	2	98	16 years
10	4	96	350 days
20	7	93	30 days
30	9	91	10 days
40	11	89	3·5 days
50	13	87	1·3 days
60	16	84	0·5 days
80	22	78	0·1 days
100	28	72	30 min
120	35	65	7 min

[a] The time necessary to reach equilibrium, starting with pure vitamin D or pure previtamin D.

reached in less than 30 min, and 28% of the mixture consists of previtamin D. At 0°C, no more than 4% previtamin D is found, and conversion is protracted over many months. When equilibrated at 20°C the ratio of previtamin D to vitamin D is 7:93. The isomerization rates of vitamins D_2 and D_3 are virtually equal (Hanewald *et al.*, 1968), and are not affected by solvent, light or catalysis (Mulder *et al.*, 1971). Because of the uncertainty of the previtamin D to vitamin D ratio, it is important in physico-chemical assays to determine the potential vitamin D, i.e. the combined value of previtamin D and vitamin D.

Apart from thermal isomerism, solutions of vitamin D in organic solvents are very stable, provided that oxygen, light and acids are excluded. Relatively dilute solutions of vitamin D_3 (10 μg/ml) could be refluxed for at least 1 h with a number of different solvents, and the solvent removed by rotary evaporation, or in a stream of nitrogen, without loss of UV absorbance. Solvents studied (with their boiling points) have been diethyl ether (34·6°C), dichloromethane (40·5°C), chloroform (61·5°C), methanol (64·7°C), ethanol (78·5°C) and isooctane (99·3°C). The deleterious effect of water has been demonstrated by the observation that 10–20 μg/ml concentrations of vitamin D_3 dissolved in water, containing 50% or less of methanol or ethanol, exhibited loss of UV absorbance as a function of time. In contrast, similar concentrations of vitamin D_3 dissolved in 80–100% alcohol exhibited long-term maintenance of UV absorbance (Chen *et al.*, 1965).

The stability of vitamin D in fats and oils corresponds to the stability of the fat itself, as described previously for vitamin A. Vitamin D is, however, more stable than vitamin A under comparable conditions.

Once freed from the protection of the food matrix, vitamin D is susceptible to decomposition by oxygen, light, acidity and water, as demonstrated by loss of UV absorbance at 265 nm. Conditions which promote destruction of vitamin D include exposure of thin films to air (especially with heat), acidic conditions, and dispersion of an alcoholic solution of the vitamin into an aqueous phase in the presence of dissolved oxygen. The decomposition products, which may be different in each case, are separable from vitamin D by some form of chromatography (Chen *et al.*, 1965).

Vitamin D will withstand smoking of fish, pasteurization and sterilization of milk, and spray-drying of eggs, although it is generally considered to be destroyed in oxidizing fats. When used to enrich infant milks, it is common practice to allow for the destruction of 25–35% of added vitamin D during the drying process (Bender, 1979).

Ultraviolet absorption

All vitamin D-active compounds possess a broad UV absorption spectrum which peaks at 265 nm (Fig. 10). The triene system, which is responsible for the absorption, is not entirely planar, thus the $E_{1cm}^{1\%}$ values of 461 and 476

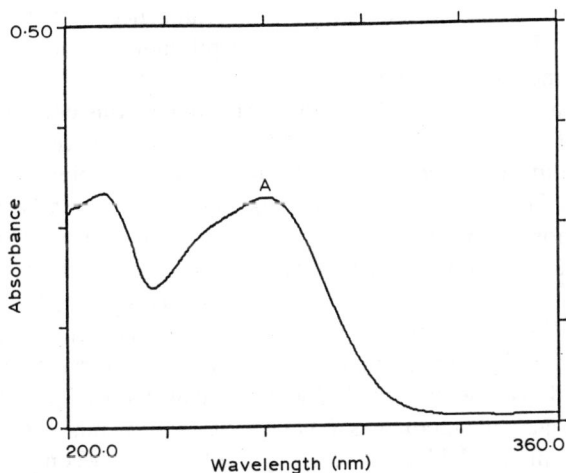

Fig. 10. UV absorption spectrum of vitamin D_2 in ethanol (λ_{max} of peak A = 265 nm).

for vitamins D_2 and D_3, respectively (Miller & Norman, 1984) are lower than might be expected.

Fluorescence
Vitamins D_2 and D_3 do not exhibit native fluoresence (Nair, 1966).

2.2.4 Biological Activity in Man

Functional metabolism
The vitamin D_3 made in the skin, or dietary vitamin D_2 or D_3 absorbed from the small intestine, must be converted to the 25-hydroxy derivative in the liver, and then to the 1,25-dihydroxy derivative in the kidney, before it can function. The renal biosynthesis of the 1,25-dihydroxy D_3 is stimulated by parathyroid hormone which, in turn, is secreted in response to a low plasma calcium concentration (hypocalcaemia).

The 25-hydroxy derivative of vitamin D_3 or D_2 is the major circulating form of the vitamin. The concentration of 25-hydroxy D_3 in foods is very low and is measured at the nanogram level. Typical values are cows' milk < 1 ng/ml; bovine muscle 2–3 ng/g; bovine liver 5–8 ng/g; bovine kidney 10–12 ng/g; chicken egg yolk 5–8 ng/g (Koshy, 1982).

Physiological role
The 1,25-dihydroxy metabolite of vitamin D_3 is the physiologically active form of the vitamin, and acts as a hormone in the regulation of calcium and phosphorus metabolism. It is now well established that the metabolite functions by increasing the intestinal absorption of calcium and phosphate by two independent mechanisms; and by mobilizing calcium, accompanied by phosphate, from the bone fluid compartment (this effect requires the presence of parathyroid hormone). There is also evidence to suggest that the metabolite improves the renal absorption of calcium, and perhaps phosphate. The maintenance of normal serum calcium and phosphorus concentrations prevents hypocalcaemic tetany, and provides for normal mineralization of bone. Vitamin D also functions in some manner to improve muscle strength and tone (DeLuca, 1978).

Vitamin D deficiency in children causes rickets, in which the bones do not develop properly through inadequate deposition of calcium and phosphorus, and become deformed. The equivalent disease in adults is called osteomalacia, in which there is a reabsorption of calcium and phosphorus from bone already laid down, causing the bones to become very brittle.

Vitamin D, in common with vitamin A, is toxic when ingested in large amounts. In adults, daily intakes of vitamin D in excess of 50 000 IU produce toxicity symptoms of anorexia, dehydration, muscle weakness, headache. nausea, vomiting, polyuria (excessive urine production) and polydipsia (frequent drinking because of extreme thirst). Serum calcium levels are increased as a result of bone demineralization, and calcium is deposited in the kidneys, causing hypertension, renal failure, cardiac insufficiency and anaemia. As in vitamin A toxicity, hypervitaminosis D results from oversupplementation with pharmaceutical products, and not from the consumption of usual diets. Hypervitaminosis D does not result from unlimited exposure to sunshine. Skin tanning or the aggregation of the pigment melanin in the skin creates a filter for UV light, and prevents conversion of the 7-dehydrocholesterol to cholecalciferol. The toxicity of excessive amounts of ingested vitamin D is attributable to the pharmacological effects of 25-hydroxycholecalciferol in high concentration; circulating concentrations of 1,25-dihydroxycholecalciferol are not greatly increased in vitamin D-intoxicated patients (Miller & Hayes, 1982; Omaye, 1984).

Biopotency
The International Unit of vitamin D is the activity of 0·025 μg of crystalline cholecalciferol. The potency of ergosterol is (for man) considered to be equivalent to that of cholecalciferol (Parrish, 1979).

The biological activity of 1 μg of vitamin D_2 or D_3 is 40 IU.

Requirement
Recommended daily amounts of vitamin D for population groups in the United Kingdom have been published (Department of Health and Social Security, 1979). No dietary sources may be necessary for children and adults who are sufficiently exposed to sunlight but, during the winter, children and adolescents should receive 10 μg (400 IU) of the vitamin daily by supplementation. Adults with inadequate exposure to sunlight, for example those who are housebound, may also need a supplement of 10 μg daily. Holmes & Kummerow (1983) emphasized the dangers of oversupplementation of vitamin D, and stated that quantities as little as 30 μg (1200 IU) per day may contribute to cardiovascular and renal damage.

2.2.5 Biological Activity in Animals
Vitamin D deficiency affects the bones, muscles and nervous system, as well as the fertility of livestock and poultry. The prominent sign is rickets in young animals, accompanied by stunted growth and weight loss.

Piglets suffer from increased irritability and convulsions due to tetany. Osteomalacia is not common in farm animals, although a similar condition can occur in pregnant and lactating animals, who require increased amounts of calcium and phosphorus. Pregnant cattle and sheep produce weak, dead or malformed offspring. Infertility in poultry is manifested by embryonic malfunctions, decreased egg production, thin-shelled eggs, and reduced hatchability (Anon., 1976).

The antirachitic activity of vitamins D_2 and D_3 is approximately equal in cattle, sheep and pigs, but vitamin D_2 has only about one-thirtyfifth of the potency of D_3 for poultry (McDonald et al., 1972).

2.2.6 Supplementation of Foods and Animal Feeds

Foods

The recommended daily allowance of vitamin D for humans exposed to inadequate sunlight is 10 μg. Except for eggs and certain salt water fish, a serving of food containing only natural sources of vitamin D would probably supply less than 1 μg of the vitamin. Fish liver oils constitute moderate to rich sources of vitamin D, but they are pharmaceuticals rather than food (Parrish, 1979).

Foodstuffs commonly enriched with vitamin D include margarine (by legislation in the United Kingdom), skimmed milk powder, evaporated milk, milk-based beverages, breakfast cereals, dietetic products of all kinds, baby foods and soup powders. Vitamin D_2 prepared commercially from bakers' yeast is either added as an oily solution, or in combination with a vitamin A formulation (Kläui et al., 1970).

Animal feeds

In grazing cattle vitamin D_3 may be synthesized by the action of sunlight upon 7-dehydrocholesterol in the skin and its secretions. Nevertheless, high yielding dairy cows and young cattle during the growing or fattening period should receive daily supplements of vitamin D in their feed rations.

Most conserved fodders have widely varying contents of vitamin D, and most concentrates contain almost none. The feeds are supplemented by using a vitamin/mineral premix or a protein concentrate with added vitamins and minerals. Since the conditions of stability and application for vitamin D closely resemble those for vitamin A, commercial forms of stabilized dry preparations have been developed (Anon., 1976; Meissonnier, 1983).

The need for supplementing the diets of pigs and poultry is greater than that for cattle and sheep.

2.2.7 Bioassays

The biological response to vitamin D, i.e. the calcification of bone, is highly specific and forms the basis of the classical assay methods. The response is also extremely sensitive; 0.1 μg of vitamin D per day is more than adequate for a white rat. The rat is most often used, as it is sensitive to both vitamins D_2 and D_3. The chick is also used, since birds respond efficiently only to vitamin D_3.

Curative methods involve feeding the test sample, and a standard preparation of the vitamin, to separate groups of rats or chicks, which have been previously subjected to rachitogenic (vitamin D-deficient) diets. The extent to which the rickets has been cured is then estimated by examination of the bones. In the line method the calcified portion of the distal end of the radius bone is measured after chemical treatment with silver nitrate. The radiographic method involves the examination of X-ray photographs of rat tibia, and is used to estimate the vitamin D activity of cod-liver oil.

In prophylactic methods the rats or chicks receive the test sample and standard preparation at the beginning of the assay, and their ability to prevent rickets is compared. The bone-ash technique has found widespread application in the testing of the cholecalciferol content of chicken feed (Kodicek & Lawson, 1967; Green, 1970; DeLuca & Blunt, 1971; Parrish, 1979).

In all vitamin D bioassays, it is essential to ensure that the reference standard solution and the sample solution are equilibrated to the same previtamin D/vitamin D ratio. This can be achieved by heating the standard and sample solutions simultaneously at 80°C for 2.5 h, then quickly cooling (Keverling Buisman et al., 1968).

2.3 VITAMIN E

Discovery. The existence of vitamin E was discovered in 1922 by Evans and Bishop, who demonstrated that pregnant rats fed on formulated diets containing all of the then known nutritional factors did not reach term. Resorption of the foetus was prevented by feeding lettuce, thus implying the addition of a hitherto unknown nutrient. The active substance was isolated in 1936 by Evans, and called tocopherol, from the Greek meaning 'to bear offspring'.

2.3.1 Chemical Structure

Eight vitamers of vitamin E occur in nature: four tocopherols and four tocotrienols (Schudel et al., 1972; Kasparek, 1980; Parrish, 1980a).

Tocopherols are methyl-substituted derivatives of tocol, and comprise a chroman-6-ol nucleus attached at C-2 to a side chain composed of three saturated isoprene units. Tocotrienols are similar structures whose side chains contain three double bonds. The tocopherols and tocotrienols are designated alpha-(α), beta-(β), gamma-(γ) and delta-(δ), and differ according to the number and position of the methyl groups in the chromanol nucleus (Fig. 11); the β- and γ-forms are positional isomers. The biological activities of the tocopherols are in the order $\alpha > \beta > \gamma > \delta$.

Vitamin E exhibits optical isomerism attributable to the asymmetric carbon atoms at C-2 and at positions 4' and 8' of the side chain, making possible eight diastereoisomers. The naturally occurring stereoisomer, d-α-tocopherol, is designated more correctly as $2R, 4'R, 8'R$-α-tocopherol or RRR-α-tocopherol; the epimer, l-α-tocopherol is designated as $2S, 4'R, 8'R$-α-tocopherol or 2-*epi*-α-tocopherol. A mixture of RRR-α-tocopherol and 2-*epi*-α-tocopherol in approximately equimolar proportions is obtained by synthesis from natural phytol as starting material. The acetate ester of this mixture formerly constituted the international standard for vitamin E and was known as 'synthetic racemic α-tocopheryl acetate'. The mixture of the

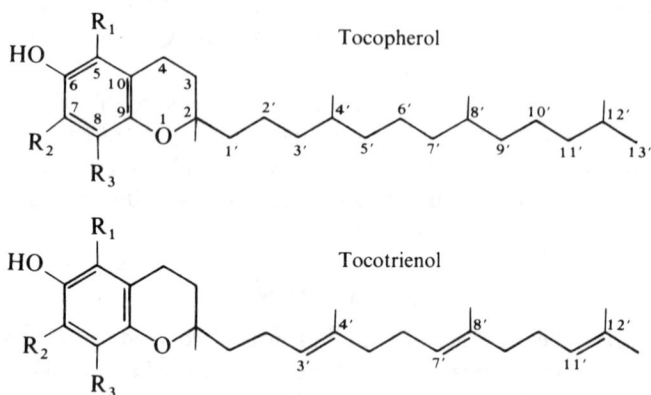

Tocopherol or Tocotrienol	R_1	R_2	R_3
α-5,7,8-Trimethyl	CH_3	CH_3	CH_3
β-5,8-Dimethyl	CH_3	H	CH_3
γ-7,8-Dimethyl	H	CH_3	CH_3
δ-8-Methyl	H	H	CH_3

Fig. 11. Chemical structures of the E vitamers.

two tocopherol epimers should be designated as 2-*ambo*-α-tocopherol. Totally synthetic α-tocopherol obtained from totally synthetic phytol or isophytol as starting material is a mixture of eight diastereoisomers as four racemates or pairs of enantiomers in unspecified proportions. It was formerly known as *dl*-α-tocopherol and should be designated as all-*rac*-α-tocopherol (AOAC, 1984*a*). The acetate ester of all-*rac*-α-tocopherol is the form usually used in the fortification of foods.

In nature, the polyene side chains of the tocotrienols have the all-*trans* configuration.

The term 'tocopherol' in this review refers specifically to the methyl-substituted tocols, whilst 'vitamin E' refers to the tocopherols and tocotrienols collectively. The different vitamin E structures are frequently, but incorrectly, referred to as homologues. In this review, the eight vitamin E structures will be referred to as E vitamers.

2.3.2 Natural Occurrence
In foods that constitute rich sources of vitamin E, the naturally occurring form of the vitamin is the free alcohol.

The richest dietary sources of vitamin E are the cereal seed oils, and the margarines, salad dressings and other products made from them. The distribution of tocopherols and tocotrienols in different plant oils varies greatly, as shown in Table 5.

Other plant sources are the lipid fraction of nuts, fruits, vegetables and

Table 5

Percentage composition of tocopherols and tocotrienols in edible oils (Taylor & Barnes, 1981)

Edible oil	% distribution of vitamin E vitamers								Total vitamin E µg/g
	Tocopherols				Tocotrienols				
	α-	β-	γ-	δ-	α-	β-	γ-	δ-	
Wheat germ	72	25	—	—	—	3	—	—	2 000
Soy bean	7	1	70	22	—	—	—	—	1 200
Corn	22	3	68	7	—	—	—	—	1 000
Cottonseed	40	—	58	1	—	—	—	—	1 000
Sunflower	96	2	2	—	—	—	—	—	700
Castor	6	6	23	65	—	—	—	—	500
Palm	25	—	—	—	30	—	40	5	500
Coconut	10	—	10	—	—	—	80	—	50

cereal grains. Nuts and seeds are particularly good sources of vitamin E. Most fruits contain relatively low amounts of vitamin E, and in apples and pears the concentration of the vitamin is greater in the skin than in the flesh. The vitamin E content of vegetables differs according to the different parts of the plant. Green leaves have low to moderate levels, whilst roots and tubers are generally low sources of the vitamin. Tocotrienols are mostly absent in nuts, fruits and vegetables, except for small amounts in carrots, sweetcorn and mushrooms (McLaughlin & Weihrauch, 1979).

Among the whole grains, maize has the highest total vitamin E content of about 8 mg/100 g. The highest levels in the different milling fractions of cereal grains are about 28 mg/100 g in wheat germ and 15 mg/100 g in rice bran. Whole wheat flour contains 4 mg/100 g of total vitamin E. More of the different vitamin E forms have been identified in cereal grains than in most other foods. Wheat is unusual in that β-tocotrienol is the most prominent form (McLaughlin & Weihrauch, 1979).

Animals store vitamin E in their fatty tissues, thus the chief animal sources of the vitamin are high-fat products such as eggs, butter, cheese and liver. In raw muscle, fat, and organs from mammals and birds vitamin E is all, or nearly all, in the form of α-tocopherol. Only small amounts of other tocopherols have been found in a few samples, and no tocotrienols have been found. Mammalian muscle generally contains less than 1 mg of total tocopherol per 100 g; liver or heart may contain slightly more. In eggs, all of the vitamin E is in the yolk. One average large chicken egg (50 g edible content) would contain 0·53 mg of total vitamin E. Chicken eggs differ from most animal products in that about one-third of the vitamin E is in the γ-tocopherol form. The concentration of vitamin E in dairy products varies with the cow's feed. The vitamin E content of fish muscle varies with the species and is mainly in the form of α-tocopherol (McLaughlin & Weihrauch, 1979).

The vitamin E contents of a wide range of raw materials and food products have been reviewed by Bunnell et al. (1965), Draper (1970), Green (1970), Ames (1972a), Bauernfeind (1977, 1980) and McLaughlin & Weihrauch (1979). A selection from the latter publication is presented in Table 6.

With regard to animal nutrition, most fresh green forage crops are a good source of vitamin E; the content of the vitamin tends to vary in parallel with that of the carotenoids. The vitamin E content of grasses reaches a peak at flowering time and then drops considerably as the plants reach maturity. Wilting destroys a certain amount of vitamin E by oxidation in the presence of heat and light. Cereals and milling by-products

Table 6

Vitamin E content of selected foods[a] (McLaughlin & Weihrauch, 1979)

Food	mg/100 g food						
	Tocopherols				Tocotrienols		Total vitamin E
	α-	β-	γ-	δ-	α-	β-	
Nuts (raw)							
Almond	23·96		0·51				24·48
Walnut	0·84		17·84	0·94			19·62
Brazil	6·5		11·0				
Peanut	8·33		8·04				16·37
Cashew	0·19		3·84	0·17			4·20
Vegetables (raw)							
Spinach	1·88		0·14	0·98			3·00
Pea	0·13		2·58				2·71
Parsley	1·74	0·18		0·61			2·53
Cabbage	1·67		trace	trace			1·67
Leek	0·92						
Lettuce	0·40		0·35				0·75
Carrot	0·44	0·02		0·01	0·04	trace	0·51
Mushroom	0·08		0·09		0·12		0·29
Potato, white	0·06	trace					0·07
Fruit (raw)							
Blackberry (wild)	3·5		4·7	4·5			
Raspberry	0·3		1·5	2·7			
Apple	0·59						0·66
Tomato	0·34	0·13		0·02			0·49
Banana	0·27						0·32
Orange	0·24						0·24
Cereal products							
Flour, whole wheat	0·82	0·66			0·27	2·20	3·95
Rice, brown	0·68		0·37	trace		0·98	2·04
Meat, poultry and fish							
Beef, lean, raw	0·41	0·02					0·43
Beef, roast	0·14						
Beef heart, raw	0·60						
Lamb, liver, raw							0·79
Bacon, fried	0·53						0·59
Chicken, cooked	0·35						0·55
Haddock, broiled	0·60						1·20

(*continued*)

Table 6—*Contd.*

Food	Tocopherols				Tocotrienols		Total vitamin E
	α-	β-	γ-	δ-	α-	β-	
Dairy products, and eggs							
Milk, cow, fluid,							
whole (USA)	0·06	0·01					0·09
Butter (USA)	1·58						1·58
Egg yolk, raw	2·05		1·03	0·03			3·12
Egg, whole, raw	0·07		0·35	0·01			1·06
Egg, whole, cooked	0·77						

[a] Data compiled from various published sources. Blanks indicate a lack of information. Brackets indicate β- and γ-tocopherols measured together.

are important sources of vitamin E in animal diets. In green fodder and cereals, losses of vitamin E occur during long-term storage, particularly if moisture is present. Silages from maize, some grasses and immature cereals are almost totally devoid of vitamin E because it is rapidly destroyed during lactic fermentation. Most conserved fodders have widely varying contents of vitamin E, whilst feed concentrates (cereals, oilseed cakes, roots) contain almost none (Meissonnier, 1983; Albers, *et al.*, 1984).

2.3.3 Physico-chemical Properties

Description
Tocopherols and tocotrienols in the pure form are pale yellow viscous oils, but darken on exposure to oxygen.

Solubility
Vitamin E is insoluble in water; readily soluble in alcohol and other organic solvents (including acetone, chloroform and ether), and in vegetable oils. Vitamin E acetates are less readily soluble in ethanol than the unesterified vitamin (Desai & Machlin, 1985).

Stability
Vitamin E in the unesterified form is slowly oxidized by atmospheric oxygen to form mainly biologically inactive quinones, such as α-tocopheryl-quinone (Fig. 12). Small amounts of various dimers and trimers are also formed. Figure 13 shows the structure of a γ-tocopherol dimer, 5-(γ-tocopheryloxy)-γ-tocopherol, formed by air oxidation when γ-tocopherol

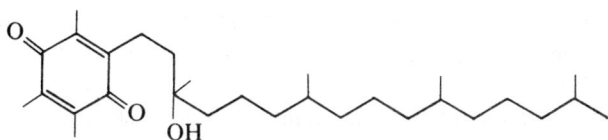

Fig. 12. α-Tocopherylquinone.

was stored for three months in a closed container in a refrigerator. This particular dimeric structure is composed of two γ-tocopherol residues joined by an ether linkage involving the phenolic oxygen of one of the γ-tocopherol moieties (Nilsson *et al.*, 1968).

Oxidation of vitamin E is accelerated by exposure to light, heat, alkaline pH conditions, and the presence of certain trace minerals, such as iron (Fe^{3+}) and copper (Cu^{2+}). Ferrous and cuprous ions, and ground-state copper, do not react with vitamin E. Ascorbic acid, if present, completely prevents the catalytic effect of ferric and cupric ions by maintaining the metals in their lower oxidation states (Cort *et al.*, 1978).

The E vitamers are stable to heat and to alkali in the absence of oxygen, and are unaffected by acids, up to 100°C. The vitamers are stable to visible light, but are destroyed by UV light, especially in the presence of oxygen (Association of Vitamin Chemists, Inc., 1966; Scott, 1978).

Vitamin E, in its antioxidant role, protects the fatty components of a food or tissue from oxidation by combining with free radicals, and stopping the chain reaction by which free radicals multiply. In combating lipid oxidation, vitamin E is itself oxidized, especially by hydroperoxides, which are oxidation products of unsaturated fatty acids (Kläui, 1971). The

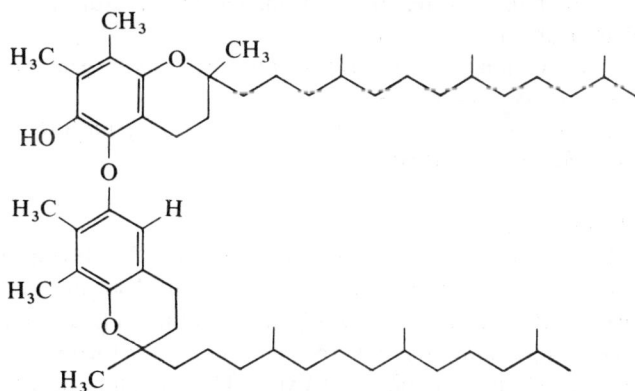

Fig. 13. 5-(γ-Tocopheryloxy)-γ-tocopherol.

oxidation products of vitamin E in natural products include quinones, hydroquinones and tocopheroxides, as well as dimers and trimers (Machlin, 1984).

Unlike the free tocopherol, the acetate ester is practically unaffected by the oxidizing influence of air, light, and UV light (Merck Index, 1983).

The influence of food processing upon the stability of vitamin E has been discussed by Bauernfeind (1980). Boiling destroys 30% of vitamin E in Brussels sprouts, cabbages and carrots (Bender, 1979), and losses of 70–90% result in the production of canned beans, sweetcorn and peas (Ames, 1972a). Frozen vegetables retain much of their vitamin E (Ames, 1972a). Much of the vitamin E loss during the processing of green vegetables is due to the discarding of the vitamin E-rich 'inedible' portions. When leaves cease growing or die, the concentration of α-tocopherol increases, thus vegetables past their prime, or wilted, are probably better sources of α-tocopherol than the preferred 'edible' portions (Ames, 1972a).

Vitamin E in grain and cereal products is unstable during storage: only 60% of the α-tocopherol of maize is retained after storage for twelve weeks at room temperature. Large losses of α-tocopherol occur during the milling of wheat flour, and in the processing of most grains to produce breakfast cereals (Ames, 1972a).

Refined corn oil contains less than half the α-tocopherol content of freshly extracted corn oil (Ames, 1972a). While there is little loss (about 10%) of vitamin E during the deep fat frying of potato crisps in fresh vegetable oil, there is a great loss (about 80%) of vitamin E in potato crisps stored at room temperature and at $-12°C$. The loss of vitamin E at freezer temperatures is due to their destruction by hydroperoxides, which are more stable at low temperatures than at higher temperatures, and hence accumulate (Bunnell et al., 1965).

Little or no vitamin E is destroyed during the hydrogenation of oils (McLaughlin & Weihrauch, 1979).

Irradiation of foods with gamma rays destroys a significant amount of vitamin E (Bauernfeind, 1980).

Ultraviolet absorption

Vitamin E exhibits a relatively low intensity of UV absorption, each vitamer being characterized by a slightly different absorption maximum within the wavelength range of 292–298 nm in ethanol (Kasparek, 1980). Figures 14 and 15 show the absorption spectra of α-tocopherol and α-tocopheryl acetate in ethanol, respectively. The $E_{1cm}^{1\%}$ and λ_{max} values of some vitamin E-active compounds are listed in Table 7.

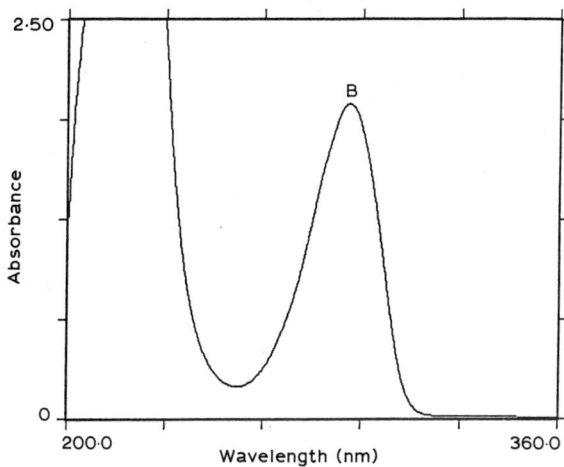

Fig. 14. UV absorption spectrum of *dl*-α-tocopherol in ethanol (λ_{max} of peak B = 294 nm).

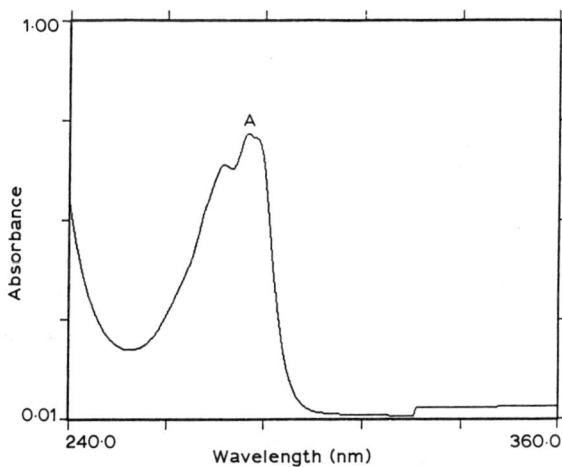

Fig. 15. UV absorption spectrum of *dl*-α-tocopheryl acetate (all-*rac*) in ethanol (λ_{max} of peak A = 285·5 nm).

Table 7
$E_{1cm}^{1\%}$ of some vitamin E-active compounds

Vitamin E vitamer	$E_{1cm}^{1\%}$	λ_{max}	Reference
d-α-Tocopherol (RRR)	71	294 nm	Scott (1978)
d-β-Tocopherol (RRR)	86·4	297 nm	Scott (1978)
d-γ-Tocopherol (RRR)	92·8	298 nm	Scott (1978)
d-δ-Tocopherol (RRR)	91·2	298 nm	Scott (1978)
d-α-Tocotrienol (RRR)	91	292·5 nm	Scott (1978)
d-β-Tocotrienol (RRR)	87	296 nm	Scott (1978)
dl-α-Tocopheryl acetate (all-rac)	40–44	285·5 nm	Machlin (1984)

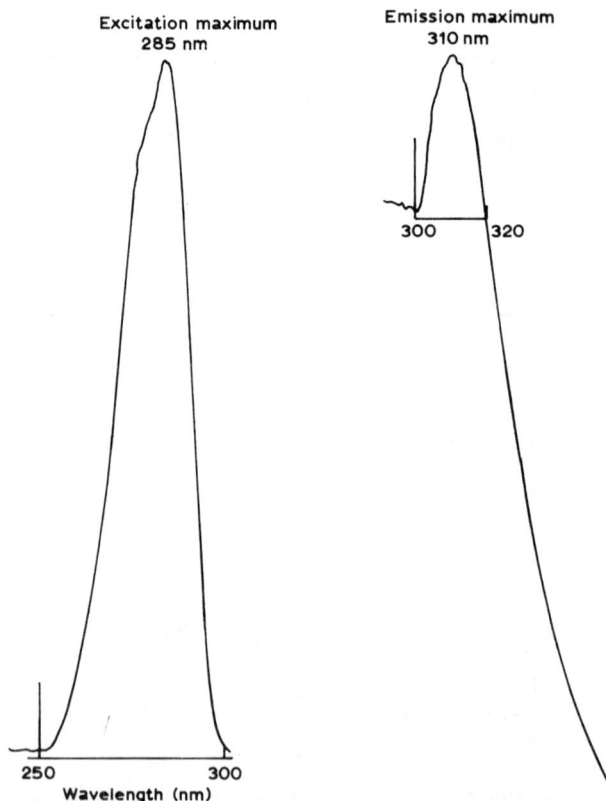

Fig. 16. Fluorescence excitation and emission spectra of α-tocopheryl acetate obtained by stop-flow scanning after passage through a silica HPLC column eluted with hexane containing 0·03% isopropanol.

Fluorescence
Non-esterified vitamin E exhibits strong native fluorescence; α-tocopherol displays excitation and emission maxima of 295 nm and 330 nm, respectively (Duggan *et al.*, 1957). Alpha-tocopheryl acetate has been generally regarded to be non-fluorescent but, with the aid of high-performance liquid chromatography used in conjunction with a suitable fluorescence detector, it has been shown to exhibit 9% of the fluorescence activity of the free tocopherol (Barnes & Taylor, 1980). The excitation and emission spectra of α-tocopheryl acetate are shown in Fig. 16.

2.3.4 Biological Activity in Man

Functional metabolism
In general, little is known about the metabolism of vitamin E. Behrens & Madère (1983) presented evidence from studies in rats that the mechanisms regulating the utilization (i.e. intestinal absorption, plasma transport and tissue uptake) of vitamin E are highly specific for α-tocopherol. Only when the concentration of dietary α-tocopherol is kept artificially low, does γ-tocopherol compete successfully for binding sites at the levels of absorption, plasma transport and tissue uptake. This could explain why the vitamin E content of meat and human plasma comprises mainly α-tocopherol, despite the fact that γ-tocopherol contributes significantly to the total vitamin E activity of the normal diet.

Dietary α- tocopheryl acetate originating from vitamin E-fortified foods is hydrolysed by esterases in the body to the free tocopherol (Cort *et al.*, 1978).

Physiological role
Owing to the prevalence of vitamin E in common foods, its widespread storage distribution throughout the body tissues, and its very slow turnover in the body, it is rare to encounter vitamin E deficiency in humans, no matter how malnourished they may be in other respects. The principal deficiency symptom in man is haemolytic anaemia (rupturing of the red blood cells), which occurs most often in premature infants, and which is due to the inefficient transportation of vitamin E across the placenta (Johnson, 1979).

It is widely believed that vitamin E functions *in vivo* mainly as an antioxidant by protecting unsaturated lipids in biological membranes from peroxidative degeneration. This concept is supported by the observation that the order of *in vivo* antioxidant activities of the tocopherols is the same as that of their biological potencies, i.e. $\alpha > \beta > \gamma > \delta$. The antioxidant activity depends on the molar ratio of antioxidant to unsaturated lipid, with one molecule each of the α-, β-, γ- and δ-tocopherol protecting, respectively, 220, 120, 100 and 30 molecules of polyunsaturated fatty acid (Fukuzawa et al., 1982).

A nutritional interrelationship exists between vitamin E and the trace element, selenium. For example, selenium substitutes completely for vitamin E in the prevention of muscular dystrophy in vitamin E-deficient sheep and cattle, whilst both nutrients are required for preventing liver necrosis in the rat. Selenium is an essential trace element because it is a constituent of glutathione peroxidase, an enzyme which protects the integrity of cell membranes by reducing fatty acid peroxides to hydroxy acids. The biosynthesis of this enzyme is prevented by a deficiency in vitamin E. At higher concentrations of selenium, where an excess remains after enzyme synthesis, the metal will act as a free-radical donor, and so may be carcinogenic. Vitamin E, being an antioxidant, will tend to counteract this free-radical damage (Johnson, 1979). These observations further support the concept that vitamin E acts to stabilize unsaturated lipids in biological membranes.

Vitamin E has also been implicated in a variety of other functions. These include the regulation of muscle metabolism and the DNA and RNA control of specific proteins in muscle cells; regulation of the development and function of the gonads; and the preparation for and protection of pregnancy (Meissonnier, 1983; Albers et al., 1984). Evidence for these functions are found in animals deprived of vitamin E (see Section 2.3.5).

More important than the absolute concentration of vitamin E in the diet is the ratio of vitamin E to polyunsaturated fatty acids (PUFA), which has been proposed as a criterion of nutritional status (Harris & Embree, 1963). Horwitt (1960) demonstrated vitamin E deficiency in adult humans by increasing the amount of PUFA relative to the amount of vitamin E in the diet. The additional antioxidizing activity required with a high PUFA diet reduced plasma tocopherol concentrations, and resulted in red cell haemolysis. Fortunately, most foods rich in PUFA also contain large amounts of vitamin E, thus deficiency will not develop under normal circumstances.

Vitamin E, being fat-soluble, accumulates in the body, especially in the liver and pancreas. Unlike vitamins A and D, however, vitamin E is regarded to be essentially non-toxic, although daily doses of 800 IU of α-tocopherol have been reported to induce severe weakness, fatigue and other side effects in otherwise healthy adults. Excess vitamin E may also interfere

Table 8
Biological activities of commercial forms of vitamin E
(Bieri & McKenna, 1981)

Form	IU/mg
dl-α-Tocopheryl acetate (all-rac)	1·00
dl-α-Tocopherol (all-rac)	1·10
d-α-Tocopheryl acetate (RRR)	1·36
d-α-Tocopherol (RRR)	1·49

with the normal blood clotting process, producing a need for more vitamin K (Omaye, 1984). Many people now take vitamin E in large doses on their own initiative. In a double blind trial this showed no benefits on work performance, sexuality, or general well being (Truswell, 1985).

Biopotency
The International Unit of vitamin E is the activity of 1 mg of dl-α-tocopheryl acetate. This is the average quantity that, administered orally, prevents resorption-gestation in fifty per cent of female rats deprived of vitamin E (Green, 1970).

The accepted biological activities, expressed in IU, of commercial forms of vitamin E are given in Table 8. The values imply that the activity of the acetate ester on a molar basis is equivalent to that of the free alcohol.

The relative percentage biological activities of the various tocopherols and tocotrienols are listed in Table 9.

Table 9
Relative percentage biological activities of vitamin E-active compounds

Vitamin E-active compound	Foetal resorption (rat)	Haemolysis (rat)	Muscular dystrophy (chick)
d-α-Tocopherol (RRR)	100	100	100
d-β-Tocopherol (RRR)	25–40	15–27	12
d-γ-Tocopherol (RRR)	1–11	3–20	5
d-δ-Tocopherol (RRR)	1	0·3–2	—
d-α-Tocotrienol (RRR)	29	17–25	—
d-β-Tocotrienol (RRR)	5	1–5	—

Reprinted from Machlin, 1984, p. 102 by courtesy of Marcel Dekker, Inc.

Requirement

In the United Kingdom a specific dietary requirement of vitamin E is not stated, but the recommended daily allowance of the vitamin for a middle-aged man in a sedentary occupation is 10 mg (Kläui *et al.*, 1970). Intakes of 1–8 mg (Losowsky, 1979) and 10 mg (Department of Health and Social Security, 1969) of α-tocopherol per day have been quoted in a typical United Kingdom diet. In the United States the values are higher owing to the larger intake of polyunsaturated fatty acids, and range from 3–18 mg of α-tocopherol per day (Losowsky, 1979). Since there appears to be an adequate concentration of vitamin E in the plasma of the general population for the prevention of haemolytic anaemia, it can be inferred that these levels of intake are normally sufficient.

2.3.5 Biological Activity in Animals

Owing to its various metabolic functions, a deficiency of vitamin E may appear in a variety of functional disorders that differ according to species, and that affect the muscular, vascular, nervous and reproductive systems.

Whilst clinical vitamin E deficiency is difficult to demonstrate in man, deficiency states in livestock are important since they frequently appear quite suddenly and with dramatic effect. In all livestock, a deficiency of vitamin E is associated with degeneration of the skeletal muscle causing muscular weakness, stiffness, and unnatural postures. The heart muscle is also affected, resulting in respiratory distress on the slightest exertion. Pigs, calves and lambs are susceptible to sudden death from heart failure. Changes in the vascular and nervous systems are most obvious in the chick. The formation of oedema in the cerebellum, owing to increased plasma exudation, leads to encephalomalacia, which is characterized by an abnormal posture of the head with uncoordinated movements. Exudative diathesis refers to oedema in the muscular tissue. Severe liver damage occurs in pigs. Reproductive disorders include testicular degeneration in piglets, calves and poultry, and foetal deaths in sheep, pigs and poultry (McDonald *et al.*, 1972; Anon., 1976).

Administration of trace amounts of selenium compounds or vitamin E prevent most of the muscular dystrophies in vitamin E-deficient sheep and cattle. Selenium can also replace vitamin E in preventing liver necrosis in the pig and exudative diathesis in the chick. Selenium, however, is ineffective in preventing encephalomalacia in the chick or muscular dystrophy induced in farm animals by dietary fats rich in unsaturated fatty acids. In preventing encephalomalacia in the chick, vitamin E appears to function as a biological antioxidant, since the condition can be completely prevented by administering synthetic antioxidants as well as by vitamin E (McDonald *et al.*, 1972).

2.3.6 Supplementation of Foods and Animal Feeds

Foods

Vitamin E, in the form of α-tocopheryl acetate, is sometimes added to whole milk powder (Indyk, 1983) and breakfast cereals (Widicus & Kirk, 1979) to supplement dietary requirements. The vitamin E requirement increases with an increased intake of polyunsaturated fatty acids, hence several types of high quality dietetic margarines are enriched with vitamin E (Kläui *et al.*, 1970).

Vitamin E can also be employed as an antioxidant to stabilize pure oils and fats. In this application the unesterified tocopherol must be used, as the ester is devoid of antioxidant activity. Animal fats, with their much lower tocopherol content than vegetable oils, can be stabilized effectively by the addition of tocopherol. Vegetable oils, which are relatively rich in natural tocopherols, can often be further stabilized by the addition of ascorbyl palmitate. The latter is a slightly fat-soluble ester of vitamin C which potentiates the antioxidant action of tocopherols (Kläui *et al.*, 1970).

There is conflicting evidence concerning the relative antioxidant effectiveness of the individual tocopherols *in vitro*. Detailed studies carried out by Burton & Ingold (1981) have revealed that the order of *in vitro* antioxidant activities of the tocopherols is the same as that of their biological activities, i.e. $\alpha > \beta > \gamma > \delta$, although there was no truly significant differences in the antioxidant activities of the β and γ isomers. According to Yamaoka *et al.* (1985), tocotrienols (α and γ forms) possess slightly superior or equal antioxidant activity to the corresponding tocopherols.

Vitamin E is claimed to help prevent the formation of harmful nitrosamines during the cooking of cured meats, such as bacon (Anon., 1985).

Animal feeds

Adult ruminants obtain sufficient vitamin E on green fodder as long as the dietary supply of selenium is adequate. Young cattle during the growing or fattening period, and all other livestock species, should receive supplemental vitamin E in their feed rations. Conserved fodders, which contain widely varying amounts of different E vitamers, are unreliable sources of vitamin E, since the important thing to know is the α-tocopherol content of the diet. Feed concentrates are almost devoid of the vitamin. The feeds are supplemented with synthetic α-tocopheryl acetate in stabilized form, either by using a vitamin/mineral premix or a protein concentrate with added vitamins and minerals (Meissonnier, 1983).

2.3.7 Bioassay

The rat foetal resorption assay has been used extensively to establish the biopotencies of the individual E vitamers, and to determine the availability of vitamin E from food sources (Ames, 1972b).

2.4 VITAMIN K

Discovery. The original coagulation factor, essential for normal blood clotting function in chicks kept on certain diets, was isolated in 1939 by the independent teams of Doisy, Dam and Karrer. Two compounds with antihaemorrhagic activity were identified; phylloquinone (vitamin K_1) from alfalfa meal, and menaquinone (vitamin K_2) from putrified fish meal.

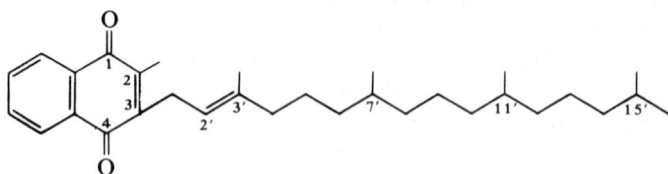

Phylloquinone (Vitamin K_1)

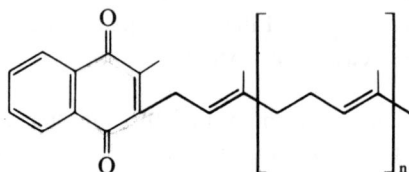

Menaquinone (Vitamin K_2)

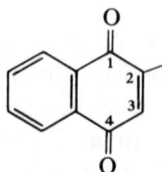

Menadione

Fig. 17.   Chemical structures of the vitamin K-active compounds.

2.4.1 Chemical Structure

Two forms of vitamin K exist in nature: vitamin K_1 is manufactured by green plants, and vitamin K_2 is synthesized by bacteria. The parent compound of vitamin K, 2-methyl-1,4-naphthoquinone, is not found as a natural product, but is available as a synthetic preparation called menadione (formerly called vitamin K_3). The chemical structures of these compounds are shown in Fig. 17.

Vitamin K_1 is called phylloquinone by nutritionists, but in the British and United States Pharmacopoeias its name is phytomenadione. Vitamin K_1 comprises a methyl-substituted naphthoquinone nucleus attached at C-3 to a side chain composed of three saturated and one unsaturated isoprene units. The natural form of vitamin K_1 is the *trans* isomer, whose stereochemistry is $2'$-*trans*, $7'R$, $11'R$. Synthetic preparations of vitamin K_1 usually contain both the *trans* and the *cis* isomers, but only the *trans* isomer is essentially responsible for the antihaemorrhagic activity of the vitamin.

Vitamin K_2 refers to a family of structural analogues called menaquinones, which have side chains composed of four to thirteen unsaturated isoprene units attached to the methyl-substituted naphthoquinone nucleus. The vitamin K_2 isoprenalogues are called menaquinone-4 (MK-4) to menaquinone-13 (MK-13), according to the number of isoprene units.

2.4.2 Natural Occurrence

Phylloquinone is found in the chloroplasts of photosynthetic plants, hence green leafy vegetables are a good dietary source of the vitamin. Most foods contribute significant amounts of the vitamin to satisfy the low dietary requirement. The data in Table 10 gives a range of values for the vitamin K content of common foods. Single values are not reported owing to the lack of a solid data base (Suttie, 1984).

Animal feed concentrates (cereals, oilseed cakes, roots) contain only small amounts of vitamin K.

2.4.3 Physico-chemical Properties

Description

Phylloquinone is a golden yellow viscous oil; the various menaquinones can be obtained in crystalline form (Suttie, 1984); and menadione is a yellow crystalline powder.

Solubility

Phylloquinone is insoluble in water; sparingly soluble in alcohol; and readily soluble in acetone, ether, chloroform, hexane, fat and oils (Anon.,

Table 10
Vitamin K content of foods (Suttie, 1984)

Food	Vitamin K (μg per 100 g)			
	< 10	10–50	50–100	> 100
Animal products				
Skeletal meats	×			
Beef liver			×	
Other liver		×		
Dairy products				
Fluid milk	×			
Butter, cheese, eggs		×		
Cereals and cereal products				
Whole corn, whole wheat	×			
Oats		×		
Bread	×			
Corn oil		×		
Vegetables				
Potatoes, carrots, tomatoes	×			
Green beans, peas		×		
Cabbage, cauliflower			×	
Broccoli, spinach, lettuce				×
Brussels sprouts				×
Fruits				
Oranges, peaches, bananas	×			
Apple sauce	×			

1976). Menadione is soluble in organic solvents and only slightly soluble in water, but the bisulphite derivatives are water soluble (Parrish, 1980*b*).

Stability
Vitamin K compounds are decomposed by UV light, alkali, strong acids and reducing agents, but are reasonably stable to oxidizing conditions and to heat (Kutsky, 1973; Parrish, 1980*b*).

Ultraviolet absorption
Phylloquinone and the menaquinones all possess the same chromophore, and exhibit identical UV absorption spectra which contain five maxima. Figure 18 shows the spectrum for phylloquinone in hexane. The $E_{1cm}^{1\%}$

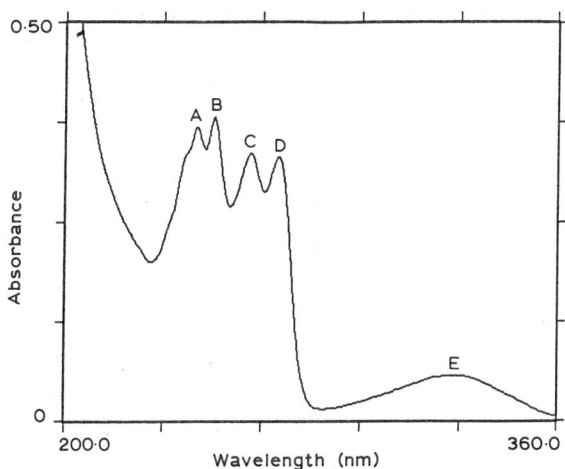

Fig. 18. UV absorption spectrum of phylloquinone (vitamin K_1) in hexane (λ_{max} of peak B = 248 nm).

value at the most pronounced absorption maximum (248 nm) is 419 (Merck Index, 1983). The $E_{1cm}^{1\%}$ values for both the vitamin K_1 and K_2 series decrease with increased length of the side chain; the molar absorptivity, however, remains constant ($\varepsilon = 18\,900$ at 248 nm) (Dunphy & Brodie, 1971). The absorption spectrum of menadione (Fig. 19) is different from that of the K_1 and K_2 vitamins, the most pronounced maximum occurring at 252 nm.

Fluorescence
Vitamin K compounds do not possess native fluorescence, but they are readily reduced or degraded to forms that do fluoresce (Shearer, 1986).

2.4.4 Biological Activity in Man
Functional metabolism
Vitamin K is absorbed from the intestine into the lymphatic system, in association with chylomicrons. It is rapidly concentrated in the liver, but has a relatively short half-life, which suggests very little long-term storage. Menaquinone-4 is the major metabolite formed, either by intestinal microorganisms or by tissue alkylating enzymes, when menadione is ingested (Suttie, 1985). Phylloquinone-2,3-epoxide is a metabolite of phylloquinone that is frequently found in biological tissues.

Physiological role
The role of vitamin K in blood coagulation lies in the biochemical synthesis

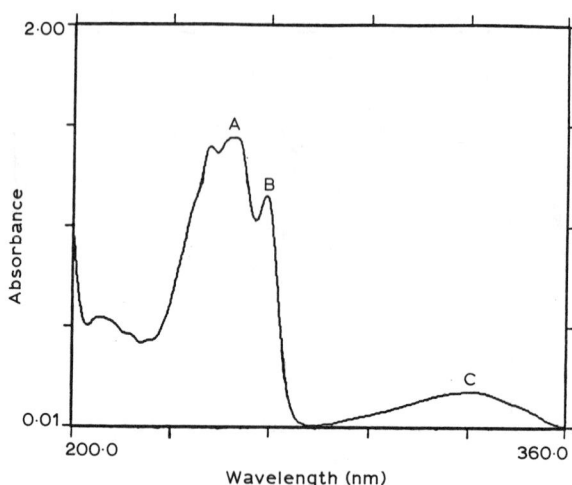

Fig. 19. UV absorption spectrum of menadione in hexane (λ_{max} of peak A = 252 nm).

and regulation of prothrombin and three other blood clotting proteins (factors VII, IX and X). In cases of vitamin K deficiency, thrombin is not generated in the plasma, and fibrinogen is not converted to fibrin (DeLuca, 1975). The vitamin acts as a cofactor for the enzymatic carboxylation of glutamic acid residues in the clotting proteins to γ-carboxyglutamic acid (GLA). The GLA residues provide the clotting proteins with the calcium-binding properties necessary for their functional activity (Lefevere *et al.*, 1985)

Phylloquinone is essentially non-toxic, but menadione is toxic to infants at excessive dose levels, producing haemolytic anaemia, liver and kidney damage, and death (Omaye, 1984). The toxic effects of large amounts of menadione are not manifestations of excessive vitamin K activity, but rather are side effects attributable to the non-physiological form of the compound (Miller & Hayes, 1982). Menadione is no longer used in human medicine or as a food supplement on account of its toxicity.

Biopotency
An official standard has not been established.

Requirement
Vitamin K is widely distributed in natural foods, and the human

requirement for the vitamin is small. Moreover, the intestinal bacteria almost always produce sufficient menaquinones to maintain normal blood clotting function, even in the absence of dietary sources. Apart from clinical and neonatal cases, a deficiency of vitamin K is therefore rare. Humans in early infancy may be at risk from the condition known as 'haemorrhagic disease of the human newborn'. The condition can be rectified by administering vitamin K either to the baby, or to the mother shortly before the baby's birth (Owen, 1971).

2.4.5 Biological Activity in Animals

Pigs and ruminants do not normally suffer from vitamin K deficiency since bacterial synthesis in the digestive tract supplies sufficient vitamin for the animal's needs.

Poultry are highly prone to a dietary deficiency of vitamin K. The symptom of vitamin K deficiency in chicks is a delayed clotting time of the blood: birds are easily injured and may bleed to death. Mature birds do not show these haemorrhagic signs. It is usually assumed that the site of vitamin K synthesis in the chick is too close to the distal end of the digestive tract to permit absorption. The rapid rate of passage of food through the intestine, and the relatively short length of large intestine in this species possibly contribute to the problem. It is also commercial practice to add antibiotics to poultry feeds, and this will decrease intestinal vitamin synthesis (Suttie, 1985).

2.4.6 Supplementation of Foods and Animal Feeds

Foods

Foods supplemented with vitamin K are confined to those infant formulae which contain phylloquinone.

Animal feeds

The requirements of adult cattle for vitamin K are largely covered by endogenous synthesis, but vitamin K supplements are advisable for calves in the early milk-feeding, rearing and fattening periods. The use of chemotherapeutic agents to combat coccidiosis and parasitic diseases in poultry inhibits the intestinal synthesis of vitamin K, and increases the requirements several-fold. Thus supplementation of poultry feeds is very important. Phylloquinone is too expensive to use for supplementing animal feeds, and various stabilized water-soluble derivatives of menadione, such as menadione sodium bisulphite, are used.

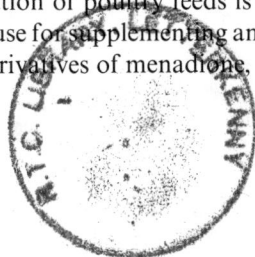

2.4.7 Bioassay

A standard bioassay for vitamin K has not been developed, but the technique most often used is the curative chick assay. Day-old chicks are placed on a vitamin K-deficient diet then separate groups are fed with the test sample, a standard menadione preparation, or continued on the same diet. Blood clotting tests are then performed and compared (Parrish, 1980*b*).

Chapter 3

Analytical Considerations

3.1 SCOPE OF ANALYTICAL TECHNIQUES

The analytical methods discussed in this literature review are physico-chemical assays for vitamins A, D, E and K in foods, infant formulae and animal feeds.

In vitamin A-fortified foods and feeds it is customary to determine either the supplemental retinyl acetate (or palmitate) or the total retinol, as well as the β-carotene. The analysis of fruits and vegetables requires the measurement of several active carotenoids for a proper evaluation of vitamin A activity; unofficial factors exist for calculating the biopotencies of carotenoid mixtures (Simpson *et al.*, 1985). It is equally important to separate inactive carotenoids, such as lycopene, so that they will not interfere with the measurements.

Vitamin D, being a highly potent nutrient, is present in foods (including fortified foods) at a much lower concentration compared with vitamins A and E. The estimation of the very low concentrations of naturally occurring vitamin D in foodstuffs is difficult, owing to the need to remove interfering substances such as cholesterol, vitamin A and vitamin E, which are invariably present in gross excess (see Table 11). In the analysis of animal products, including meat products, dairy products and eggs, a proper evaluation of the natural vitamin D content must include the 25-hydroxy metabolite of vitamin D. The determination of supplemental vitamin D_2 or D_3 is relatively more straightforward, but it is still necessary to remove the bulk of the interfering lipids prior to measurement. In practice, the estimated vitamin D value represents potential vitamin D, i.e. the sum of vitamin D and previtamin D.

In vitamin-E fortified foods and feeds, it is usually sufficient to determine

Table 11

Ratios of vitamins A, E and cholesterol to vitamin D in some foodstuffs
(Osborne & Voogt, 1978)

Foodstuff	Ratio relative to vitamin D on a weight basis			
	D	A	E	Cholesterol
Whole milk	1	1 500	5 000	600 000
Ox liver	1	6 000	1 400	300 000
Whole egg	1	75	500	80 000
Cod liver oil	1	120	60	10 000

either the supplemental α-tocopheryl acetate or the total α-tocopherol. Chromatographic techniques are available for determining, simultaneously, all of the natural tocopherols and tocotrienols present, as well as supplemental α-tocopheryl acetate. Knowledge of the concentration of naturally occurring non-esterified vitamin E provides an indication of the stability of fatty foods towards oxidative rancidity. The analysis of vegetable oils is discussed, since the tocopherols and tocotrienols are present in characteristic proportions in a given oil. The vitamin E profile of a vegetable oil therefore provides a possible means of detecting the adulteration of one vegetable oil with another.

Infant formula foods are supplemented with synthetic preparations of phylloquinone (vitamin K_1) which often contain some of the biologically inactive *cis* isomer with the active *trans* isomer. Analytical techniques are available that can distinguish between these isomers of vitamin K_1. The various derivatives of menadione, which are used to supplement animal feeds, can be determined chemically.

Before commencing the analysis, one must decide what is supposed to be measured, and how the results are to be expressed. Ideally, this information should be defined unambiguously in the instructions relating to the analysis. In the absence of clear-cut instructions concerning definitions and units, it is advisable to express results separately, in μg or mg, for each vitamin or vitamer measured in the analysis, and to refrain from calculating International Units or 'equivalents' (Thompson, 1986).

The first step in the determination of fat-soluble vitamins in foods is to isolate a vitamin-rich fraction using a suitable extraction procedure. This may involve saponification, enzymatic hydrolysis, or direct solvent extraction of the total lipid component. The bulk of the cholesterol and other sterols, where present, can be removed by precipitation from a freezing methanol solution, or by co-precipitation with digitonin. The analysis of the enriched fraction may then proceed according to one of the following techniques.

Ultraviolet-visible spectrophotometry facilitates the determination of the fat-soluble vitamins at around the 1 ng level, provided that the vitamin is isolated from the interfering substances that accompany it in the food matrix. Spectrophotometry is best utilized as a means of detection in high-performance liquid chromatography.

Fluorometry provides a detection limit of around the 1 pg level and is thus more sensitive, and also more selective, than absorption spectro-photometry. Fluorometry has been exploited as a detection method in high-performance liquid chromatography for measuring the native fluorescence of vitamins A and E. This technique has also been used to determine vitamin K after reduction to its fluorescent hydroquinone form.

Voltammetry (polarography) has been employed in the electrooxidative determination of vitamin E. The technique is limited in that it cannot distinguish the tocopherols from their corresponding tocotrienols; neither can it differentiate between their respective β- and γ-isomers.

Colorimetry is a non-specific measurement technique, and therefore necessitates prior purification of the vitamin-rich fraction by means of open-column or thin-layer chromatography. Depending on the purity of the isolated vitamin, the limit of detection is around the 1 μg level. The technique cannot distinguish between the various forms of a particular vitamin unless the vitamers are separated beforehand; this can often be achieved by means of thin-layer chromatography.

Gas–liquid chromatography (GLC) is a combined separation and measurement technique that relies upon the vitamins or chemical derivatives of the vitamins being volatile at elevated temperatures without decomposing. The flame ionization detector, which is the most suitable type of detector for the purpose, is non-selective, hence the extract to be analysed must be free from lipids (including sterols) and other interfering substances. GLC, using so-called 'packed' columns, provides a useful, but somewhat limited, knowledge of vitamin E activity, whilst high resolution open-tubular capillary columns enable all eight of the E vitamers to be individually determined. GLC methods have been used in the past for determining vitamins A, D and K but, owing to the need for extensive sample purification, followed by chemical reaction to produce stable derivatives, have been superseded by HPLC.

High-performance liquid chromatography (HPLC) is a combined separation and measurement technique that can be carried out at ambient temperature, and that does not rely upon derivatization of the vitamins. The technique, with absorbance detection, provides the most practical means of determining the fat-soluble vitamins in foods and feeds in terms of accuracy, precision, speed, and ease of operation. Fluorescence detection provides additional selectivity for vitamins A, E, and the reduced form of vitamin K, whilst electrochemical detection offers high sensitivity and selectivity for vitamin E. The high degree of resolution and selectivity provided by the column and detector, respectively, permits the simultaneous determination of the various vitamers of a particular parent vitamin, provided that interfering substances are removed beforehand. For example, supplemental and naturally occurring vitamin A can be determined, as can various combinations of carotenoids; vitamins D_2 and D_3 can be resolved from their respective previtamins and provitamins; the E vitamers, together with supplemental α-tocopheryl acetate, can be determined; and vitamin K_1 isomers can be separated from the various vitamin K_2 analogues. Various combinations of fat-soluble vitamins within a given food can also be determined simultaneously.

Depending upon the chromatographic conditions employed, the vitamins can be determined in the presence of certain other components, which therefore need not be removed beforehand. Vitamins A and E can often be measured by direct injection of a vitamin-rich fraction onto the HPLC column. Additional purification of vitamin D extracts is required to remove the relatively large amounts of interfering substances, particularly sterols. Vitamin K extracts, too, often demand a preliminary clean-up, depending upon the type of food under analysis.

3.2 APPRAISAL OF ANALYTICAL TECHNIQUES

The main criteria by which a measured value is judged are accuracy and precision. The accuracy of a measurement describes the difference between an observed value and the true value. A method is said to have high accuracy if the observed value is close to the true value. The precision of a set of measurements on the same quantity describes the differences among the individual measurements themselves; if they are close together, the measurements have high precision. Precision deals only with random errors that cannot be eliminated. These errors follow the normal distribution curve, hence can be expressed in units of standard deviation.

The repeatability of a method refers to the intra-laboratory precision, and is defined as the precision of a single operator repeating the same analysis on the same apparatus. The reproducibility of a method refers to the inter-laboratory precision, and refers to the precision of a number of operators performing the same analysis with different equipment.

Accuracy and precision can be expressed in terms of systematic error and statistical error. Systematic error refers to the difference between an ideal value and the true value. An ideal value can be estimated by taking the average result of a series of analyses performed on the same sample by the same person with the same equipment in the same laboratory. The statistical error refers to the standard deviation of this set of results. Accuracy is high if the systematic error is small, and the precision is high if the statistical error is small.

Since it is impossible to determine the true value of the concentration of a component in a natural product, it follows that there is no method of measuring the systematic error. Accuracy can only be assessed by comparing the results obtained from various independent methods. If two independent methods give the same result it is more probable that the measured value is near to the true value than that both methods have the same systematic error by chance. The accuracy of a method can be maximized by using an internal standard, performing a recovery experiment, and checking the purity of reference standards.

The relative standard deviation (RSD) can be calculated from the mean ($\bar{x}$) and the standard deviation (SD) of a set of replicate results as follows:

$$\text{RSD} = \frac{\text{SD} \times 100}{\bar{x}}$$

The RSD allows the analyst to tell quickly if the observed measurement falls within the acceptable precision of the method, independent of the size of the measurement. The precision depends on the concentration range of the analyte. Under optimal conditions the SD should increase linearly with the concentration, while the RSD should remain more or less constant. The detection limit of the method corresponds to the concentration when the RSD exceeds a certain value, which is generally about 25–50% (Brubacher et al., 1985).

In cases of official analyses, where the method is defined by law, the accuracy is of secondary importance to precision.

Vitamins, among other substances, are unevenly distributed in foods and the 'concentration' of a nutrient is actually a mean value with an associated uncertainty (Thompson, 1986). Therefore, before a food sample can be analysed, consideration must be taken to obtain a representative sample in order to reduce this uncertainty.

Liquid processed foods and dairy products will be reasonably homogeneous in nature, but solid processed foods will be relatively heterogeneous. The problem of inhomogeneity is probably greatest in those foods and animal feeds in which the supplemental vitamins are added in the form of gelatin-coated beadlets. The beadlets are not of uniform size or vitamin content; moreover, they tend to separate during mixing and handling, and then to agglomerate if exposed to moisture. The analysis of several randomly selected containers provides useful information concerning the homogeneity of the original food or feed, and is preferable to subsampling a large quantity of pooled material. Techniques have been described for sampling various types of food products (Lento, 1984; Elkins & Dudek, 1985) and animal feeds (HMSO, 1982; Thompson, 1986).

It is very important that the method employed is reproducible, or rugged, and gives good agreement between results from different laboratories. This means that small changes in the conditions of the analytical procedure (pH, purity of the analytical reagents, storage time of the sample, wavelength, etc.) result in insignificant changes in the measured result. A measure of the ruggedness of a method is its reliability; a reliable method exhibits a low variation of errors with time, and a low number of anomalous values.

3.3 GENERAL PRECAUTIONS AGAINST DESTRUCTION OF THE FAT-SOLUBLE VITAMINS DURING THE ANALYSIS

Great care must be taken throughout vitamin A assays to prevent oxidation and isomerization of the vitamin and carotenoids. During the extraction and subsequent purification stages, the retinol, if liberated from the ester by saponification, becomes increasingly sensitive to oxidation and destruction by light. Direct sunlight must be avoided and, if possible, illumination must be provided by gold fluorescent tubes which exclude light of less than 500 nm wavelength. Extractions should be performed in amber or low actinic glassware, and solvents should be de-oxygenated. Chlorinated solvents must not be used, and any diethyl ether used must be peroxide-free. Saponifications must be performed in an inert (oxygen-free) atmosphere. Antioxidants such as sodium ascorbate or pyrogallol may be added during both extraction and saponification. Evaporation of solutions containing vitamin A or carotenoids should be carried out under vacuum using a rotary evaporator, or under an inert gas at temperatures not exceeding 50°C. Chromatographic columns must be protected from light.

Retinol and the carotenoids can withstand boiling in strong alkali, provided that oxygen is excluded. However, these compounds are extremely sensitive to acid conditions below pH 4·5, which cause some degree of *cis-trans* isomerization.

In carotenoid assays, some plants must be blanched in boiling water to inactivate lipoxidase enzymes that would otherwise accelerate destruction of carotenoids during storage and mixing (Thompson, 1986).

Standards for vitamin A analysis are less stable than vitamin A extracts of samples where accompanying lipids and antioxidants provide protection. According to Thompson (1986) most of the commercially available standard retinol preparations are less than 60% pure, and further deterioration occurs soon after a container is opened. Dilute solutions of retinol and carotene undergo oxidation within minutes if exposed to even small amounts of air. The instability of vitamin A standards requires that they be prepared freshly each day, and that their concentrations be determined spectrophotometrically (see Section 6.1).

Thompson (1986) recommended preparing solutions of retinol in cottonseed oil at a concentration of about 2 mg/g; such solutions are stable for months, even when handled frequently. The oil solutions can be used daily to prepare standards for HPLC by weighing a few drops of the oil and dissolving them in an appropriate solvent. The concentration of retinol in the oil can be measured spectrophotometrically by dissolving the oil in isopropanol; the cottonseed oil does not interfere in this measurement.

Similar precautions to those described for vitamin A must be taken throughout the assay to avoid destruction of vitamin D by oxygen, light and acidity. Vitamin D should be maintained in an organic solvent solution whenever possible, as contact with water causes decomposition. Heating organic solutions of vitamin D promotes reversible thermal isomerization to previtamin D but, providing oxygen and light are excluded, does not degrade the vitamin.

Oxygen and light must be avoided in vitamin E assays, especially during the alkaline conditions of saponification.

Vitamin K compounds are rapidly decomposed in alkali, and thus it is not expedient to isolate them from fat by saponification. Enzymatic hydrolysis in a neutral medium offers an alternative to saponification, but solvent extraction is generally preferred. Vitamin K is destroyed by UV radiation, therefore exposure of the vitamin to daylight should be avoided during the analysis.

Chapter 4

Extraction of the Fat-Soluble Vitamins

The lipid fraction of foods containing the fat-soluble vitamins is composed mainly of triglycerides, with much smaller amounts of sterols, carotenoids, phospholipids, mono- and diglycerides, free fatty acids, hydrocarbons, etc. The amounts of fat-soluble vitamins in the lipid fraction may be very small. For instance, in whole milk fortified with 10 μg of vitamin D/g, it has been estimated that the vitamin D is present within a 3·5 million-fold excess of fat (Sertl & Molitor, 1985). The lipid material exhibits similar solubility properties to the fat-soluble vitamins, and can therefore interfere with the separation and measurement of the vitamins.

Some of the natural vitamin content of a food is bound up with a lipoprotein complex and, in milk, emulsifiers cause the fat and protein to interact strongly. The first task in the analytical procedure is, therefore, to break the fat/protein bonds, and to release the vitamins from any combined form in which they may exist. A vitamin-rich fraction is then isolated for subsequent analysis.

In the analysis of animal feeds, the protective gelatin coating surrounding the beadlets of stabilized vitamin preparations must be dissolved. This is most conveniently achieved by alkaline hydrolysis (saponification).

Extraction methods involve either, or both, of the following techniques:

(i) Release of the vitamins from the sample matrix by saponification, and extraction of the unsaponifiable matter containing the vitamins. Saponification is an economical way of digesting a large amount of material for analysis. Enzymatic hydrolysis may be used as an alternative to saponification. Either saponification or enzymatic hydrolysis facilitate the estimation of total retinol and total tocopherol by hydrolysing the esters of each vitamin to their respective alcohols.

(ii) Extraction of the total lipid from the sample with a suitable solvent or solvent system.† This technique allows the individual esters of vitamins A and E to be subsequently determined.

4.1 ALKALINE HYDROLYSIS (SAPONIFICATION)

Saponification involves the release of the vitamins from the sample matrix using a mixture of ethanol and 60% w/v aqueous potassium hydroxide (KOH) solution. The hydrolysis reaction attacks ester linkages, and releases the fatty acids from the glycerol moiety of glycerides and phospholipids, and from sterol esters. The reaction also breaks down a large number of pigments, and other substances that might otherwise interfere in vitamin measurements, into small, water-soluble fractions. The sterols, carotenoids, fat-soluble vitamins, etc., which constitute the unsaponifiable matter, are extractable into organic solvents from the alkaline solution: the fatty acids, which are precipitated as soaps, and the glycerol are not extractable under alkaline conditions.

Food products may be saponified directly, but prior solvent extraction of the sample may be employed as a means of preparing a concentrated vitamin extract for saponification. Samples containing starch have been digested with the enzyme takadiastase before saponification so as to avoid the formation of lumps in solution (Bui, 1987).

Saponification is conventionally carried out by refluxing the suitably prepared sample, or sample extract, with ethanolic KOH and added antioxidant for 30 min. Alternatively, prolonged alkaline digestion at ambient temperature may be carried out. The amount of ethanolic KOH solution required is dependent on the fat content of the sample. A rough guide is to use 5 ml of 60% w/v aqueous KOH and 15 ml of ethanol per 1 g of fat. If fat globules are still visible after the saponification period, the procedure should be repeated with an increased amount of KOH/ethanol reagent (Reynolds, 1984). About 25 mg of pyrogallol or 250 mg of sodium ascorbate is sufficient as antioxidant per 1 g of sample (Desai, 1980).

The fat-soluble vitamins are extracted from the diluted saponified solution with a 1:1 mixture of diethyl ether and petroleum spirit.‡ The

†The proportions of solvents in the various extracting solutions and mobile phases quoted throughout the entire text are by volume.
‡'Petroleum spirit' refers to petroleum spirit (petroleum ether) of boiling range between 30–60°C.

soaps are soluble in diethyl ether, and thus must be washed from extracts obtained with this solvent. The use of hexane as an extracting solvent has been reported, and is advantageous in that soaps are not extracted. However, with hexane, the minimum number of extractions needed is affected by the amount of fatty acids in the digest, and this, in practice, is not always easy to predict (Thompson, 1986).

The diethyl ether/petroleum solution is washed free of soaps and alkali, and carefully reduced to dryness on a rotary evaporator. The residue can now be redissolved in an appropriate solvent for analysis.

The following example of a saponification procedure was designed for saponifying 10 g amounts of skimmed milk powder (Reynolds & Judd, 1984). Different foods may require different amounts of sample, or may require preliminary solvent extraction.

A 10 g quantity of the suitably prepared, homogeneous food sample is weighed into a round-bottomed flask fitted with a side-arm. The anti-oxidant and about four-fifths of the ethanol are added, and the mixture is swirled to ensure that all the sample is wetted. The 60% w/v aqueous KOH solution is added and carefully mixed with the ethanol, followed by the remainder of the ethanol to wash down the sides of the flask. A slow stream of nitrogen is introduced via the side-arm, and the contents are boiled gently under reflux for 30 min.

When saponification is complete, the resultant solution is cooled as quickly as possible, then quantitatively transferred into a separating funnel using two 25 ml portions of distilled water to rinse out the flask. The unsaponifiable matter is extracted by adding 125 ml of diethyl ether:petroleum spirit (1:1), and shaking the funnel vigorously for 1 min. A further 125 ml of extracting solvent is added, and the funnel is re-shaken vigorously for a further 1 min. The layers are allowed to separate completely, and the lower aqueous layer is discarded. The organic layer is washed carefully with successive 100 ml portions of distilled water until the washings are free from alkali, and impart no coloration to phenolphthalein solution. Gentle swirling should be employed during the washing procedure to avoid the formation of emulsions which, if not broken, retain some of the vitamin, and result in poor recoveries. The substitution of water with saturated sodium chloride solution minimizes emulsion formation: persistent emulsions may be broken by centrifugation.

The solvent extract is dried over anhydrous sodium sulphate, and transferred into a 500 ml rotary evaporation flask, using 5 ml of methanol to rinse the separating funnel. The extract is then evaporated to dryness using a rotary evaporator at 50°C. During evaporation under vacuum, the flask is rapidly filled with inert solvent vapour, but nitrogen should be introduced during the last stages of evaporation. The residue is dissolved in a measured volume of solvent, the choice of solvent depending upon subsequent operations.

Special modifications for the saponification of the different fat-soluble vitamins are considered below.

Vitamin A and carotenoids

DeVries *et al.* (1979) compared the effectiveness of ascorbic acid and pyrogallol as antioxidants on vitamin A recovery after saponification. All-*trans*-retinyl acetate (equivalent to 58·6 μg of retinol) was added to each of six 3 g samples of a food product having a peroxide value of 45·5 milli-equivalents/kg. No antioxidant was used in two of the samples; ascorbic acid was used in another two samples; and the same amount of pyrogallol was used in the remaining two samples. The samples were run through the entire analytical procedure, which entailed saponification and precipitation of the fatty acid salts, followed by HPLC. The amounts of 13-*cis*- and all-*trans*-retinol, and recoveries of total vitamin A are shown in Table 12. It is evident that the unprotected sample exhibited significant isomerization and degradation of the vitamin A. Ascorbic acid reduced the loss somewhat, but was not fully effective. Pyrogallol was most effective, allowing only a small loss due to degradation, although some isomerization occurred.

Another experiment was set up to investigate whether refluxing the pyrogallol with the sample under nitrogen, before the KOH was added, would destroy the peroxides. Four samples of food product were spiked with all-*trans*-retinyl acetate (equivalent to 19·1 μg of retinol). Potassium hydroxide was added to two of the samples before bringing the samples to reflux; the other two samples were brought to reflux before the KOH was

Table 12

Effects of antioxidants on vitamin A recovery after saponification (DeVries *et al.*, 1979)

Antioxidant used in sample	μg 13-cis recovered	μg all-trans recovered	Total μg vitamin A recovered	Total vitamin A recovery (%) and SD[a]
No antioxidant	16·4	12·6	29·0	49·5 ± 18·4
Ascorbic acid	16·4	29·8	46·2	78·8 ± 4·6
Pyrogallol	6·9	50·9	57·8	98·6 ± 2·7

[a] Recoveries are based on the average of duplicate analysis.

Table 13
Effect of base (KOH) addition on vitamin A recovery after saponification (DeVries
et al., 1979)

Sample	µg vitamin A recovered	Vitamin A recovery (%)
KOH added before heating	19·4	101·6
KOH added after bringing sample to reflux	13·4	70·0

added. The results shown in Table 13 indicate that the pyrogallol functions
more effectively as an antioxidant when it is in the phenoxide form in
alkaline media (DeVries et al., 1979).

According to Thompson (1986), there is no evidence to support the
implication that vitamin A is destroyed during saponification: retinol will
survive at least a week while steeping in ethanolic KOH containing
pyrogallol.

Overnight alkaline digestion at ambient temperature has been proposed
for the determination of carotenes and xanthophylls in dried plant
materials and mixed feeds (AOAC, 1984b), provided that xanthophyll
esters are not present; hot saponification is employed for samples
containing xanthophyll esters (Quackenbush, 1973).

For the efficient extraction of vitamin A from the saponified sample with
organic solvent, the aqueous ethanol phase should contain at least 40% of
water, as retinol is relatively soluble in ethanol:water (80:20) mixtures
(Christie & Wiggins, 1978). Care should be taken not to shake vitamin
solutions too vigorously in the presence of oxygen, otherwise vitamin A
may be converted to the 5,6-epoxide (Hubbard et al., 1971).

Vitamin D
Conventional saponification by refluxing at the boiling temperature of the
saponification mixture incurs the thermal isomerization of vitamin D to
previtamin D, and the consequent need to determine the potential vitamin
D content. Colorimetric and gas–liquid chromatographic techniques
measure the potential vitamin D directly, unless previtamin D and vitamin
D are separated beforehand in the clean-up procedures using open-column
or thin-layer chromatography. In HPLC, however, the vitamin D peak is
well separated from the previtamin D peak, and in food analysis it is
generally not possible to measure the latter because of interference from
coeluting contaminants. Saponification of milk by refluxing for 30 min at
83°C in the presence of pyrogallol resulted in a 10–20% loss of added

vitamin D due to thermal isomerization (Thompson *et al.*, 1977). To compensate for the loss of vitamin D, the previtamin D and the vitamin D can either be converted to a common derivative prior to HPLC or, more commonly, the potential vitamin D is calculated after measuring the vitamin D peak alone.

There are several possible ways of compensating for the loss of vitamin D by thermal isomerization incurred by hot saponification. Correction factors can be applied on the basis that the saponification conditions employed (30 or 45 min at 75–80°C) result in a constant ratio of previtamin D/vitamin D (de Vries & Borsje, 1982; de Vries *et al.*, 1983; Sertl & Molitor, 1985). Alternatively, a standard solution of authentic vitamin D can be subjected to the entire procedure, and the peak height of the sample compared with that obtained from the standard solution (Okano *et al.*, 1981; Kobayashi *et al.*, 1986). If the HPLC technique is capable of separating vitamin D_2 from vitamin D_3, one of the two vitamins can be added to the sample at the start of the analytical procedure to act as an internal standard for the other. Measuring the two vitamin D peaks and using the internal standardization equation gives the potential vitamin D content of the sample (van Niekerk & Smit, 1980; Jackson *et al.*, 1982; Reynolds & Judd, 1984).

The complication of thermal isomerization of vitamin D during hot saponification can be eliminated by employing 'cold' saponification, i.e. alkaline digestion at ambient temperature overnight with slow constant stirring. Thompson *et al.* (1977) reported that saponification of a 50 g milk sample was complete under such conditions, and losses of vitamin D were negligible. Alkaline digestion has been adopted in vitamin D assays in the presence (Thompson *et al.*, 1982; Wickroski & McLean, 1984) and absence (Muniz *et al.*, 1982) of pyrogallol. As an additional step, the saponification vessel has been flushed with nitrogen, and then sealed prior to overnight digestion; the omission of nitrogen during this stage was reported to reduce vitamin D recoveries by 10–20% (Indyk & Woollard, 1984). A similar procedure, using ascorbic acid as antioxidant instead of pyrogallol, has been published (Zonta *et al.*, 1982).

With regard to the extraction of vitamin D from the saponification mixture, the inclusion of diethyl ether in the extracting solvent improves the recovery of vitamin D by up to 10%, and reduces any tendency for emulsion formation during extraction (Indyk & Woollard, 1984). The liberated vitamin D should be quickly partitioned from the saponifying medium into the immiscible organic solvent, in which it is relatively stable (Chen *et al.*, 1965). Thompson *et al.* (1982) washed the extracting solvent (hexane) with 55% aqueous ethanol, after the initial KOH and water washes, in order to remove lipids that were more polar than vitamin D.

Vitamin E

In vitamin E assays, the extraction recoveries of tocopherols with hexane are affected by the concentration of ethanol in the saponification medium. Extraction is complete with ethanol concentrations up to 40%, but at higher concentrations the recoveries are reduced. For instance, only 50% of the δ-tocopherol present is recovered at 60% ethanol (Ueda & Igarashi, 1987).

Saponification has been reported to destroy a significant amount of tocotrienols (Chow *et al.*, 1969), and has also been shown to reduce certain vitamin E metabolic dimers, which do not interfere in colorimetric determinations of vitamin E, to other dimers which do interfere (Igarashi *et al.*, 1973).

Krukovsky (1964) demonstrated that the addition of ascorbic acid protects vitamin E from oxidation during saponification. The recovery data revealed that pure tocopherols, in the absence of ascorbic acid, are much more readily decomposed in alkaline media by heat than are the natural tocopherols of milk fat. Buttriss & Diplock (1984) reported that adding a freshly prepared 1% pyrogallol solution resulted in a higher recovery of α-tocopherol after saponification at 70°C than adding a 1% ascorbic acid solution.

Several authors have recommended saponification in methanolic solution, as opposed to ethanolic solution, in order to reduce the risk of decomposition of vitamin E by lowering the saponification temperature (methanol boils at 65°C; ethanol at 78°C). However, this necessitates extending the saponification time in order to compensate for the lower rate of hydrolysis, and this is considered to be undesirable in view of the susceptibility of vitamin E to light and oxygen (Strohecker & Henning, 1966).

Vitamin K

Vitamin K compounds are rapidly decomposed in alkali and thus it is not expedient to isolate them from fat by saponification.

4.2 ENZYMATIC HYDROLYSIS

Enzymatic hydrolysis using lipase has been employed as an alternative to saponification to reduce the risk of vitamin degradation. In a HPLC method for determining supplemental vitamins A, D, E and K in milk and dairy products, Barnett *et al.* (1980) incubated the lipid component of the sample with lipase for 1 h at 37°C, and then made the hydrolysate alkaline in order to precipitate the fatty acids as soaps. The solution was then diluted with ethanol, and extracted with pentane. A final water wash yielded an organic phase containing, primarily, the fat-soluble vitamins and cholesterol. Similar procedures have been employed in HPLC methods for vitamin K_1 in infant formula foods (Bueno & Villalobos, 1983) and soy bean oil (Zonta & Stancher, 1985).

4.3 SOLVENT EXTRACTION

Direct extraction of the total lipid can be accomplished by selecting proper solvent(s), depending on the nature of the sample and the amount of lipid to be extracted. Solvents must be capable of effectively penetrating the tissues and breaking lipoprotein bonds, whilst minimizing oxidative destruction of the lipid or vitamins. The more polar the solvent, the more efficient is the extraction but, simultaneously, more of the interfering materials are extracted. For example, hot ethanol will extract all of the vitamin E and fat from the food matrix, but also some phospholipids and glucosides (Ames, 1972*b*). A mixture of chloroform and methanol (2:1), using a blender or homogenizer, is a generally effective means of extracting foods (Desai, 1980). Another method entails initial extraction of the sample with acetone, followed by addition of water to remove the acetone, any added antioxidant, and other water-soluble substances, then re-extraction with hexane (Ames, 1972*b*). Dried foods can be extracted in a Soxhlet apparatus with acetone (Desai, 1980) or isopropanol/chloroform mixtures (Christie & Wiggins, 1978). Mechanical shaking with diethyl ether can also be used to extract dried foods (Desai, 1980). Håkansson *et al.* (1987) obtained good recoveries ($>95\%$) of tocopherols from wheat product after Soxhlet extraction with hexane containing added BHT (butylated hydroxytoluene). Soft tissues, such as liver, can be ground with sodium sulphate until a dry mix is obtained; this can then be extracted in a Soxhlet apparatus with acetone (Bunnell, 1967). For the determination of vitamin E by HPLC, vegetable oils are simply dissolved in hexane (Carpenter, 1979; Taylor & Barnes, 1981; Gertz & Herrmann, 1982) and analysed directly.

Chow *et al.* (1969) proposed the following low temperature crystallization technique for the removal of glycerides in vitamin E assays. Dried foods, such as breakfast cereals, are ground, then extracted with acetone in a Soxhlet apparatus. The extract is evaporated to dryness under vacuum at 50°C, and samples of the dried extract are dissolved in acetone, and immersed in a solid carbon dioxide-acetone bath at −70°C for 10 min. The samples are then filtered using a Pyrex funnel cooled to the same temperature. The filtrate contains the free tocopherols and tocotrienols, whilst any vitamin E esters present remain in the crystallization fraction. Similar extraction techniques have been employed in vitamin E assays as a means of avoiding losses of tocotrienols incurred during saponification (Müller-Mulot, 1976; Zandi & McKay, 1976).

Liquid–liquid extraction can provide a useful clean-up step after direct solvent extraction. A typical application is the partitioning of the lipids, including the fat-soluble vitamins, from a crude organic solvent extract into a more selective immiscible organic solvent. The transfer is based on the preferential solubility of the lipid in the second solvent.

Precautions against vitamin degradation during extraction include the use of amber- or foil-covered glassware, and the addition of antioxidants to the solvent mixture.

Specialized methods of extracting the lipid from milk, margarine and animal feeds are discussed below.

For the extraction of milk prior to the determination of vitamin A by HPLC (Thompson et al., 1980), sufficient ethanol was added so that the constituents of the milk would be suspended in 71% aqueous ethanol; this solvent denatures the proteins and fractures the fat globules. The mixture was shaken vigorously with hexane so that the lipid was completely partitioned into this hydrophobic solvent. Water was then added to induce the aqueous and organic phases to separate, and the process was accelerated by centrifugation. The final mixture thus consisted in total of equal parts of water, ethanol and hexane. After separation, the upper phase was a hexane solution of the milk lipids containing a trace of ethanol, and the lower phase was aqueous ethanol in which were dissolved salts, proteins, polar lipids and a trace of hexane. The interface contained a mixture of upper and lower phases plus insoluble protein. Grace & Bernhard (1984) employed a similar technique in HPLC methods for vitamins A and D in fortified non-fat milk and whole milk, respectively, using an extracting mixture of saturated sodium chloride solution, acidified ethanol, and hexane. BHT was added as an antioxidant in the vitamin A assay.

For the determination of vitamin D in full cream dried milk by GLC (Bell & Christie, 1974), the sample was mixed with hot water to form a creamy paste, then treated with a mixture of ethanol, sodium hexametaphosphate and a surface-active agent (Triton X-100), followed by extraction with diethyl ether:petroleum spirit (1:1). In another GLC method for vitamin D, the milk protein from non-fat dried milk was precipitated with an acetone: ethanol mixture (1:1) containing ascorbic acid as antioxidant. The solvent was concentrated by rotary evaporation, followed by extraction of the fat with chloroform (Panalaks, 1970).

Dispersion of milk powder in a non-aqueous solvent (dimethyl-sulphoxide:dimethylformamide:chloroform; 2:2:1 containing ascorbic acid) released vitamin A esters, native vitamin E and supplemental α-tocopheryl acetate, if present. The lipid fraction was then partitioned into hexane for HPLC (Woollard & Woollard, 1981; Woollard & Blott, 1986).

For the subsequent determination of vitamin D in non-fat dried milk by HPLC, the lipid fraction was extracted with dichloromethane containing sodium phosphate tribasic solution and BHT (Cohen & Wakeford, 1980). In another HPLC method for vitamin D, the lipid fraction of low fat milk was extracted by homogenization in isopropanol/dichloromethane, with magnesium sulphate added to remove water, and BHT (Landen, 1985).

Vitamin K was extracted from infant formula foods by liquid–liquid partition with a mixture of petroleum spirit:diethyl ether (1:1) after precipitation of the protein with aqueous ethanol (Manes et al., 1972). Infant formula foods could also be diluted with concentrated ammonium hydroxide, followed by methanol, prior to extraction with dichloro-methane:isooctane (2:1) (Hwang, 1985), or extracted directly with chloroform:methanol (2:1) (Haroon et al., 1982). Milk was extracted with hot isopropanol, followed by acetone extraction, and partitioning of the vitamin K and accompanying lipids into hexane (Thompson et al., 1979).

In HPLC methods for vitamin A in margarine, the margarine was dissolved in hexane (Thompson & Maxwell, 1977), heptane containing BHT and α-tocopherol as antioxidants (Aitzetmüller et al., 1979), dichloromethane containing tricthylamine and BHA (butylated hydroxy-anisole) (Landen & Eitenmiller, 1979) or 60% aqueous ethanol (Thompson et al., 1980).

For the simultaneous determination of vitamins A, D and E in animal feeds by HPLC, feed samples were extracted with a mixture of isooctane: dioxan (80:20), filtered, then shaken with 0·3 ml of tetraethylene pentamine to render the chlorophyll partly insoluble before rotary evaporation to near dryness. The residue was extracted with acetonitrile, and the filtered extracts were evaporated to 60–80 ml. The acetonitrile solution was then extracted with isooctane. As a result of this liquid partition step, the chlorophyll and certain other interfering substances remained in the acetonitrile phase, whilst the lipids and accompanying vitamins were transferred to the isooctane phase. The latter phase was shaken with sodium phosphate tribasic to precipitate inorganic salts and to remove any traces of amine (Cohen & Lapointe, 1978).

A non-aqueous solvent mixture composed of dimethylsulphoxide: dimethylformamide:chloroform (2:2:1) containing ascorbic acid has also been found suitable for the analysis of animal feeds (Blott & Woollard, 1986). The dimethylsulphoxide component is included in the extracting solution primarily because of its ability to dissolve the gelatin coating on encapsulated vitamin additives.

In the AOAC (1984c) spectrophotometric method for the determination of carotene in fresh plant materials and silages, the extraction procedure entails blending the sample with a mixture of acetone, hexane and magnesium carbonate. The residue is washed with acetone followed by hexane, and the combined extracts are washed with water to remove the acetone. The hexane layer is purified by open-column chromatography before spectrophotometry.

The following methods have been proposed (AOAC, 1984d,e) for the extraction of foods and feeds prior to saponification and colorimetric determination of the natural α-tocopherol or total α-tocopherol (natural α-tocopherol plus supplemental α-tocopheryl acetate). Milk and milk products are mixed successively with ethanol, diethyl ether and petroleum spirit. The ether layer is removed and the extraction is repeated twice. The combined ether layers are evaporated to 50 ml, a 10 ml aliquot is evaporated, and the lipid is weighed. The analysis is performed on an aliquot containing approximately 1 g of lipid. Wet products are ground with two to three times their sample weight of anhydrous sodium sulphate, then extracted with ethanol in a Soxhlet apparatus for 16 h; dry products are Soxhlet-extracted directly. The alcohol extract is shaken with petroleum spirit, which is then evaporated to obtain a lipid sample for analysis. Dry products supplemented with α-tocopheryl acetate in gelatin, vegetable gum, or dextrin matrix are Soxhlet-extracted with ethanol, and the ethanol extract is shaken with petroleum spirit. The contents of the extraction thimble are re-extracted with 2·5 N sulphuric acid, then diluted with ethanol and extracted with petroleum spirit. The petroleum spirit extract is combined with the extract obtained from the hot ethanol extraction, evaporated, and the lipid is weighed for analysis.

Water-soluble derivatives of menadione were extracted from premixes and animal feedstuffs, and converted to the free menadione, by agitating a sample weighing between 1 and 10 g sequentially with chloroform, dilute ammonia solution, and a Celite/sodium sulphate mixture in a 100 ml centrifuge tube, and then centrifuging. The chloroform extract was diluted or concentrated to give a suitable concentration of menadione for measurement by HPLC (Manz & Maurer, 1982). In the Feeding Stuffs Regulations (HMSO, 1982) method for determining menadione in animal feeds, samples are extracted with diluted ethanol, clarified with tannin solution, and centrifuged. The supernatant is treated with a solution of sodium carbonate, and the menadione is extracted with 1,2-dichloroethane for colorimetric assay.

Chapter 5

Purification of Vitamin-Rich Extracts

Purification of the unsaponifiable matter, or other form of vitamin-rich extract, is necessary before the fat-soluble vitamins can be measured by the techniques of spectrophotometry, fluorometry, colorimetry and GLC. HPLC, itself, constitutes an effective purification step and, in vitamin A and vitamin E assays, can often be applied directly to the vitamin-rich extracts.

The purification technique usually involves some form of liquid chromatography, in which the sample is applied to a solid stationary phase (adsorption chromatography) or solid support coated with a liquid stationary phase (partition chromatography), and eluted with a liquid mobile phase. Separation of sample components depends upon the different affinities of each component for the mobile and stationary phases.

The liquid chromatographic techniques employed in the purification of vitamin extracts are open-column and thin-layer chromatography. A more recent innovation is the use of silica-packed disposable plastic cartridges connected to a syringe, which acts as a low-pressure pump.

GLC and HPLC combine separation and measurement, and are discussed separately in Chapters 7 and 8.

Before liquid chromatography can be applied, it is often necessary to remove the bulk of the sterols from the vitamin-rich extract by precipitation. Hydrolysis of milk yields an unsaponifiable fraction that constitutes 0·3–0·45% by weight of the total fat, and is composed largely of cholesterol (Muniz *et al.*, 1982). In vegetable products the larger part of the unsaponifiable material is composed of the phytosterols, which are predominantly β-sitosterol, stigmasterol and campesterol; only trace amounts of cholesterol are generally present (Itoh *et al.*, 1973).

Typical sterol contents of vegetable oils, margarines and milk are given in Tables 14–16.

Table 14
Typical sterol content of vegetable oils

Oil	$(mg/100 g \ oil)^a$			
	β-Sitosterol	Stigmasterol	Campesterol	% fat
Corn	587	68	149 ⎫	
Olive	157	3	7 ⎪	
Peanut	171	26	43 ⎬ 99.9[b]	
Safflower	129	18	27 ⎪	
Soy bean	177	67	76 ⎪	
Sunflower	210	33	31 ⎭	

[a] Slover et al. (1983).
[b] Paul & Southgate (1978).

5.1 PRECIPITATION OF STEROLS

The bulk of the sterols may be removed from the unsaponifiable matter by precipitation from a methanolic solution at $-12°C$, followed by recrystallization to release any entrapped vitamin (Russell Eggitt & Ward, 1953). Alternatively, digitonin may be added to the vitamin-rich extract, and the vitamin re-extracted from the digitonide complex (Morris & Haenni, 1962; Osborne & Voogt, 1978). According to Green (1951), 72% aqueous ethanol is the best solvent from which to precipitate cholesterol with digitonin.

Table 15
Typical sterol content of UK packet and tub margarine

Type of margarine	$(mg/100 g \ lipid)^a$						
	Choles- terol	β-Sitos- terol	Stig- masterol	Campes- terol	Brassi- casterol	Other	% fat
Mixed oils (animal, fish, vegetable)	130–260	25–80	0–15	20–60	0–20	0–30 ⎫	
Vegetable oils	6–26	80–200	0–35	30–70	0–10	0–25 ⎬ 81[b]	
Vegetable oils high in PUFA	0–5	130–200	20–50	30–50	0	20–35 ⎭	

[a] Egan et al. (1981).
[b] Paul & Southgate (1978).
PUFA = polyunsaturated fatty acids.

Table 16
Typical cholesterol and fat content of cows milk (Paul & Southgate, 1978)

Type of milk	Cholesterol (mg/100 g)	% fat
Fresh, whole	14	3·8
Fresh, skimmed	2	0·1
Condensed, whole, sweetened	34	9·0
Condensed, skimmed, sweetened	3	0·3
Evaporated, whole, unsweetened	34	9·0
Dried, whole	120	26·3
Dried, skimmed	18	1·3

Eisses & de Vries (1969) devised a colorimetric assay for vitamin D in evaporated milk whereby cholesterol was removed from the unsaponifiable matter by precipitation with digitonin. Panalaks (1971) employed a similar step in the analysis of whole and partially skimmed milk. For the determination of vitamin D in fortified milk by HPLC, the cholesterol present in the dry unsaponifiable matter was removed by digitonin precipitation at −20°C, followed by further purification on an alumina column (Muniz et al., 1982), or simply dissolved in methanol to precipitate the sterols, which were then removed by filtration (Jackson et al., 1982; Indyk & Woollard, 1984, 1985a,b).

For the determination of vitamin E in various foods by GLC, the unsaponifiable matter was subjected to open-column chromatography on alumina, followed by precipitation of the cholesterol with digitonin solution at −15°C overnight, and further purification on a Celite–digitonin column (Christie et al., 1973). Pickston (1978) removed the sterols from the unsaponifiable fraction of milk and milk substitutes by precipitation from a methanolic solution at −20°C prior to the determination of vitamin E by HPLC.

5.2 OPEN-COLUMN CHROMATOGRAPHY

Open-column chromatography refers to the use of gravity-flow and low-pressure liquid chromatography as opposed to HPLC. Two distinct mechanisms are involved: adsorption (liquid–solid) chromatography and partition (liquid–liquid) chromatography.

5.2.1 Adsorption Chromatography

Chromatographic adsorbents are porous solids whose large surface areas are covered with terminal hydroxyl (—OH) groups that are highly polar, and function as the active sites. Separations are based on the competition between the solute molecules and the organic solvent molecules in the mobile phase for the active sites. Fully active adsorbents, in which all the active sites are available, are too strong, and must be partially deactivated by mixing with a known amount of water. Adsorbents include fuller's earth, magnesium (or calcium) hydrogen phosphate, Florisil, alumina, magnesia, and silica gel. Adsorption chromatography is useful for preparative separations owing to the relative cheapness of the adsorbents, high sample loading capacity, and stability toward pH extremes. Open columns packed with the above adsorbents are usually used only once, then discarded.

Adsorption chromatography is best suited for compounds of low or intermediate polarity, where the energy of binding of solute and organic solvent to the adsorbent is similar. The most satisfactory adsorption occurs from a non-polar solvent in which the solute is poorly soluble (DeLuca et al., 1969). When components are dissolved in the mobile phase and passed over the adsorbent, the more polar compounds are adsorbed more strongly than the less polar compounds, and a separation results. Adsorption chromatography primarily separates compounds according to the type and number of functional groups. Different degrees of resolution are due to variables such as water content and particle size of the adsorbent, size of column, purity of preparation analysed, and type of mobile phase used. Some adsorbents have been employed in open columns to fractionate different vitamins and their vitamers, but HPLC has superseded this particular application.

The deactivated adsorbent may be packed into the column as a slurry with a suitable organic solvent; alumina and silica gel columns may also be dry-filled.

Dry-column chromatography enables separations directly comparable with those obtained by TLC to be carried out rapidly in a column on a preparative scale. The column is filled with dry adsorbent, either alumina or silica gel, and loaded by depositing the semi-purified vitamin extract on a small quantity of adsorbent, which is then poured on top of the column and covered with a little more adsorbent. The chromatography is achieved by maintaining a column head of only 1–2 cm of mobile phase, and allowing the mobile phase to move down the column by capillary action aided by gravity. Since there is essentially no liquid flowing down the column, channelling does not occur and zone separation is usually sharp and straight. The chromatography is complete when the solvent front reaches the bottom of the column; this usually takes 15–30 min (Loev & Snader, 1965; Loev & Goodman, 1967).

Fuller's earth

The term fuller's earth is applied to any clay that has adequate decolorizing and purifying capacity to be used commercially in oil refining without chemical treatment (Merck Index, 1983). Florex earth is the brand name of a Florida fuller's earth, which is marketed by Floridin Co., USA; it is also referred to as Floridin earth.

The activity or adsorptive power of fuller's earth depends upon the fineness of the particles, and the extent of dehydration produced by washing with ethanol; the earth is deactivated by adding water (Russell Eggitt & Ward, 1953). Fuller's earth adsorbs carotenoids, vitamin A and its derivatives, and some sterols (provided the quantities of the latter are not excessive) from unsaponifiable extracts of biological material, and has been used to purify extracts in colorimetric assays for vitamins D and E.

In vitamin E assays, the fuller's earth must be boiled before use with stannous chloride and hydrochloric acid to reduce its iron content from the ferric to the ferrous state, since ferric iron can cause oxidation of vitamin E (Brown, 1952). Stannous chloride-treated fuller's earth can reduce substances such as ubiquinone (Coenzyme Q), vitamin K and tocopheryl-quinone, so that they are reactive with ferric chloride in the Emmerie–Engel colorimetric reaction for vitamin E; subsequent purification by thin-layer chromatography will separate these contaminants (Bunnell, 1967). Fuller's earth chromatography incurs no significant losses with large (1000 µg) applications of vitamin E, but if very low (10 µg) amounts are applied to the column, only about 6 µg is recovered (Booth, 1961).

Adsorption chromatography on fuller's earth has been used in the United States Pharmacopoeia (USP) colorimetric assay of vitamin D applied to evaporated milk, following the removal of vitamin A by partition chromatography (Jones *et al.*, 1965). The adsorption column was found to be necessary to remove vitamin A decomposition products and other interfering impurities.

Fuller's earth has been employed in the determination of supplemental α-tocopheryl acetate in premixes, feeds and pet foods (Ames & Tinkler, 1962). A solvent extract of the material is evaporated to dryness and the residue, dissolved in petroleum spirit, is applied to a column of fuller's earth treated with ceric sulphate, a strong oxidizing agent. Naturally occurring reducing substances, including the unesterified tocopherols, are oxidized and adsorbed. The stable α-tocopheryl acetate is quantitatively eluted from the column with benzene, then saponified to release the free α-tocopherol, which is determined colorimetrically. This procedure has been adopted by the Association of Official Analytical Chemists, Inc. (AOAC, 1984e).

Magnesium (or calcium) hydrogen phosphate
Open-column chromatography on magnesium hydrogen phosphate (MgHPO$_4$) or calcium hydrogen phosphate (CaHPO$_4$) provides an extensive purification of unsaponifiable extracts, and is capable of separating β-carotene, vitamin E, sterols, vitamin D and vitamin A. The technique was originally developed for vitamin E assays, but it has also been used for purifying extracts in the determination of vitamins A and D.

Magnesium hydrogen phosphate facilitates a partial fractionation of the E vitamers according to the number of methyl groups in the tocol molecule. Unsaponifiable extracts of foods dissolved in petroleum spirit are applied to the column, and the mono-, di-, and trimethyl derivatives of tocol are eluted with petroleum spirit containing progressively increasing amounts of diethyl ether (Bro-Rasmussen & Hjarde, 1957a,b). β-Carotene is removed with pure petroleum spirit prior to elution of the E vitamers, and other carotenoids may be eluted with 0·5% diethyl ether (Ames, 1972b). A mobile phase containing 2·0% diethyl ether specifically elutes α-T (tocopherol) and α-T3 (tocotrienol); 4·0% diethyl ether elutes β-T, γ-T and β-T3; and 6–7% diethyl ether elutes δ-T. Sterols are distributed among the fractions containing more than 2% diethyl ether, whilst vitamin A is washed off the column with 10–15% diethyl ether (Strohecker & Henning, 1966). A 98–100% recovery of α-tocopherol from the magnesium hydrogen phosphate column is possible, but it has been found difficult to achieve a constant degree of deactivation of the adsorbent between different batches (Dicks-Bushnell, 1967). Hence it is essential to check the elution properties of each batch with a mixture of α- and γ-tocopherols to ensure reliable results (Ames, 1972b).

Hjarde *et al.* (1973) obtained a similar, but more distinct, separation of E vitamers using CaHPO$_4$ instead of MgHPO$_4$. Quinones and the oxidation products of α-tocopherol were eluted before α-tocopherol; γ-tocopherol dimers and plastochromanol appeared in the fractions containing α-T3 and γ-T, respectively. The duration of the chromatographic separation, however, was very long: α-T was eluted in 90 min and the last vitamer, δ-T3, in 170 min.

Florisil
Florisil is a hard, porous, granular form of activated magnesium silicate (Merck Index, 1983) and exhibits similar chromatographic properties to magnesium hydrogen phosphate in the separation of tocopherols. Unsaponifiable extracts of foods dissolved in petroleum spirit are applied to the column, and the three fractions of tocopherols (α-, $\beta + \gamma$- and δ-tocopherol) are eluted with petroleum spirit containing increasing amounts of diethyl ether. Vitamins A and K, and most (about 90%) of the β-carotene present, are retained.

The correct degree of hydration is essential in quantitative analysis. Hydration to 20% water is optimum, and yields an average 95% recovery of the tocopherols; 15% hydration yields low recoveries of 72%, while untreated Florisil retains the tocopherols completely. Large amounts of non-tocopherol reducing substances appear in the α-tocopherol fraction, hence further purification of the tocopherols by thin-layer chromatography is necessary before they can be measured colorimetrically (Dicks-Bushnell, 1967). Florisil chromatography has also been used to fractionate the unsaponifiable matter of vegetable oils prior to the determination of tocopherols by GLC (Eisner *et al.*, 1966).

Alumina
Alumina (aluminium oxide, $Al_2O_3.xH_2O$) is presumed to be a basic adsorbent owing to the presence of oxide ions. It preferentially retains acidic compounds, such as carboxylic acids and phenols. Acid treatment, however, reduces this basic behaviour (Majors, 1976). Alumina must be partially deactivated by mixing a fully active preparation of the adsorbent with a known amount of water in the presence of a large volume of hexane. Preparations that are too active or too weak fail to provide the necessary chromatographic resolution, and may also cause decomposition of the fat-soluble vitamins. The practical working range for alumina is 2–10% water-deactivated, i.e. where the adsorbent is fully activated by driving out the water at 600°C, and then deactivated by shaking with 2–10% of its weight of water. The deactivated alumina is stored in hexane and packed wet into a column; alternatively, dry-packed columns may be used.

The relative retentions of vitamin A-active compounds on alumina are shown in Table 17. Mobile phases used with slurry-packed alumina columns include petroleum spirit containing progressively increasing amounts of diethyl ether; and hexane containing progressively increasing amounts of acetone.

In the AOAC (1984*f*) method for the determination of vitamin A and

Table 17
Relative retentions of vitamin A-active compounds on
alumina (DeLuca *et al.*, 1969)

Weakly adsorbed	Anhydroretinols
↑	Carotenes; food dyes
	Retinyl esters
	Retinaldehydes
↓	Retinols
Strongly adsorbed	Vitamin E; quinones

Reprinted from DeLuca *et al.*, 1969, p. 360 by courtesy of
Marcel Dekker, Inc.

carotene in margarine, the unsaponifiable fraction is applied to a 3% water-deactivated sandwich column of neutral and alkaline alumina, and the carotene is eluted with 16% diethyl ether in petroleum spirit. The carotene eluate is evaporated, and the residue is dissolved in petroleum spirit for spectrophotometric measurement of the yellow colour. Elution is continued with 16% or 25% diethyl ether in petroleum spirit to elute the vitamin A, which is finally determined spectrophotometrically.

In the AOAC (1984g) assay for vitamin A and carotene in mixed feeds, premixes and foods, the unsaponifiable fraction in hexane solution is applied to a neutral 5% water-deactivated alumina column. Carotene is eluted with 4% acetone in hexane, followed by retinol with 15% acetone in hexane. Carotene, if present, is determined spectrophotometrically, whilst vitamin A is measured colorimetrically.

The Feeding Stuffs Regulations (HMSO, 1982) method for determining retinol in animal feeds utilizes a column of neutral, deactivated alumina to fractionate the unsaponifiable matter of feeds that contain less than 200 000 IU (60 000 μg) of retinol per kg. The column is slurry-packed with petroleum spirit, and is eluted successively with 10 ml lots of petroleum containing 0, 4, 8, 12, 16 and 20% diethyl ether. The carotene is eluted with the pure petroleum, and the retinol is usually eluted with the 20% diethyl ether eluent. The elution is followed by brief irradiation of the column with a mercury UV lamp. The fluorescent vitamin A zone is clearly separated from the yellow xanthophyll zones following it. The vitamin A content of the eluate is determined colorimetrically.

The irradiation products of provitamin D have been separated into three distinct bands on activated alumina using a mixture of petroleum spirit and acetone as the mobile phase. Previtamin D and lumisterol were included in the first band; vitamin D and tachysterol were in the second band; and provitamin D (ergosterol or 7-dehydrocholesterol) were eluted in the third band (Shaw & Jefferies, 1957).

Alumina adsorption columns have been used in the colorimetric determination of vitamin D in fortified whole and partially skimmed fluid milk (Panalaks, 1971). In this method, the cholesterol was first removed from the unsaponifiable matter by column chromatography on Celite/digitonin, followed by the removal of vitamin A by partition column chromatography. The carotenoids and decomposition products of vitamin A were removed from the semi-purified extracts on slurry-packed columns of alkaline, 12% water-deactivated alumina by elution with 6% chloroform in isooctane; the vitamin D was eluted with diethyl ether. A further purification on a silica micro-column was necessary to eliminate colorimetric interfering substances.

Two dry-packed columns of neutral, 8% water-deactivated alumina columns were used to remove cholesterol, vitamin A, and other interfering substances from the unsaponifiable matter of fortified full cream, dried milk (Bell & Christie, 1974), fatty fish, freeze-dried eggs and margarine (Wiggins, 1978) prior to the determination of vitamin D by GLC. The first column, developed with chloroform, isolated a fraction containing vitamin D, vitamin A, cholesterol, and other sterols. The fraction was treated with antimony trichloride to convert vitamin D into isovitamin D before application to the second column, which was also eluted with chloroform. Vitamin A, as its anhydro derivative, eluted with the solvent front, and was followed by isovitamin D, well separated from cholesterol and other sterols. In this way, isovitamin D was substantially freed from sterols without recourse to precipitation with digitonin, and an extract was obtained that was suitable for the determination of vitamin D by GLC.

Dry-column chromatography using neutral, 8% water-deactivated alumina with chloroform elution has been used to remove cholesterol and carotenes from the unsaponifiable fraction of fortified milk in the assay of vitamin D by HPLC (Wickroski & McLean, 1984). Thompson et al. (1982) dissolved the unsaponifiable fraction of margarine in hexane: isopropanol (99:1), and passed it through a column of neutral, 5% water-deactivated alumina contained in a Pasteur pipette prior to the determination of vitamin D by HPLC. Muniz et al. (1982) reported that cholesterol is not quantitatively removed from alumina columns; some of the cholesterol is eluted with the vitamin D. These authors described an HPLC method for vitamin D in fortified milk, in which a dry column of neutral, 8% water-deactivated alumina was used to purify the unsaponifiable fraction of milk, after precipitation of the cholesterol with digitonin. The vitamin D fraction was eluted from the alumina column with hexane:acetone (85:15). In another HPLC method, de Vries *et al.* (1983) used a column of neutral alumina deactivated with petroleum spirit to remove carotenes and vitamin E from the unsaponifiable material obtained from animal feeds and pet foods. Carotenes were removed from the column by elution with hexane; vitamin E and the antioxidant ethoxyquin (if present) were removed by elution with hexane:diethyl ether (92:8). The column was then eluted with hexane:diethyl ether (60:40), and the eluate containing vitamins A and D was collected when the front of the fluorescent vitamin A band (located by means of a portable UV lamp) reached 3 cm from the bottom of the column.

The E vitamers are fractionated on alumina according to the number of methyl groups in the tocol molecule using a mobile phase of petroleum spirit containing progressively increasing amounts of diethyl ether. Although similar in this respect to magnesium hydrogen phosphate, alumina is usually preferred because the adsorbent does not take so long to prepare, and the filtration rate is more rapid. However, alumina columns that are too active can cause significant losses of vitamin E in natural products whose vitamin content is already low, thus magnesium hydrogen phosphate is more suitable for unfortified foods (Strohecker & Henning, 1966).

Using columns of deactivated alumina, subjected to gradient elution with petroleum spirit containing increasing amounts of diethyl ether, the following vitamin E fractions may be obtained from unsaponifiable lipid: α-T, α-T3, β-T + γ-T, β-T3 + γ-T3, and δ-T; sterols are eluted after δ-T. Triglycerides, if they were present, would coelute with α-T (Laidman & Hall, 1971). Alternatively, alumina columns can be eluted with pure petroleum spirit to remove the β-carotene, and the combined tocopherols and tocotrienols eluted with 10% diethyl ether in petroleum spirit; vitamin A is eluted with 15–20% diethyl ether in petroleum spirit (Strohecker & Henning, 1966). Elution of 10% water-deactivated alumina columns with hexane, followed by 5% diethyl ether in hexane, removed α-tocopherol from the unsaponifiable matter of margarine; γ-tocopherol was eluted with 15% diethyl ether in hexane (Lambertsen *et al.*, 1964). Elution of 10% water-deactivated alumina columns with cyclohexane, followed by 7% diethyl ether in cyclohexane, removed α-tocopherol or the total tocopherols and tocotrienols, according to the volume of mobile phase, from the unsaponifiable matter of foods (Christie *et al.*, 1973). In this method the alumina column separated the tocopherols from carotenoids, retinol and

cholesterol fairly well, and allowed the subsequent colorimetric determination of vitamin E to be made without serious interference. The
antioxidants BHA and BHT, and any tocopherol dimers present, were
retained on the column (Christie & Wiggins, 1978).

Vitamin K has been separated from interfering neutral and polar lipids
using gravity-flow columns packed with 8% water-deactivated neutral
alumina and eluted stepwise with 0–12% benzene in petroleum spirit
(Manes *et al.*, 1972) or 0–6% diethyl ether in hexane (Seifert, 1979). Freshly
distilled diethyl ether is a suitable substitute for benzene as a polar solvent.
Petroleum spirit or hexane alone elutes interfering carotenoids, if present,
while successive elution with mobile phases of increasing polarity removes
the vitamin K_1. Seifert (1979) reported that most of the vitamin K_1 was
eluted with 1·5% diethyl ether in hexane. Zonta & Stancher (1985) used an
alumina column to purify pentane extracts of soy bean oil obtained after
removal of the triglycerides by enzymatic hydrolysis. The column was eluted
with 7% diethyl ether in hexane, and the eluate was suitable for
measurement of vitamin K_1 by HPLC.

Magnesia

Magnesia (magnesium oxide, $MgO \, . \, xH_2O$) possesses the ability to separate
α- and β-carotene, which is useful in margarine analysis to determine
whether red palm oil or β-carotene has been used in the manufacturing
process.

Open columns packed with heat-activated magnesia and eluted with
petroleum spirit containing diethyl ether facilitate the separation of α- and
β-carotene from carotene fractions obtained from alumina column
chromatography. Mobile phases ranging from 4, 8 and 12% diethyl ether in
petroleum spirit remove α-carotene from the magnesia column; β-carotene
is eluted with 20, 24, 36 and 50% diethyl ether in petroleum spirit (Osborne
& Voogt, 1978). A similar procedure has been described by Usher *et al.*
(1968). The two carotenes can be measured spectrophotometrically.

Silica gel

Silica gel is a polymer of silicic acid and has a general formula $SiO_2 \, . \, xH_2O$.
The internal structure of the silica gel particle comprises a lattice of SiO_4
tetrahedra. At the surface of the particle, where the lattice is abruptly
terminated, the valencies of the surface silicon atoms can be satisfied either
by forming silanol groups ($\equiv$Si—OH) or siloxane bridges ($\equiv$Si—O—Si$\equiv$).
It is the slightly acidic silanol groups which are considered to be of

Table 18

Relative retentions of vitamin A-active compounds and other vitamins on silica gel
(DeLuca *et al.*, 1969)

Weakly adsorbed	Anhydroretinol; retinyl esters; β-carotene; vitamin K_1
	α-Tocopherol
	Retinoic acid and its isomers; 13-*cis*-retinaldehyde
	All-*trans*-retinaldehyde
	Vitamin D_2
	13-*cis*-retinol; 9,13-di-*cis*-retinol
Strongly adsorbed	All-*trans*-retinol; 9-*cis*-retinol

Reprinted from DeLuca *et al.*, 1969, p. 371 by courtesy of Marcel Dekker, Inc.

importance in the separation of solutes by adsorption at the silica surface; the siloxane groups give rise to weak, non-specific interactions.

The relative retentions of vitamin A-active compounds and other vitamins on silica gel are given in Table 18. Chromatography of vitamin A compounds on open columns packed with untreated silica gel is seriously hampered by degradation of the compounds, leading to recoveries of only 48–60%. In the case of retinyl esters, the degradation has been attributed to acid-catalysed dehydration reactions, as alkali-treated (basic) silica gel columns eluted with 1–8% diethyl ether in hexane yield good (>94%) recoveries of retinyl palmitate. Retinol, retinaldehyde and retinoic acid are quite stable, especially when protected by antioxidants during the chromatographic process (DeLuca *et al.*, 1969).

Regular straight-bore gravity-flow silica gel columns are incapable of separating previtamin D from vitamin D, but the separation of previtamin D, vitamin D, tachysterol and provitamin D (7-dehydrocholesterol or ergosterol) has been achieved using a four-stage multi-bore column eluted with a diethyl ether/petroleum spirit gradient (DeLuca & Blunt, 1971).

Panalaks (1970) devised a procedure for purifying non-fat dried milk prior to the determination of supplemental vitamin D by GLC. The residue obtained from chloroform extracts of the milk (after precipitation of the milk protein with acetone/ethanol) was dissolved in hexane and loaded onto a multi-bore column slurry-packed with 15% water-deactivated silica gel. Elution was carried out using a diethyl ether/petroleum spirit gradient, and the eluate was treated with antimony trichloride reagent to convert the vitamin D to isovitamin D. The cholesterol was then removed using disposable Pasteur pipettes dry-filled with silica gel, and eluted with chloroform. The final eluate was suitable for GLC. Panalaks (1971) used similar silica gel micro-columns as a final purification step in the colorimetric determination of vitamin D in fortified whole and partially skimmed milk.

Adsorption chromatography on silica gel has been used to purify unsaponifiable extracts for the subsequent determination of vitamin E, but the correct activity, achieved by hydration, is essential to ensure a good recovery of the vitamin (Dicks-Bushnell, 1967). Nair et al. (1965) used 8 cm × 1 cm silica gel columns slurry-packed with isooctane. Elution with 5% ethyl acetate in isooctane removed the vitamin E, whilst 10% ethyl acetate in isooctane removed the sterols; vitamin A was retained on the column indefinitely.

Vitamin E dimeric and trimeric oxidation products detected by TLC can be removed on dry columns (300 mm × 15 mm i.d.) of silica gel. This purification step has been performed prior to the colorimetric determination of vitamin E in foods (Dean, 1971; Christie et al., 1973). The dimers and trimers are collected in the first 15 ml of eluate, and the tocopherols are collected in the next 75 ml.

Gravity-flow columns of silica gel have been used to purify lipid extracts of milk and infant formula foods in HPLC methods for vitamin K_1. Haroon et al. (1982) removed the non-polar hydrocarbons from a slurry-packed silica gel column by elution with petroleum spirit, after which the vitamin K fraction was eluted with petroleum spirit: diethyl ether (97:3). Hwang (1985) eluted the vitamin K fraction from a dry-packed silica gel column with a predetermined amount of isooctane:dichloromethane: isopropanol (85:15:0·02).

Mixed adsorbents

The AOAC (1984c) spectrophotometric procedure for determining carotenes in fresh plant materials and silages entails chromatography of hexane/acetone extracts on a dry-packed column of magnesia: diatomaceous earth (1:1, w/w) eluted with hexane:acetone (9:1). Carotenes are eluted rapidly, leaving the xanthophylls, carotene oxidation products and chlorophylls on the column.

The AOAC (1984b) spectrophotometric procedure for determining carotenes and xanthophylls in dried plant materials and mixed feeds involves chromatography of the unsaponifiable matter on silica gel:diatomaceous earth (1:1, w/w). Total carotenes are eluted with hexane:acetone (96:4), whilst monohydroxy- and dihydroxy-xanthophylls are eluted with hexane:acetone (9:1), followed by hexane:acetone (8:2). Total xanthophylls can be determined by chromatography of the unsaponifiable matter on a magnesia:diatomaceous earth (1:1, w/w) column. Carotenes are eluted with hexane:acetone (9:1) and total xanthophylls with hexane:acetone:methanol (8:1:1).

5.2.2 Partition Chromatography

In partition chromatography a glass column is packed with an inert, finely divided, porous solid (the support) that has been impregnated with the liquid stationary phase. The mobile phase is a second liquid that is immiscible with the stationary phase. Separation is achieved by distribution (partition) of sample molecules between the mobile and stationary phases, according to their relative solubilities in the two phases.

Partition clean-up columns are usually operated in the 'normal' mode in which a polar (hydrophilic) stationary phase is used in conjunction with a relatively non-polar mobile phase. Normal-phase partition chromatography is suitable for separating hydrophilic compounds of moderate to strong polarity. Solute elution order is similar to that observed in adsorption chromatography: non-polar solutes prefer the mobile phase and elute first; polar solutes prefer the polar stationary phase and elute later.

The alternative to the 'normal' mode is the 'reversed' mode in which a non-polar stationary phase is used in conjunction with a polar mobile phase. Reversed-phase partition chromatography is generally used to separate samples with poor solubility in water. Solute elution order is the reverse of that observed in the normal mode, i.e. polar compounds are eluted before non-polar compounds.

Partition chromatography exhibits several advantages over adsorption chromatography. Partition columns are easier to prepare and use; the chromatography is independent of concentration; there is a logical relationship between the chemical structure of a substance and its chromatographic behaviour; it is possible to resolve isomers and to separate polar substances; there is less chance of loss or chemical alteration (especially of vitamin A) during development; and smaller quantities of substances can be separated (DeLuca et al., 1969).

Diatomaceous earth

Partition columns of diatomaceous earth (Celite 545) impregnated with polyethylene glycol (PEG 600) and eluted with hexane removed β-carotene, vitamin A decomposition products, anhydrovitamin A, and vitamin E from unsaponifiable extracts of margarine, leaving an almost pure fraction of vitamin A for spectrophotometric determination. The mean recovery of vitamin A from the column was 99% (Murray, 1962).

A column of Celite 545 impregnated with PEG 600 was used to remove vitamin A from unsaponifiable extracts of evaporated milk (Eisses & de Vries, 1969), whole milk and partially skimmed milk (Panalaks, 1971) following the removal of cholesterol by digitonin precipitation, in the colorimetric assay of vitamin D.

Disadvantages of Celite columns are that they can only be used a few times before renewal; the carotene and retinol fractions are only just separated; and some of the PEG stationary phase is removed during elution, which can cause some interference during spectrophotometry (Christie, 1975).

5.2.3 Gel Chromatography

Sephadex (a cross-linked dextran gel) and its derivatives exhibit adsorption properties in addition to their size-exclusion properties. Unlike the adsorption chromatography columns mentioned previously, dextran gel columns can be used repeatedly. Thorough washing with methanol after each sample purification prevents the accumulation of material in the column packing.

Sephadex LH-20 (an hydroxypropyl derivative of Sephadex) columns with chloroform elution have been shown to separate β-carotene, α-tocopherol and retinol; and retinyl palmitate or retinyl acetate from retinol (Holasová & Blattná, 1976).

Sephadex LH-20 has been utilized to separate retinol from retinyl palmitate in unsaponified pork liver extracts; and retinol from α-tocopherol in the unsaponifiable fraction of margarine fortified with vitamins A and E (Holasová & Blattná, 1976). The elution time was about 3 h for these samples. LH-20 columns eluted with chloroform:hexane:methanol (65:30:5) are capable of separating sterols from carotenes, thus providing a sterol-free carotene preparation from biological materials (Hasegawa, 1980).

Hydroxyalkoxypropyl Sephadex (HAPS) columns eluted with hexane facilitate the separation of α-tocopherol and α-tocotrienol from each other, and from other E vitamers, in unsaponified extracts of various foods (Thompson et al., 1972a). HAPS/hexane has also been used to purify unsaponifiable extracts of fortified milk prior to the determination of vitamin D by HPLC. The HAPS column removes highly polar lipids from the sample, and prevents their accumulation on the HPLC column (Thompson et al., 1977). Recovery experiments, however, indicated a 10–20% loss of vitamin D which was eventually attributed to its separation from previtamin D on the HAPS column.

In an HPLC method for vitamin K_1 in fruit, vegetables and milk, a short (3 cm × 1 cm) HAPS column, eluted with hexane containing 1% isopropanol, was used to eliminate polar lipids and chlorophylls from the lipid fraction. A longer (120 cm × 1 cm) HAPS column, eluted with hexane and monitored photometrically at 254 nm, was used after the short column in the analysis of milk to separate vitamin K_1 and lower menaquinones from the triglycerides (Thompson *et al.*, 1979).

Sephadex LH-20 has also been used as the inert support packing for partition chromatography by treatment with 90% aqueous methanol as the stationary phase and elution with a mobile phase of isooctane. In the analysis of margarine, β-carotene travels with the solvent front, followed closely by anhydrovitamin A, if present. Vitamin A then begins to appear, well separated from all interfering substances. Vitamin A is fluorescent, hence its elution position on the column can be followed with the aid of a low power UV lamp. A 500 mm × 20 mm LH-20 column is capable of isolating vitamins A and D, but vitamin E is incompletely resolved from β-carotene (Bell, 1971). Partition chromatography on 250 mm × 20 mm columns of LH-20 has been used to purify unsaponifiable extracts in the colorimetric determination of vitamin A in a wide range of foods (Paul & Southgate, 1978).

The LH-20/methanol system with isooctane elution has also been applied to remove retinol in the determination of vitamin D in cod liver oil, which contains about 2 μg/g of vitamin D. Despite losses at some stages of the procedure, sufficient of the vitamin D remains to provide a satisfactory result (Bell & Christie, 1973). However, when the technique is applied to fortified dried milk containing only 0·1 μg/g of vitamin D, losses are excessive and the amount of vitamin D that remains is insufficient for quantitative measurement (Bell & Christie, 1974).

In addition to a greatly improved separation of β-carotene and retinol, within a shorter time, the LH-20/methanol partition system is easier to prepare and operate than Celite/PEG, and can be easily regenerated by washing with methanol. The system has the further advantage that there is no interference from material removed from the column by the mobile phase, as sometimes occurs with Celite/PEG (Christie, 1975).

5.3 THIN-LAYER CHROMATOGRAPHY (TLC)

TLC is a planar form of adsorption chromatography in which the solid stationary phase, either silica gel or alumina, is coated as a thin layer onto a glass plate or some other backing material. A suitable sample extract is applied to the plate as a spot or band, and the plate is placed vertically into a closed vessel containing sufficient solvent (mobile phase) to reach a level just below the applied sample. Solvent flow proceeds up the plate by capillary action, and the separation is stopped before the sample components leave the plate.

TLC serves a dual purpose in removing interfering substances, and separating different vitamins and their vitamers, in a single operation. Detection of the separated spots can be accomplished *in situ* by spraying the plate with a selected chromogenic reagent; some reagents permit the quantification of the vitamin by densitometric measurement. Another quantitative method is to use fluorescein-impregnated silica gel or alumina as the adsorbent. The separated vitamins appear as quenched purple spots against a green fluorescent background when viewed by UV light at 254 nm. The spots, thus located, can be scraped off the plate, and subjected to colorimetric measurement by reaction with a suitable reagent.

Preparative TLC has been used to purify vitamin D and E extracts prior to determination of these vitamins by GLC or HPLC. In this technique the sample is applied to the plate as a band, which permits the loading of a relatively large amount of material. After chromatographic separation, the purified vitamin band is scraped off the plate; eluted from the adsorbent; concentrated by evaporation of the eluting solvent; and analysed by GLC or HPLC. Preparative TLC plates have thicker adsorbent layers than analytical TLC plates, which permits a higher sample loading capacity.

TLC enhances the risk of oxidative losses by exposing the vitamins on large surface areas to air for prolonged times. The damaging effect of light can be minimized by developing the plates in the dark.

Retinol, retinyl acetate, retinyl palmitate and β-carotene can be separated on silica gel TLC plates, and visualized by spraying the plate with the Carr–Price reagent. Quantitative TLC is not possible, however, owing to the unavoidable decomposition of vitamin A compounds and carotenoids on dry silica gel or alumina layers (Strohecker & Henning, 1966).

TLC on fluorescein-impregnated silica gel plates has been employed as a means of separating vitamin D from vitamins A and E. The main difficulty arises from the instability of vitamin D on dry chromatographic adsorbents, although the vitamin is stable as long as solvent is present. For quantitative assay, the vitamin D spots are located under UV irradiation (254 nm) while the plate is still damp with solvent. The spots are scraped off the plate and immediately eluted with chloroform for colorimetric determination with Nield's reagent. The minimum detection limit is $0.5 \mu g$ of vitamin D applied to the plate (Strohecker & Henning, 1966). Attempts to reduce the decomposition of vitamin D during TLC have included the addition of squalene to the sample extract, and BHT to the mobile phase (Hanewald *et al.*, 1968).

Of the many different mobile phases that have been reported to develop silica gel plates, cyclohexane:diethyl ether (1:1) (Bolliger & König, 1969a) has been widely used. This solvent system separates vitamin D ($R_f = 0.4$) from cholesterol ($R_f = 0.3$), α-tocopheryl acetate ($R_f = 0.8$) and vitamin A esters ($R_f = 1.0$) in crude, unsaponified lipid extracts. In unsaponifiable lipid extracts, the retinol spot moves with the vitamin D spot, and it is therefore necessary to remove the retinol by partition column chromatography before TLC (Strohecker & Henning, 1966). Benzene:diethyl ether (4:1) permits the separation of vitamin D ($R_f = 0.29$) from previtamin D ($R_f = 0.42$) on silica gel plates, thus differentiating between the actual vitamin D content (vitamin D *per se*) and the potential vitamin D content (the sum of vitamin D and previtamin D) (Hanewald *et al.*, 1968). The separation of cholesterol, vitamin D and previtamin D has been achieved using alumina containing fluorescent indicator as an adsorbent with pure chloroform as the mobile phase (Ponchon & Fellers, 1968).

Preparative TLC has been used to further purify unsaponifiable extracts of butter and margarine after open-column chromatography in the determination of vitamin D by GLC (Christie, 1975). The technique has also been used to clean up the unsaponifiable fraction obtained from eggs, butter, milk and cheese, following the removal of sterols by precipitation from a methanolic solution at $0°C$ (Jackson *et al.*, 1982). Silica gel plates were developed with hexane:ethyl methyl ketone:dibutyl ether (34:7:6) containing 0.5% BHA, and the extracted vitamin D_3 bands were analysed by HPLC.

Grace & Bernhard (1984) used preparative TLC to separate triglycerides (transformed to their methyl esters) from vitamin D in hexane extracts of whole milk. The TLC plates were coated with silica gel containing a chemically inert indicator (manganese-activated zinc silicates) with an activation peak of $254\,nm$. The plates were developed in hexane:ethyl acetate (80:20), which separated vitamin D from the triglyceride methyl esters. Partial development in a second mobile phase, hexane:isopropanol (85:15), was employed to narrow the vitamin D band on the plate. The band containing the vitamin D was visualized under UV light and extracted with ethyl acetate; this solvent yielded the highest recovery (82%) of vitamin D from the plate from over thirty solvent combinations tested. The ethyl acetate solution was evaporated to dryness, and the residue was dissolved in methanol for analysis by HPLC.

Vitamins D_2 and D_3 are inseparable by the TLC procedures described above, but can be separated from each other by argentation TLC. Sklan & Budowski (1973) used an adsorbent of silica gel impregnated with 5% (w/w) silver nitrate, with chloroform:acetone (9:1) as the mobile phase. After development, the plates were kept in the development tanks under nitrogen, until they were ready for spraying with fluorescein, and visualization under UV light. The following R_f values were obtained: retinol (0·17), vitamin D_2 (0·35), vitamin D_3 (0·42), ergosterol (0·64), α-tocopherol (0·69), cholesterol and other sterols (0·71), anhydroretinol (0·97). Chromatographic losses of vitamin D_3 were about 4% as determined by the radioactivity of $[4-^{14}C]$ cholecalciferol.

TLC is used frequently to separate and purify the E vitamers in the glyceride-free fraction of foods prior to the colorimetric determination of the tocopherols and tocotrienols. In a typical procedure, oils and fats are purified by low temperature crystallization of the glycerides (Chow et al., 1969), and the E vitamers are separated into bands by TLC on fluorescein-impregnated silica gel. The individual bands are located under UV light, scraped off the TLC plate, eluted with chloroform, then evaporated to dryness. The residue is finally redissolved in ethanol for reaction with the Emmerie–Engel reagent (Müller-Mulot, 1976). Alternatively, the TLC bands are eluted directly with ethanol prior to similar colorimetric measurement (Zandi & McKay, 1976).

Many different TLC mobile phases have been published for the determination of vitamin E (Bolliger & König, 1969b). Whittle & Pennock (1967) used two-dimensional TLC to separate seven out of the eight possible E vitamers (β-tocotrienol overlapped with γ-tocopherol); vitamin E dimers were also separable. Müller-Mulot (1976) reported a one-dimensional system which separated the same seven vitamers after triple development. The AOAC (1984d) colorimetric method for natural and total vitamin E (natural vitamin E plus supplemental α-tocopheryl acetate) in food involves extraction, saponification and two-dimensional TLC on sheets coated with alumina. After development in the first mobile phase (benzene:ether) the sheets are dried with nitrogen, then turned 90° and developed in the second mobile phase (petroleum spirit:isopropyl ether). The proportions of solvents in each mobile phase are dependent upon the ambient humidity. After development in the second mobile phase, the sheets are dried with nitrogen, then sprayed with alcoholic dichloro-fluorescein solution. When the sheets are completely dry, the α-tocopherol spots are located under UV light, then cut out and measured colorimetrically.

Christie et al. (1973) detected tocopherol dimers in purified unsaponifiable extracts of foods by TLC on silica gel plates developed with chloroform. Upon spraying with the Emmerie–Engel reagent, the tocopherols and dimers appear as red spots, with R_f values of 0·3–0·5, and 0·7–0·8, respectively. A similar TLC system separates BHT and tocopherols, but BHA has the same mobility as γ-tocopherol in a wide range of mobile phases (Christie, 1975).

Among the many TLC spraying reagents, potassium ferricyanide/ferric chloride and DPPH (1,1-diphenyl-2-picrylhydrazyl)/sulphuric acid have proved useful for the qualitative determination of vitamin E (Ball, unpublished). Gibbs' reagent (2,6-dichloro-p-benzoquinone-4-chlorimine) permitted the densitometric quantification of the separated E vitamers (Ball & Ratcliff, 1978).

Erickson et al. (1973) employed preparative TLC to purify the unsaponifiable fraction of cocoa lipids prior to the determination of the tocopherols by GLC. The TLC plates were coated with silica gel containing a fluorescent indicator. The vitamin E-rich fraction was dissolved in benzene and applied as a band across the bottom of the TLC plate; solutions of α- and δ-tocopherol reference standards were spotted along the side of the plate as markers. The plates were developed in benzene: methanol (98:2); the vitamin E band was scraped off into a 25 cm × 1 cm glass column; and the column was eluted with diethyl ether. The solvent was removed under nitrogen, and the extract was analysed by GLC.

Similar preparative TLC techniques have been used to remove the sterols from the unsaponifiable material of palm oil prior to the determination of the tocopherols and tocotrienols by GLC (Mordret & Laurent, 1978; Meijboom & Jongenotter, 1979; Lercker & Caboni, 1985).

Johnson & Vickers (1973) described a TLC procedure for the identification and semi-quantitative assay of vitamins A, D and E, and certain antioxidants on fluorescein-impregnated silica gel plates developed with hexane:ethyl methyl ketone:dibutyl ether (34:7:6). Decomposition of vitamins A and D was inhibited by the addition of triethylamine to the spotting solvent. As a general spray reagent, ferric chloride–potassium hexacyanoferrate reacted with the vitamins and antioxidants, and was one of the few reagents that could detect α-tocopheryl acetate without the need for a preliminary hydrolysis. Vitamins A and D could be more specifically visualized by spraying with antimony trichloride. The antioxidants, including α-tocopherol, were best visualized by the Emmerie–Engel reagent. The following R_f values were obtained: retinol (0·17), vitamin D (0·22), previtamin D (0·30), BHA (0·32), ethoxyquin (0·42), α-tocopherol (0·51), vitamin A acetate (0·58), α-tocopheryl acetate (0·66), BHT (0·75), anhydrovitamin A (0·81), vitamin A palmitate (0·85) and β-carotene (0·88). The limits of detection (amounts applied to the plate) using antimony trichloride were 0·1 μg of retinol and vitamin D, 0·25 μg of retinyl acetate and 0·5 μg of retinyl palmitate. The detection limit for α-tocopherol, as visualized with the Emmerie–Engel reagent, was 0·4 μg.

TLC on silica gel has been used extensively for the purification of vitamin K from natural sources. Phylloquinone, menaquinones—1, 2, 4, 6 and 9, and also menadione, are separated with chloroform as the mobile phase. The *cis* and *trans* isomers of phylloquinone can be separated using 10% diisopropyl ether in petroleum spirit as the mobile phase. Argentation TLC (silica gel:silver nitrate, 90:10, w/w) with diisopropyl ether as the mobile phase separates phylloquinone, menaquinones—3, 4, 5, 6 and 7, and menadione (Dunphy & Brodie, 1971; Christie & Wiggins, 1978).

TLC, using silica gel and a two-step development with carbon tetrachloride and benzene, was used to purify vitamin K_1 in the analysis of infant formula foods previously subjected to gravity-flow column chromatography on neutral alumina (Manes *et al.*, 1972). The vitamin K_1 spots were measured by reflectance densitometry using a detection wavelength of 275 nm, and the amount of vitamin in the sample was determined by reference to a standard curve.

5.4 SILICA-PACKED 'CLEAN-UP' CARTRIDGES

Disposable pre-packed cartridges containing silica provide a quick and simple means of removing much of the interfering polar material from a lipid extract. The sample extract, dissolved in a non-polar solvent, is passed through the cartridge by means of a glass hypodermic syringe, and the purified eluate is collected.

Indyk & Woollard (1985a) used a special manifold containing a dry-packed cartridge of 40 μm silica to clean up the unsaponifiable extract of fortified milk powders and infant formula foods prior to the determination of vitamin D by HPLC. The extract, dissolved in 1 ml of hexane, was applied to the top of the silica cartridge and eluted with hexane:chloroform (21·5:78·5) to remove vitamin E and other interfering substances. The vitamin D was removed from the column by elution with 10 ml of methanol.

Silica-packed cartridges eluted with isooctane:dioxan in proportions of 95:5 and 98:2 have been employed to purify dichloromethane extracts of fortified instant non-fat dried milk (Cohen & Wakeford, 1980) and saponified animal feedstuffs (Cohen & Lapointe, 1980a) in HPLC methods for vitamins D and E, respectively. In another vitamin D assay using HPLC, a silica cartridge, eluted with 0·4% isopropanol in hexane, was used to remove an unknown contaminant that occurred in large amounts in the unsaponifiable fraction of fatty fish and egg yolk. Non-removal of this contaminant would have necessitated its removal from the subsequent semi-preparative HPLC column by continuous elution for 1 h (Takeuchi et al., 1984).

Chapter 6

Non-Chromatographic Measurement of the Fat-Soluble Vitamins

6.1. SPECTROPHOTOMETRIC METHODS

Molecules will exhibit absorption in the UV or visible region of the spectrum when radiation causes an electronic transition within its structure. The degree of absorbance is proportional to the concentration of irradiated compound over a certain concentration range.

The specific extinction coefficient ($E_{1cm}^{1\%}$) is defined as the absorbance of a 1% w/v sample concentration in a 1 cm path at a given wavelength. The molar absorptivity ε is the absorbance of a sample concentration of 1 gram molecule/litre in a 1 cm path at a given wavelength. The relationship between ε and $E_{1cm}^{1\%}$ is:

$$\varepsilon = E_{1cm}^{1\%} \times \frac{\text{Molecular weight}}{10}$$

Absorbance and quantity are related by the equation:

$$\text{mg} = \frac{A \times D \times V \times 10}{E_{1cm}^{1\%}}$$

where A is the absorbance; D is the dilution factor; and V is the total volume of sample (ml).

Purified solutions of vitamins A, D, E and K in suitable solvents may be assayed spectrophotometrically in the UV region, and solutions of carotenoids in the visible region. The radiation wavelength selected is usually at the λ_{max} of the vitamin or carotenoid in question, i.e. the wavelength at the peak of the absorption spectrum. Absorbance measurement provides a rapid and accurate means of determining the concentration of vitamin in a standard solution.

In food analysis, spectrophotometry has been applied to the determination of vitamins A and E following the removal of interfering substances by some form of liquid chromatography, other than HPLC. The technique has not found application for determining vitamins D and K, owing to the relatively low concentrations of these vitamins in foods, and the consequent need for extensive chromatographic purification of sample extracts.

HPLC methods for determining the fat-soluble vitamins using absorbance detection are discussed in Chapter 8.

Spectral interference in spectrophotometric assays depends upon the wavelength employed in the measurement and the strength of absorbance of the vitamin in question relative to the absorbance of accompanying substances. Most fats and oils contain at least trace amounts of conjugated ethylenic double bonds formed by autoxidation or bleaching. Free or esterified conjugated fatty acids exhibit very strong UV absorption within wavelength maxima of 230–235 nm (dienes) and 260–280 nm (trienes) (Gunstone & Norris, 1983). Apart from conjugated lipids, most lipids found in foodstuffs do not have chromophores which absorb strongly in the UV region above 220 nm. Saturated free fatty acids exhibit virtually no UV

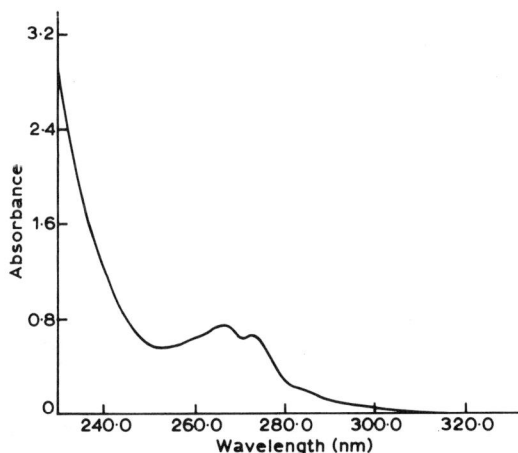

Fig. 20. UV absorption spectrum of triolein in hexane ($E_{1cm}^{1\%}$ at 265 nm = 0·74).

absorption, whilst monoenoic and non-conjugated polyenoic free fatty acids do not absorb sufficiently within the wavelength range used in vitamin assays to constitute an interference.

Triglycerides and sterols exhibit weak, but measurable, UV absorbance at the λ maxima for vitamins D and K, hence constitute a potential source of interference in the spectrophotometric determination of these vitamins. The absorption spectra of vitamins A and E lie beyond those for triglycerides and sterols. The absorption spectrum for triolein (Fig. 20) yielded an $E_{1cm}^{1\%}$ of 0·74 at 265 nm. Spectra for cholesterol (Fig. 21) and cholesteryl acetate (Fig. 22) yielded $E_{1cm}^{1\%}$ values of 0·68 at 266 nm, and 1·22 at 241 nm, respectively.

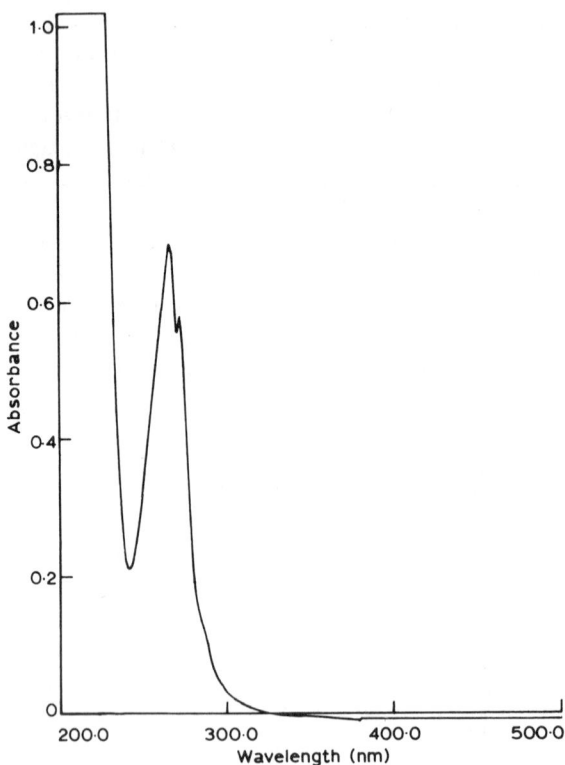

Fig. 21.   UV absorption spectrum of cholesterol in chloroform ($E_{1cm}^{1\%}$ at 266 nm = 0·68).

Saponification will remove the fatty acids, leaving other fat-soluble vitamins, vitamin decomposition products, carotenoids and sterols as sources of spectral interference in the unsaponifiable matter.

Vitamin A

Spectrophotometric assays of vitamin A demand the removal of the various lipids, sterols, and vitamins D and E that absorb in the same general region of the spectrum. The amount of retinol in sufficiently pure extracts dissolved in isopropanol can be calculated from the $E_{1\,cm}^{1\%}$ value of 1830 for all-*trans*-retinol in isopropanol at λ_{max} 325 nm.

If interfering substances that absorb light between 300 nm and 350 nm are present in the sample solution, a false value of vitamin A content is

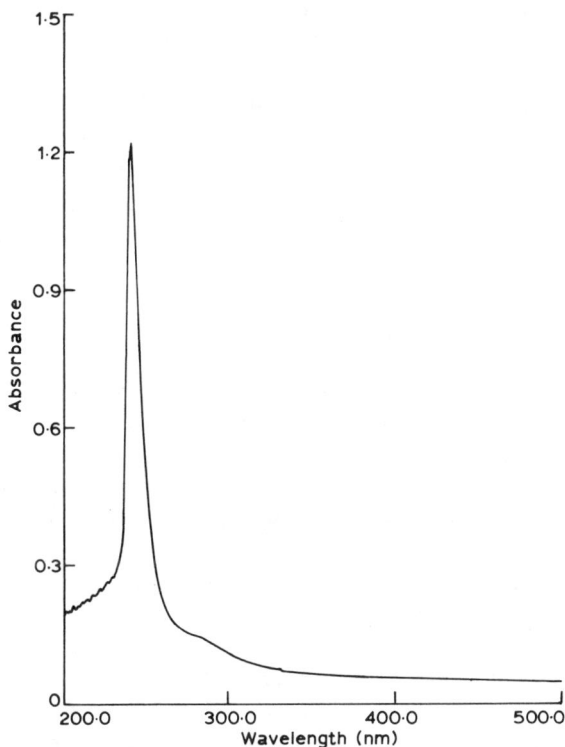

Fig. 22. UV absorption spectrum of cholesteryl acetate in chloroform ($E_{1\,cm}^{1\%}$ at 241 nm = 1·22).

obtained due to 'irrelevant absorption'. This problem can be overcome by applying the Morton and Stubbs equation, which entails measuring the absorbance at 325 nm (λ_{max}) and at 310 nm and 334 nm. The correction is calculated thus:

$$A_{325(corrected)} = 6.815A_{325} - 2.555A_{310} - 4.260A_{334}$$

The correction should only be applied when the corrected absorbance at 325 nm differs by more than 3% from the uncorrected value (Parrish et al., 1985). In the analysis of margarine, interference can be eliminated more reliably by using a solution of the unfortified margarine as a blank, should such material be available (Thompson, 1986).

The Feeding Stuffs Regulations (HMSO, 1982) stipulate spectrophotometry for the determination of vitamin A in animal feeds that contain amounts equal to or greater than 200 000 IU (60 000 μg) per kg. The unsaponifiable matter is extracted with 1,2-dichloroethane, the solvent is evaporated, and the residue is dissolved in petroleum spirit. An aliquot of the petroleum solution containing approximately 200 IU of retinol is evaporated to dryness, and the residue is dissolved in isopropanol. The absorbance of this solution is read at the three wavelengths of 310, 325 and 334 nm. The ratios of the absorbances A_{310}/A_{325} and A_{334}/A_{325} must be 0.857. If one of these ratios differs appreciably from this value (< 0.830 or > 0.880) the measurement of the absorbances must be preceded by alumina column chromatography. If the ratios calculated after chromatography still differ appreciably from the value of 0.857, the determination must be carried out colorimetrically by the Carr–Price method.

Spectrophotometry is used in the current AOAC method for the assay of vitamin A in margarine, after purification of the unsaponifiable fraction on an alumina column (AOAC, 1984f).

Indyk (1982) devised a simple spectrophotometric method for measuring vitamin A in fortified whole milk powder products that allowed rapid on-site analysis at the manufacturing plant. Samples of the powder (0.5 g) were saponified at 70°C for 6 min with intermittent swirling. The unsaponifiable matter was extracted with petroleum spirit:diisopropyl ether (3:1), and a portion of the upper organic phase was read in a spectrophotometer at 325 nm against the extracting solvent (blank). The ability to directly measure the absorbance of the unsaponifiable lipid, without involving chromatographic purification, was attributed to the fact that milk powder is nowadays fortified with all-*trans*-retinyl esters (palmitate or acetate). In the past, dairy products have been fortified with vitamin A preparations that included 3-dehydroretinol (vitamin A_2), carotenes, sterols, and vitamins D and E. This additional unsaponifiable material allegedly caused the spectral interference experienced in the earlier analysis of dairy products. Indyk (1983) adopted a similar procedure for the simultaneous determination of vitamin A, β-carotene and vitamin E in whole milk powder products fortified with vitamins A and E. A mathematical correction was applied to compensate for the spectral interference by β-carotene on the vitamin A measurement.

A modification of the spectrophotometric method for estimating vitamin A is based on the conversion of retinol to anhydroretinol using p-toluenesulphonic acid in benzene as the dehydrating agent (Budowski & Bondi, 1957). Anhydroretinol exhibits well-defined absorption maxima at 377 nm and 399 nm, with a higher extinction value than retinol. The determination is carried out at 399 nm because pure retinol, retinol oxidation products, and carotenoids do not absorb in this region. Thus the method can be applied directly to unsaponifiable extracts of foods without the need for further purification by chromatography.

Vitamin D

Spectrophotometry facilitates the detection of as little as 2 μg of vitamin D but, because of interference from substances with similar absorbances (these include vitamins A, E and decomposition products of vitamin A), UV assays for vitamin D are only possible after extensive chromatographic purification. In food analysis, the necessary degree of purification can only be achieved by HPLC, following some form of sample clean-up.

Vitamin E

Many substances that accompany vitamin E in unsaponifiable fractions contribute to its absorbance, and some substances, including vitamin A and sterols, completely mask the vitamin E spectrum (Olson, 1965). A spectrophotometric method has been proposed for the determination of supplemental α-tocopheryl acetate in whole milk powder products also fortified with vitamin A (Indyk, 1983). Absorbance measurements are made directly upon the unsaponifiable lipid, without involving chromatographic purification. A mathematical correction is applied to compensate for the spectral interference by retinol and β-carotene on the tocopherol measurement. Most foods demand extensive chromatographic purification prior to spectrophotometry, hence the technique (apart from HPLC with absorbance detection) has not been widely used in food analysis.

Vitamin K

Vitamins K_1 and K_2 exhibit absorption spectra which contain five maxima. Spectrophotometric assays may be carried out by reducing the quinone structure to the quinol, and stabilizing the latter as the diacetate. Completion of this reaction results in a single major peak at 230 nm. The $E_{1\,cm}^{1\%}$ value at 230 nm of K_1 dihydro-*O*-diacetate is 1720. The reduction reaction may be carried out with potassium borohydride after chromatographic purification of the sample extract (Olson, 1965). Since the change in absorbance is proportional to the amount of naphthoquinone present, the vitamin may be assayed by measuring either the increase in absorbance at 245 nm or the decrease in absorbance at 270 nm.

Carotenoids

Before 1960, very little synthetic β-carotene was available, and red palm oil was used as the source of colour in margarine. Red palm oil consists of a mixture of α- and β-carotene, and inactive carotenoids. α-Carotene has only about one-half of the provitamin A activity of β-carotene, hence it was necessary to separate and measure both carotenoids. Nowadays, the colouring matter used in margarine is predominantly synthetic β-carotene,

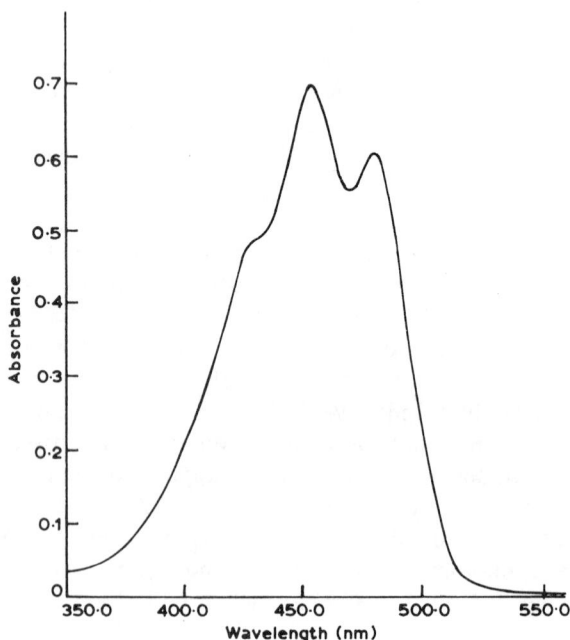

Fig. 23. Absorption spectrum for β-carotene (from De Ritter & Purcell, 1981).

which precludes the need to separate and measure α- and β-carotene (Christie, 1971).

β-Carotene, by virtue of its deep orange colour, exhibits very strong absorption in the visible region of the spectrum ($E_{1cm}^{1\%} = 2590$ at λ_{max} 450 nm in hexane; Brubacher *et al.*, 1985). The absorption spectrum for β-carotene is shown in Fig. 23. In the analysis of margarine by the AOAC (1984*f*) method, the carotene in the unsaponifiable fraction is separated from vitamin A by open-column chromatography, before spectrophotometric determination.

De Ritter & Purcell (1981) described a simpler method for determining synthetic β-carotene in margarine, where it is the only added colouring agent. For margarine containing . 5000 IU of β-carotene per pound (11023/kg), a 10 g sample is shaken with 50–60 ml of petroleum spirit in a 100 ml measuring cylinder, then diluted to 100 ml with petroleum ether. The emulsion is allowed to settle and the volume of the aqueous layer in the bottom is subtracted from 100 ml to obtain the volume of the solvent layer. The extract is clarified by treating a portion with filter aid (diatomaceous earth), and centrifuging. The absorbance of the solution is read at 454 nm against a blank of margarine containing no β-carotene, or an uncoloured oil solution. The concentration of β-carotene in the tube is determined by comparison with a standard curve of pure all-*trans-β*-carotene. Identification of the carotene is carried out by comparing the absorption spectrum with that of the pure compound.

Procedures for separating β-carotene from other food colours, i.e. anatto and turmeric, have been described (De Ritter & Purcell, 1981).

The AOAC (1984*c*) procedure for determining carotene in fresh plant materials and silages entails hexane/acetone extraction of the ground sample, followed by open-column chromatography, and spectro-photometric measurement of the eluate at 436 nm. The AOAC (1984*b*) procedure for determining carotene and xanthophylls in dried plant material and mixed feeds entails saponification, followed by fractionation of the carotenes and the monohydroxy—and dihydroxy—xanthophylls, or total xanthophylls, by open-column chromatography. The carotene and xanthophyll fractions are measured spectrophotometrically at 436 nm and 474 nm, respectively.

6.2 FLUOROMETRIC METHODS

Fluorescence is a form of luminescence, and refers to the long-wave radiation energy emitted from certain compounds excited by UV irradiation. Fluorescence activity may be expressed in terms of quantum efficiency, which is the ratio between the number of photons emitted and the number of photons absorbed during fluorescence (Rhys Williams, 1980). In general, compounds that fluoresce contain either an electron-donating group (e.g. amines, alcohols) or multiple conjugated double bonds; the presence of a rigid planar aromatic ring is particularly favourable to fluorescence.

In a typical fluorescence spectrometer the sample is irradiated with UV light, and the desired excitation wavelength is isolated by means of filters or by a monochromator. The fluorescence emission, which is also isolated by filters or by a monochromator, is detected by a photomultiplier at right-angles to the incident beam, thus the emitted radiation is detected against a relatively dark background.

Fluorometry is more selective than absorption spectrophotometry because the former uses two wavelengths in the measurement, and certain structural features are required in a molecule for fluorescence to occur. Glycerides and sterols, for example, do not fluoresce, whilst vitamin A and its esters, and non-esterified vitamin E possess strong native fluorescence. Maximum sensitivity is obtained by selecting the wavelengths corresponding to the intensity maxima in the excitation and emission spectra. At other wavelengths the sensitivity, although reduced, may still be adequate for measurement purposes. The sensitivity of the fluorometer also depends upon the width of the slits, the age of the lamp, and the performance of the photomultiplier amplifier. The limit of detection with fluoromethyl, given a pure sample and optimum instrumental settings, is at the 1 pg level compared with 1 ng obtained with absorption spectrophotometry.

Under commonly used conditions, the observed fluorescence signal is directly proportional to the concentration up to an absorbance value of $0 \cdot 01\ A$ when measured in a 1 cm cuvette. If a 1 mm pathlength cuvette is used (as in an HPLC detector) the range increases to $0 \cdot 1\ A$. Above these values the fluorescence decreases due to quenching effects whereby the excited molecules lose their excess energy through a variety of inter-molecular processes. The inner filter effect is a type of concentration quenching that refers to an attenuation of the excitation beam and also to the absorption of the emitted beam within the solution (Rhys Williams, 1988; private communication). Impurities can cause several types of quenching, and the presence of dissolved oxygen causes pronounced collisional quenching. Other factors that affect quenching include temperature, viscosity, pH and ionic strength (Guilbault, 1973; Lakowicz, 1983).

Vitamin A

Retinol and retinyl esters fluoresce very strongly upon excitation with long wave UV light at 330–360 nm (maximum 325–330 nm) and emit between 470 nm and 490 nm (maximum 480 nm). The fluorescence of retinol is a linear function of concentration until self-absorption becomes significant at concentrations of 0·25 µg/ml (Hubbard *et al.*, 1971; Christie & Wiggins, 1978). Fluorometry therefore provides a potentially highly sensitive method for the determination of vitamin A with a reported detection limit of 0·01 ppm (Senyk *et al.*, 1975). Specificity, too, is high since compounds such as sterols, vitamin D and low concentrations of carotenoids, which can severely interfere with the spectrophotometric and colorimetric methods, do not affect the fluorometric determination of vitamin A (Christie & Wiggins, 1978). However, different vitamin A isomers do not exhibit the same degree of fluorescence: Lawn *et al.* (1983) demonstrated that the quantum efficiency of the 13-*cis* isomer was only 33% of that of the all-*trans* isomer, compared with a UV absorptivity of 92%. Thus in foods with a relatively high 13-*cis* isomer content, the total vitamin A concentration measured by fluorometry will be less than that measured by spectrophotometry.

Exposure of retinol or retinyl ester standards to UV radiation must be avoided as irradiation will result in the formation of fluorescent retro-vitamin A derivatives, which interfere with the measurements. The use of chlorinated solvents must also be avoided, since they tend to increase the rate of formation of retro derivatives (Thompson *et al.*, 1971).

A fluorometric method for the determination of vitamin A in foods has been described (Erdman *et al.*, 1973). Convenience foods, which contain low amounts of carotenoids, were analysed directly after saponification and extraction of the unsaponifiable matter with hexane. High-carotenoid foods, such as fortified vegetable entrees and some margarines, were further purified on a column of deactivated alumina prior to fluorometric measurement. Both procedures involved a correction formula to compensate for the presence of the fluorescent carotenoid, phytofluene, which is found predominantly in carrots and tomatoes.

Rapid methods for the assay of retinol in milk and dairy products (Thompson *et al.*, 1972*b*; Senyk *et al.*, 1975) involve saponification and extraction, but not chromatography, as studies have shown that there is no significant interference from phytofluene. Since the fluorometric method does not measure the provitamin A carotenoids, the methods are applicable to skimmed milk fortified with vitamin A.

Fluorescence detection in conjunction with HPLC has been used in the determination of vitamin A in breakfast cereals and other foods (Egberg *et al.*, 1977), milk (Woollard & Woollard, 1981; Woollard & Fairweather, 1985) and in feedstuffs (Lawn *et al.*, 1983). These methods are described in Section 8.3.1.

Vitamin D
Underivatized vitamins D_2 and D_3 do not exhibit fluorescence, but a number of published colorimetric reactions for vitamin D produce fluorescence as well as colour. The most sensitive reaction studied has been produced by acetic anhydride–sulphuric acid in trichloroethane, which has been utilized for the colorimetric or fluorometric determination of cholesterol. The excitation/emission wavelengths for vitamins D_2 and D_3 (475/510 nm) are different from those of cholesterol (350/415 nm) (Chen *et al.*, 1964). No applications of this technique have been found for the assay of vitamin D in foods or feedstuffs.

Vitamin E
Solutions of non-esterified vitamin E in pure solvents exhibit strong native fluorescence. The response of a spectrofluorometric detector after separation of seven of the E vitamers by HPLC was quantitatively similar for the tocopherols and tocotrienols; BHA was detected among the vitamin E peaks (Thompson & Hatina, 1979). The excitation and emission maxima for α-tocopherol at 295 and 330 nm, respectively, are relatively close together so that a dual monochromator spectrofluorometer, rather than a filter fluorometer, may be necessary to measure the fluorescence. Vitamin A quenches the fluorescence because its absorption maximum at 325 nm is in the range of the emission wavelength of vitamin E. The fluorescence of vitamin E is abolished by even traces of chlorinated hydrocarbons (Thompson, 1982).

Thompson *et al.* (1972*a*) used gel chromatography to purify unsaponifiable extracts of foods, with spectrofluorometric monitoring of the column effluent at 290 nm excitation and 340 nm emission. This technique allowed the separation and detection of α-tocopherol and α-tocotrienol from the remaining E vitamers.

Fluorescence detection has been used in the determination of naturally occurring tocopherols and tocotrienols in oils and foods by HPLC (see Section 8.3.4). The sensitivity of a fluorescence detector towards E vitamers was found to be at least ten times superior to that of a variable wavelength absorbance detector (Thompson & Hatina, 1979). The high selectivity of a fluorescence detector permits the measurement of E vitamers in crude lipid extracts. Alpha-tocopheryl acetate is only weakly fluorescent but, owing to its relatively high concentration in fortified foods, it can be determined fluorometrically under defined HPLC conditions.

Vitamin K
Vitamin K has been determined by HPLC using fluorescence detection after reduction to its hydroquinone form.

6.3 VOLTAMMETRIC METHODS

Voltammetry (or polarography) is an electroanalytical technique which can be applied to the determination of oxidizable or reducible compounds. The technique is based on the principle that when a voltage is applied to a polarizable electrode immersed in an electrolyte solution, any electroactive solute in contact with the electrode will undergo electrolysis and produce an electric current. In linear-sweep voltammetry, a voltammogram for an electroactive solute in a stationary solution is obtained by scanning the voltage in a positive or negative direction, and measuring the peak current as the solute is oxidized or reduced. At a certain potential value electrolysis of the solute will begin to occur at the electrode, and a small current will flow. As the potential is made still more positive (or negative) the current increases sharply as more solute is oxidized (or reduced) until a point is reached at which the solute is oxidized (or reduced) as fast as it arrives at the electrode surface by diffusion from the bulk of the solution. At this point the current becomes independent of the scanning potential, and is called the limiting current.

In a diffusion-controlled electrolytic process, quantification of the electroactive solute is based on the measurement of the wave height; that is, the difference between the limiting current and the residual current before the wave rise. Qualitative results can be obtained because the potential at which the current reaches half the total wave height (half-wave potential) is characteristic for each solute in a given electrolyte solution and electrode system. If more than one electroactive compound is present in the solution, the recorded voltammogram consists of superimposed voltammetric waves of the individual compounds. The wave heights and half-wave potentials are, in principle, independent of each other.

Voltammetry is most suitable for the detection of electrooxidizable compounds; the monitoring of electroreducible compounds is complicated by the high background currents generated by dissolved oxygen.

Linear sweep voltammetry has been carried out to determine tocopherols in fats, oils and foods after saponification (Atuma & Lindquist, 1973; Atuma, 1975) and in unsaponified vegetable oils (McBride & Evans, 1973; Waltking *et al.*, 1977; Deldime *et al.*, 1978). The technique involved the electrooxidation of tocopherols to tocopherylquinones using positive potentials. Voltammetric waves were obtained for α-, $\beta + \gamma$- and δ-tocopherols, which were quantified by measuring the peak heights. Further voltammetric investigations carried out by Podlaha *et al.* (1978) revealed detection limits of $10\,\mu g/g$ of oil for α- and $(\beta + \gamma)$-tocopherols and $20\,\mu g/g$ of oil for δ-tocopherol. The value for each tocopherol is, in fact, a sum of the tocopherol and the corresponding tocotrienol. Carotenoids, vitamin A, sterols and other reducing substances are completely inactive electrochemically in the potential range of operation.

6.4 COLORIMETRIC METHODS

Colorimetry involves the reaction of the vitamin with a reagent to form a coloured compound, the absorbance of which is proportional to the concentration of vitamin over a certain range. The technique, as applied to the fat-soluble vitamins is non-specific, and therefore necessitates prior chromatographic purification of the vitamin-rich fraction to eliminate interfering substances. Colorimetric methods cannot distinguish between the various forms of a particular vitamin unless the vitamers are separated beforehand.

Vitamin A
Vitamin A and other polyenes containing at least three double bonds react with a group of acidic reagents known as Lewis acids (e.g. antimony trichloride, trifluoroacetic acid and trichloroacetic acid) to give an intense blue colour of maximum absorbance within the range 616–620 nm. Antimony trichloride in chloroform is known as the Carr–Price reagent, and was introduced in 1926. The colour reaction (λ_{max} 620 nm) is 2·5 times more sensitive than spectrophotometry for the determination of retinol, and is relatively free from interference by non-polyenic contaminants. Polyunsaturated fatty acids, carotenoids and sterols form coloured products with Lewis acids, and must therefore be removed before estimation of retinol (Christie & Wiggins, 1978). The reaction must be carried out after saponification, which removes polyunsaturated fatty acids. Some form of chromatography is then required to remove

carotenoids, sterols and other interfering substances from the unsaponifiable matter.

The *cis* isomers of vitamin A produce the same reaction to the Carr–Price reagent as all-*trans*-retinol. Since the *cis* isomers are markedly less potent than all-*trans*-retinol in inducing a growth response in animals, this can result in an overestimation of the biological value of fish oils and other food supplements which contain significant amounts of *cis* isomers. Maleic anhydride reacts with 13-*cis* and 11,13-di-*cis*-isomers, and prevents them from reacting with the Carr–Price reagent. Thus two Carr–Price values may be obtained; one of the mixture of isomers, and the other after elimination of the two *cis* isomers. The difference between the two values provides an estimate of the isomer composition of the sample and its biological potency (Association of Vitamin Chemists, Inc., 1966; Roels & Mahadevan, 1967; Hashmi, 1973).

Several difficulties are inherent in the Carr–Price reaction. The colour is extremely transitory, and the absorbances must be read within 5–10 s of addition of the reagent. In the presence of traces of water, insoluble antimony hypochlorite forms, which causes turbidity as well as opaque films on the glass cuvettes. Acetic anhydride is added to act as a water scavenger, but it may also influence the colour reaction (Olson, 1965; Strohecker & Henning, 1966; Association of Vitamin Chemists, Inc., 1966; Roels & Mahadevan, 1967; Brubacher, 1968).

Trifluoroacetic acid (TFA) (Dugan *et al.*, 1964; Olson, 1965; Roels & Mahadevan, 1967; Hashmi, 1973) and trichloroacetic acid (TCA) (Grys, 1975, 1980; Kamangar & Fawzi, 1978; Bayfield & Cole, 1980) react with vitamin A in a similar manner to antimony trichloride. However, the colours produced by TFA and TCA are much less susceptible to interference by traces of water, and it is also easier to clean the cuvettes. These reagents are more stable in dichloromethane than in chloroform or 1,2-dichloroethane (Subramanyam & Parrish, 1976). Grys (1975, 1980) improved the technique by using a fast-measurement accessory and a chart recorder so that readings could be obtained at the maximum colour intensity of the reaction.

The blue colour produced with TFA decays to a more stable pink colour within 1·5–2 h, but the intensity of this pink colour is less than one-third of that of the blue colour. Gharbo & Gosser (1975) proposed a method for determining retinol based on the discovery that a mixture of TFA and 0·1 N perchloric acid (5:1) added to a dichloromethane solution of vitamin A increases the speed of development and the sensitivity of the pink colour. Maximum absorbance of the pink colour with λ_{max} at 502 nm is attained within 7–12 min, and the colour remains stable for at least 30 s. The intensity of the pink colour is equivalent to 45% of the intensity of the blue colour produced by the Carr–Price reaction. The pink colour is destroyed within 2–4 min by the addition of pentane-2,4-dione followed by hydrogen peroxide, and this reaction is used in the blank determination.

The Feeding Stuffs Regulations (HMSO, 1982) utilizes the Carr–Price reaction to determine vitamin A in animal feeds that contain < 200 000 IU (60 000 μg) per kg. The unsaponifiable material is fractionated on an alumina column, and the colorimetric reaction, including the acetic anhydride addition, is performed on the concentrated vitamin A fraction. The Carr–Price or TFA reaction is also employed in the current AOAC method for the assay of vitamin A in mixed feeds, premixes and foods, after column chromatography on alumina (AOAC, 1984g).

Vitamin D

Vitamin D compounds with three conjugated double bonds (i.e. vitamins D_2 and D_3, and their corresponding previtamins and tachysterols) give an identical reaction with Nield's reagent (antimony trichloride and acetyl chloride in chloroform) to produce a pink colour of λ_{max} 500 nm (Nield *et al.*, 1940). Measurement of the absorbance of the pink colour provides a means of determining the potential vitamin D content of a suitably purified solution. The reaction attains maximum intensity in 1 min at 20°C, and the use of 1,2-dichloroethane, rather than chloroform, stabilizes the chromophore. Other polyenes, including vitamin A and its decomposition products, carotenoids, and vitamin E, interfere with the reaction; the interference by vitamin A is due to the immediate formation of an intense blue colour, i.e. the Carr–Price reaction. Residual amounts of cholesterol do not interfere with the vitamin D determination since the absorptivity of cholesterol at 500 nm with Nield's reagent is less than 0·1% of that of vitamin D (de Vries *et al.*, 1969).

A colorimetric method using Nield's reagent, in combination with purification by open-column chromatography, has been adopted by the Pharmacopoeia of the United States in 1970 as an official method for vitamin D. The method, modified by Mulder & de Vries (1974), is applicable for the assay of vitamin D in fortified foods, e.g. dried milk, evaporated milk, and cereals. Acetic anhydride specifically inhibits the reaction time between vitamin D and Nield's reagent, and is used in the blank determination. The vitamin D content is calculated by means of internal standards and a calibration curve. A correction factor derived from absorbance measurements at two wavelengths is applied as a further attempt to eliminate colorimetric interfering substances. At least 5 μg of vitamin D must be present in the final 2 ml of solution, after removal of interfering substances by chromatography (Olson, 1965; Strohecker & Henning, 1966). The specificity of the method is improved by eliminating two of the biologically inactive isomers, tachysterol and *trans*-vitamin D; this is achieved by reacting the sample solution with maleic anhydride for 30 min at room temperature (Mulder *et al.*, 1971).

Vitamin D in chloroform solution reacts with TFA to give an immediate pink colour, which changes to a yellow colour with maximum absorption at 403 nm after 3–4 min, and is suitable for the quantitative determination of the vitamin (Hashmi, 1973). The blue colour of maximum absorption 616 nm, obtained by reaction of vitamin A with TFA, does not interfere with the determination of vitamin D (Dugan *et al.*, 1964). The stability and sensitivity of the yellow colour may be improved by mixing the sample with hydroquinone, which prevents loss of colour due to oxidation by air (Gharbo & Gosser, 1974). The blank is prepared by measuring the test solution after decolorization with hydrogen peroxide.

Vitamin D is a highly potent factor, and effective fortification levels are often below the minimum concentration necessary to apply the colorimetric assay successfully. Colorimetric assays, using Nield's reagent, have therefore been confined to relatively highly fortified foods, such as evaporated milk. As the ratio of cholesterol and vitamin A to vitamin D tends to be high in the unsaponifiable extracts of such foods, colorimetry can only be applied after the removal of cholesterol and vitamin A. Eisses & de Vries (1969) estimated the vitamin D content of evaporated milk following two successive saponification treatments, precipitation of the cholesterol with digitonin, removal of retinol by partition chromatography on a Celite–polyethylene glycol column, and removal of carotenoids and decomposition products of vitamin A on an alumina column. Panalaks (1971) determined vitamin D in fortified whole milk and partially skimmed fluid milk by using similar purification techniques. The sample blank was determined by measuring the absorbances of the chromophore at the wavelength minima (435 nm and 550 nm) of the spectrum (λ_{max} 500 nm), which eliminated the use of the acetic anhydride colour inhibitor.

Vitamin E

The Emmerie–Engel colorimetric method has been widely used for estimating vitamin E in oils, foods, and animal feedstuffs since its introduction in 1939. The reagent used in this procedure is a mixture of ferric chloride and 2,2′-bipyridyl in ethanolic solution. Tocopherols and tocotrienols reduce the iron to the ferrous state, which then combines with the bipyridyl to form an intense red complex, the absorbance of which is measured at 520 nm. The reaction must be carried out under dim artificial light, since the excess ferric ions are subject to photo-reduction.

The Emmerie–Engel method gives a high degree of accuracy and precision with pure tocopherols, but is not specific. Synthetic antioxidants (e.g. BHA and BHT), and naturally occurring reducing agents (e.g. vitamin A, carotenoids, some sterols and biologically inactive tocopherol dimers and trimers) that accompany vitamin E in the unsaponifiable fraction, give a similar colour reaction. Furthermore, individual E vitamers react at different rates, and produce different intensities of colour. The validity of the reaction depends, therefore, upon the degree of purity of the final vitamin E extract. Vitamin E esters do not exhibit reducing activity, hence must be hydrolysed to the alcohol forms before they can be determined by the Emmerie–Engel method.

The sensitivity of the original Emmerie–Engel method can be increased 2·5-fold by using bathophenanthroline in place of 2,2′-bipyridyl (Tsen, 1961). In this method excess ferric ions are complexed with phosphoric acid, hence the possibility of photo-reduction is eliminated. Erickson & Dunkley (1964) used the bathophenanthroline reagent in the determination of tocopherol in milk and milk lipids after extraction of the vitamin with ethanol and hexane, and purification by adsorption column chromatography. A correction was made for the interference of carotenoids by measuring at two absorbance wavelengths. Christie *et al.* (1973) also utilized the bathophenanthroline reaction to determine total vitamin E in various foods after purification of the unsaponifiable matter by adsorption column chromatography.

Colorimetry is most frequently performed on vitamin E extracts purified by TLC. Using this approach, total vitamin E, α-tocopherol alone, or the individual E vitamers have been determined using the Emmerie–Engel reagent (Analytical Methods Committee, 1959; Association of Vitamin Chemists, Inc., 1966; Strohecker & Henning, 1966; Bunnell, 1967; Brubacher, 1968; Müller-Mulot, 1976; Zandi & McKay, 1976).

The AOAC (1984*d*) procedure for determining natural α-tocopherol or total α-tocopherol (natural plus supplemental) in foods or feeds entails solvent extraction of the sample, followed by saponification, isolation of α-tocopherol by TLC and colorimetric determination using bathophenanthroline. To specifically determine supplemental α-tocopheryl acetate (all-*rac* form) (AOAC, 1984*e*), the sample is extracted and the reducing substances, including natural α-tocopherol, are removed by oxidative column chromatography. The α-tocopheryl acetate is then saponified, and the resulting α-tocopherol is determined colorimetrically.

Vitamin K

In the Irreverre–Sullivan reaction, vitamin K is reacted with sodium diethyldithiocarbamate and sodium ethylate in ethanolic solution to give a cobalt blue colour, which develops to a maximum within 5 min and then fades to reddish orange after 8 min. The highest reading obtained at 575 nm is used. Colour development is proportional to the concentration of vitamin K_1 over a certain concentration range, and the test is sensitive to 35 μg of vitamin K_1 per ml. The colour developed with ubiquinones and plastoquinones differs from that obtained with vitamin K_1 regarding shade, intensity and speed of development. The reaction is not suitable for the determination of menadione (Dam & Søndergaard, 1967).

In the Schilling–Dam procedure for vitamin K, the sample in ethanol is treated with 80% saturated xanthine hydride in ethanol in the presence of KOH, and the solution is heated at 50°C for 10 min. A transient blue–violet colour which cannot be stabilized appears; this then fades to a stable orange colour which absorbs at 410 nm. The $E_{1cm}^{1\%}$ of this orange product at 410 nm is about 70 for vitamin K. Tocopherylquinone gives only a slight colour (Olson, 1965). A major disadvantage of the Schilling–Dam assay is the narrow range of validity of the calibration curves, which extend only from 25–80 μg/ml for vitamin K_1 and from 10–200 μg/ml for menadione (Aaron, 1980).

The Feeding Stuffs Regulations (HMSO, 1982) method for determining menadione in animal feeds involves extraction with diluted ethanol, clarification with tannin solution and centrifugation. The supernatant is treated with sodium carbonate solution and the menadione is extracted with 1,2-dichloroethane. The dichloroethane extract is treated, according to its menadione content, either directly or after evaporation with 2,4-dinitrophenylhydrazine in acidified ethanolic solution. The resulting hydrazone is treated with excess ammonia to form a blue–green complex, the absorbance of which is measured at 635 nm. The lower limit of the determination is 1 mg/kg.

Chapter 7

Gas–Liquid Chromatography (GLC)

7.1 GENERAL ASPECTS OF GLC RELEVANT TO FAT-SOLUBLE VITAMIN ASSAYS

7.1.1 Principle of GLC

GLC relies upon the volatilization of the sample components of interest within a heated column, hence the components must be sufficiently volatile without decomposing under the conditions of separation.

In GLC the stationary phase is an organic liquid which is involatile at the column operating temperature; the mobile phase is an inert gas. Separation of the various sample components results from intermolecular forces that occur between the solute and the stationary liquid phase. For non-polar solutes (e.g. hydrocarbons) the interaction is due solely to non-selective dispersive forces. The elution of non-polar solutes from any chromatographic column occurs, therefore, in order of increasing boiling point. For the separation of polar solutes the important interactions are orientation and induction forces, the sum of which constitutes a measure of the polarity of that phase with respect to that solute. The magnitude of the individual interaction energies is a measure of phase selectivity, thus two solutes of equal polarity can be separated by a selective stationary phase.

In packed column GLC the stationary phase is coated upon granules of an inert porous material (the support), which is usually diatomaceous earth. The coated granular material is packed into a glass column of typical dimensions 1·8 m length × 4 mm internal diameter to form a homogeneous bed that completely fills the column. The surface silanol ($\equiv$Si—OH) groups of untreated diatomaceous earth function as active sites in promoting severe peak tailing of polar solutes. Sample components may also undergo decomposition, structural rearrangement, and even complete adsorption.

116

The diatomaceous earth is therefore deactivated by converting the surface silanol groups to silyl ethers by reaction with dimethyldichlorosilane (DMCS) or some other silylating reagent.

Open-tubular capillary columns (nowadays commonly referred to as simply 'capillary' columns) provide superior separation efficiencies compared with packed columns, and the sharper peaks facilitate a more accurate integration as well as a greatly improved sample detectability. In open-tubular columns the stationary liquid phase is chemically bonded as a thin film upon the inner surface of a glass or fused silica capillary column, leaving a lumen throughout the length of the column. Fused silica columns are coated on the outside with a protective layer of polyimide to impart mechanical strength and flexibility. Capillary columns of 15 m, 20 m or 50 m length and 0·25 mm or 0·4 mm internal diameter have found applications in vitamin E assays.

Compounds that would produce interfering peaks in the chromatogram obtained from a packed column can often be separated on a capillary column, and thus need not be removed from the sample extract. 'Column bleed' caused by volatilization of the liquid phase of packed columns during temperature programming is not a problem with capillary columns. On the demerit side, the injection systems required for use with narrow bore capillary columns are more complicated in design and operation compared with the simple packed column injectors.

7.1.2 GLC Stationary Phases

GLC methods using packed columns have been published for the assay of vitamins D, E and K in foods. The earliest methods have utilized stationary phases of silicone rubber gums that are either non-polar (e.g. SE-30) or possess intermediate polarity (e.g. SE-52).

Apiezon greases have also been used as non-polar stationary phases. The more recent polysiloxanes of the OV series of stationary phases owe their popularity to their high thermal stability, wide liquid range, and wide range of polarities. A representation of the siloxane backbone is shown in Fig. 24 in which R can be; methyl, phenyl, 3,3,3-trifluoropropyl, cyanopropyl, or some other group.

Terminal silanol ($\equiv$Si—OH) groups are end-capped to maximize thermal stability. OV liquid phases that have been used in vitamin assays have included OV-1 (R = methyl), which is non-polar, and OV-17 (R = 50% methyl; 50% phenyl), OV-210 (R = 50% methyl; 50% trifluoro-propyl) and OV-225 (R = 50% methyl; 25% phenyl; 25% cyanopropyl), which all possess intermediate polarity.

$$\left[\begin{array}{ccc} R & & R \\ | & & | \\ \text{Si} & \text{—O—} & \text{Si} & \text{—O—} \\ | & & | \\ R & & R \end{array}\right]$$

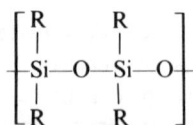

Fig. 24. Representation of the siloxane backbone of a polysiloxane GLC stationary phase.

Only a few stationary phases are required for most capillary column applications because column efficiency, rather than phase selectivity, determines the separation.

7.1.3 Detection Systems
In GLC the detection of the separated components is carried out by continuous monitoring of the gaseous column effluent. Detection of the fat-soluble vitamins is achieved, in most cases, by hydrogen flame ionization (FID). The FID works on the principle that when organic compounds are burned in a hydrogen and air flame, ions are produced. The ions are collected by a pair of polarized electrodes inside the detector, and the current produced is amplified before being passed to a recorder or integrator. The FID is regarded as a universal detector since it responds to virtually all organic compounds; formaldehyde, formic acid and compounds containing a single carbon atom bonded to oxygen or sulphur (e.g. CO_2, CS_2) do not provide a significant response. The detector combines a low detection limit of approximately 1 ng with an exceptional linear response range of up to seven orders of magnitude of solute concentration.

The electron capture detector (ECD) is selective for electrophilic compounds, and is capable of detecting halogenated compounds at the 1 pg level. It is used mainly in the analysis of herbicide and pesticide residues, but has also been applied to halogenated derivatives of vitamin D. Quinones are strongly electrophilic, hence the ECD has been used for the determination of vitamin K. The linear range of an ECD with pulse-modulated operation is four orders of magnitude.

7.1.4 Quantification
In vitamin assays by GLC, quantification is usually performed by internal standardization, which is a technique designed to compensate for analyte (vitamin) losses incurred during the sample preparation and final chromatographic analysis. The internal standardization method involves adding a known amount of a suitable internal standard to the sample at the

earliest possible point in the analytical procedure, and measuring the peak heights or areas of the analyte and internal standard in the chromatogram. The quantification is based upon the comparison of the ratio of the internal standard peak size to analyte peak size in the sample with that ratio in a standard solution containing known amounts of the analyte and internal standard. As the calculation involves ratios of peak sizes, and not the absolute peak size, the injection volumes need not be constant. The concentrations of the analyte and internal standard must, however, remain within the linear range of the detector. A major advantage of the internal standardization procedure over other methods of quantification (e.g. normalization) is that there is no assumption that all sample components have been eluted and detected.

The ideal internal standard conforms to the following requirements:

(i)   it must never occur naturally in the original sample;

(ii) it must elute near to the analyte;

(iii) it must be completely resolved from the analyte and from other neighbouring components;

(iv) it must be added at a concentration that will produce a peak height or area ratio of about unity with the analyte;

(v) it must resemble the analyte as closely as possible in terms of chemical and physical properties (including stability), so that it is incorporated into the sample matrix in the same way as the analyte, and it behaves in a similar manner to the analyte during all steps in the analytical procedure (extraction, derivatization, etc.);

(vi) it should not react with any components of the sample or with the column packing;

(vii) it must be commercially available in high purity.

A satisfactory internal standard is usually a compound that is structurally related to the analyte (e.g. an isomer or close homologue). In the determination of supplemental vitamin D_2 in foods, vitamin D_3 can be used as an internal standard, and vice versa. This technique is not ideal, however, since trace amounts of naturally occurring vitamin D_2 and/or D_3 may be present in the sample. In vitamin E assays that involve saponification, the use of tocol as an internal standard is precluded as it undergoes up to 85% loss during a 70°C saponification compared with losses of 5% and 15% for α- and γ-tocopherol, respectively (Buttriss & Diplock, 1984).

The internal standardization procedure is performed as follows:

A standard solution containing a known concentration (W_A) of the analyte (A) and a known concentration (W_S) of the internal standard (S) is chromatographed. Let the peaks for A and S have peak heights of h_A and h_S, respectively. The electrical signal from the detector is proportional, over a certain concentration range, to the amount of detected component in the sample.

Peak size $\propto$ component concentration

The response of the detector varies from one component to another.

$$h_A = K_A \times W_A \tag{1}$$

where K_A is the response factor of the detector to analyte A. Similarly,

$$h_S = K_S \times W_S \tag{2}$$

where K_S is the response factor of the detector to the internal standard S. Combining eqns (1) and (2),

$$\frac{h_A}{h_S} = \frac{K_A}{K_S} \times \frac{W_A}{W_S} \tag{3}$$

$$\frac{K_A}{K_S} = \frac{h_A}{h_S} \times \frac{W_S}{W_A} \tag{4}$$

where K_A/K_S is the relative response factor. To the sample solution containing an unknown concentration (W'_A) of analyte (A) is added a known concentration (W'_S) of the internal standard (S). Let the peaks for A and S in the resultant chromatogram have peak heights of h'_A and h'_S, respectively. Then

$$\frac{h'_A}{h'_S} = \frac{K_A}{K_S} \times \frac{W'_A}{W'_S} \tag{5}$$

Substituting the relative response factor K_A/K_S from eqn (4),

$$\frac{h'_A}{h'_S} = \frac{h_A}{h_S} \times \frac{W_S}{W_A} \times \frac{W'_A}{W'_S} \tag{6}$$

$$W'_A = \frac{h_S}{h_A} \times \frac{W_A}{W_S} \times \frac{W'_S \times h'_A}{h'_S} \tag{7}$$

$$W_S = W'_S$$

where the same amount of S is added to the sample and to the standard solution, thus these values cancel out.

The internal standardization equation then becomes:

$$\text{Conc. A in sample} = \frac{\text{Peak size S in standard}}{\text{Peak size A in standard}}$$

$$\times \frac{\text{Peak size A in sample}}{\text{Peak size S in sample}} \times \text{Conc. A in standard}$$

The above procedure is applicable for peak areas as well as for peak heights.

The inherent errors of the internal standardization procedure will be minimized if the analyte and internal standard yield peaks of similar size, since errors in measuring peaks of about the same size will tend to cancel out. The effect of changing the peak size ratios can be ascertained by chromatographing a series of standard solutions containing different concentrations of analyte and a fixed concentration of internal standard. A calibration plot is then constructed in which the analyte to internal standard peak height (or peak area) ratios are plotted against the concentration of analyte, i.e.

$$\frac{h_A}{h_S} \text{ versus } W_A.$$

A linear calibration plot which intercepts the origin is evidence that the relative response factor is constant at all concentration ratios of internal standard and analyte over the concentration range of analyte to be used.

7.2 VITAMIN ASSAYS BY GLC

7.2.1 Vitamin A and the Carotenoids

Retinol and its acetate and palmitate esters undergo thermal decomposition on conventional GLC columns to produce multiple tailing peaks that are attributable to the formation of anhydroretinol (Sheppard *et al.*, 1972). Vecchi *et al.* (1973) established that anhydroretinol could not be determined quantitatively by GLC as it undergoes isomerization on the column. The thermal decomposition of vitamin A is due to the lability of the conjugated system of double bonds in the polyene side chain. Evidence for this is the stability of the saturated form of vitamin A (perhydrovitamin A) toward GLC. If retinol or retinyl acetate are converted to their respective perhydro forms by catalytic hydrogenation with hydrogen gas and platinum dioxide prior to GLC, two distinct and well separated peaks of similar area are

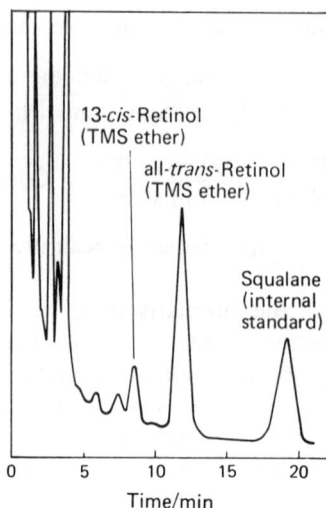

Fig. 25. GLC of TMS ethers of vitamin A (13-*cis*- and all-*trans*-retinol) obtained from a multivitamin tablet. Column packing, 1% SE-30 on Gas Chrom Q; glass column, 2 m × 4 mm i.d.; oven temp., 175°C; FID (from Wiggins, 1976).

obtained. Gas chromatography–mass spectrometry (GC–MS) has confirmed that one peak is the saturated alcohol or ester form of vitamin A, while the other peak is the saturated hydrocarbon, i.e. perhydroretinol, but with a hydrogen atom replacing the alcohol group. This technique, reported by Fenton *et al.* (1973), has been suggested as a possible method of determining vitamin A.

Retinyl ethers are more stable thermally than retinol or retinyl esters. All-*trans*-retinol and 13-*cis*-retinol have been completely separated as their trimethylsilyl (TMS) ethers using a GLC stationary phase of SE-30 (Fig. 25). The separation of the 9-*cis*- and 13-*cis*-retinol isomers as their TMS ethers could not be achieved, whilst 11-*cis* and 11.13-di-*cis* isomers partially rearranged into each other. In order to prepare a retinyl ether from a retinyl ester it is necessary to saponify beforehand, or to quantitatively convert the ester to the alcohol (i.e. retinol) by reduction with lithium aluminium hydride (Vecchi *et al.*, 1973).

As vitamin A can be assayed more easily by other means, such as HPLC, GLC has not been utilized for such assays in food analysis.

Carotenoids undergo cracking and polymerization at the temperatures necessary to achieve sufficient volatilization in the gas chromatograph (De Ritter & Purcell, 1981). Catalytic hydrogenation of carotenoids to their

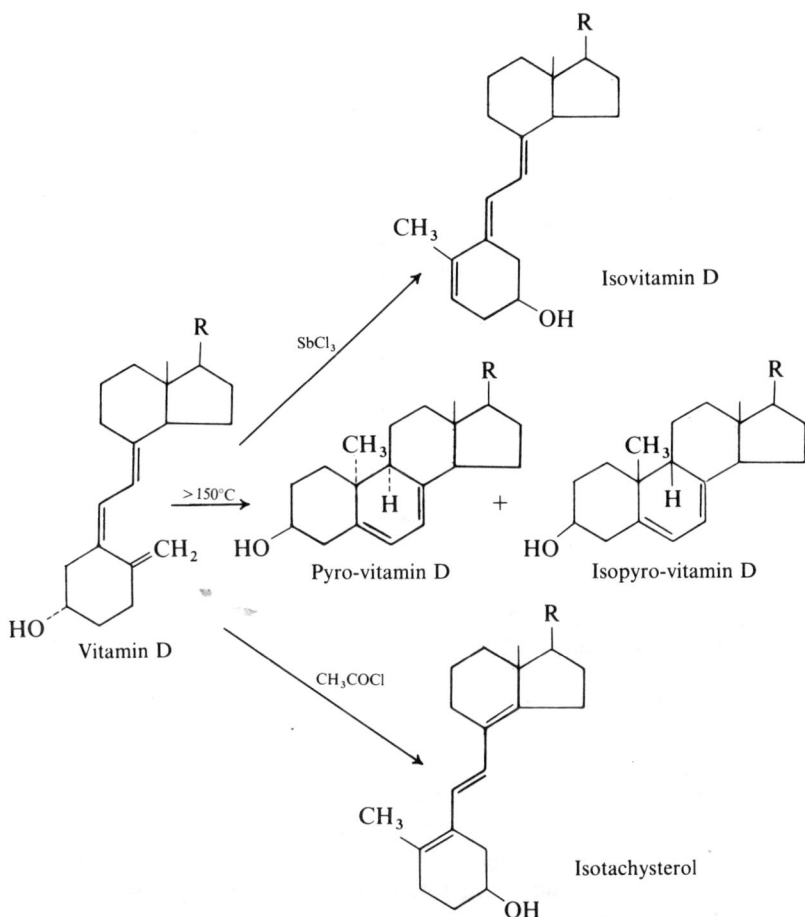

Fig. 26. GLC on-column thermal cyclization of vitamin D to pyro- and isopyro-vitamin D; and chemical conversion of vitamin D to isovitamin D and isotachysterol D with antimony trichloride (SbCl₃) reagent and acetyl chloride (CH₃COCl) (reprinted from Koshy, 1982 p. 106, by courtesy of Marcel Dekker, Inc.

stable perhydro forms has been employed in GC–MS analysis of carotenoids for the purposes of identification (Taylor & Ikawa, 1980).

7.2.2 Vitamin D

The possibility of applying GLC to the determination of vitamin D was first investigated by Ziffer *et al.* (1960), and later applied to the assay of rat liver by Nair *et al.* (1965).

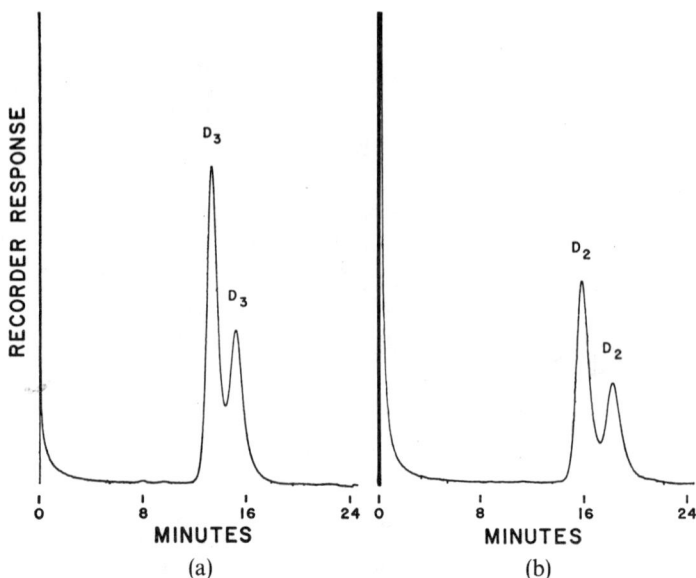

Fig. 27. GLC of vitamins D_3 (a) and D_2 (b) illustrating the pyro and isopyro thermal cyclization products. The pyro peak is the larger of each pair. Column packing, $3 \cdot 8\%$ SE-30 on Diatoport S; glass column 4 ft $\times$ 3/16 in o.d.; oven temp., $215°C$; sample size 25 ng each of vitamins D_3 and D_2; FID (from Avioli & Lee, 1966).

Vitamins D_2 and D_3 are converted at temperatures greater than about $150°C$ to the so-called pyro and isopyro isomers (Fig. 26), which appear as twin peaks in the chromatogram (Fig. 27). For each D vitamin the pyro peak is eluted earlier, and is larger, than the isopyro peak. If both vitamins D_2 and D_3 are present only three of the four peaks are usually resolved; isopyro-D_3 and pyro-D_2 display similar retention times. The pyro and isopyro isomers of vitamins D_2 and D_3 are resolved from their respective provitamins (ergosterol and 7-dehydrocholesterol), but not from cholesterol. The thermal reaction involves ring closure, which proceeds quantitatively to give a constant 2:1 peak area ratio of pyro- to isopyro-vitamin D for both D_2 and D_3. The 2:1 ratio remains constant, irrespective of sample size and GC operating temperature (Nair *et al.*, 1965), hence the area of the larger peak can be quantitatively related to the parent vitamin D.

GLC is applicable to the determination of vitamin D in foods after the removal of cholesterol and other interfering substances by appropriate purification techniques. The hydroxyl group in the 3β position confers upon vitamin D a slightly polar character, which causes some adsorptive loss of the vitamin and peak broadening during gas chromatography (De Leenheer & Cruyl, 1980). The formation of the less polar TMS ether derivatives of vitamins D_2 or D_3 overcomes these effects, but does not prevent the formation of the pyro and isopyro isomers. The gas chromatographic behaviour of the TMS ethers of vitamins D_2 and D_3 on OV-17 is illustrated in Fig. 28. The TMS derivatives of vitamin D are unstable, even under refrigeration, hence quantitative analysis is valid only if the interval between derivatization and injection is standardized (Fisher *et al.*, 1972).

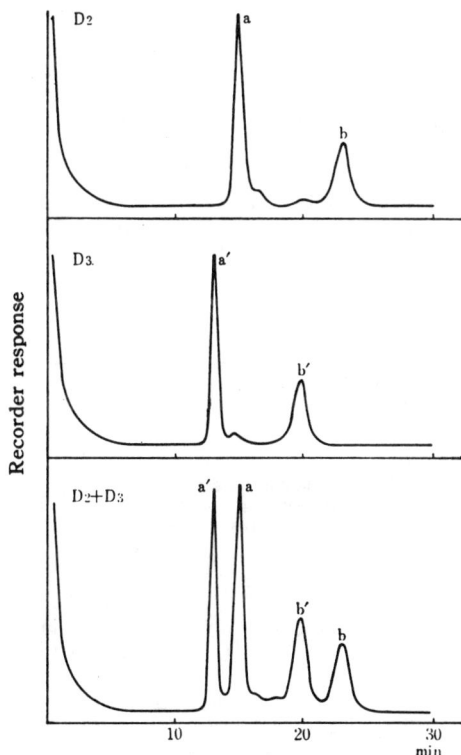

Fig. 28. GLC of TMS ethers of vitamins D_2 and D_3 illustrating the derivatized pyro and isopyro thermal cyclization products. Peaks: (a') pyro-D_3; (a) pyro-D_2; (b') isopyro-D_3; (b) isopyro-D_2. Column packing, 1·5% OV-17 on Shimalite W; glass column, 1 m × 4 mm i.d.; oven temp., 240°C; FID (from Tsukida & Saiki, 1970).

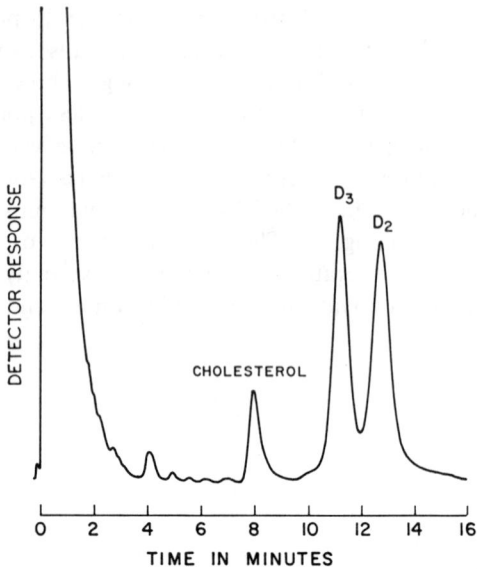

Fig. 29. GLC of isovitamins D_2 and D_3, illustrating their separation from cholesterol. Column packing, 3% OV-1 on Gas Chrom Q; glass column, 4 ft × 1/8 in i.d.; oven temp., 220°C; FID (from Murray *et al.*, 1968).

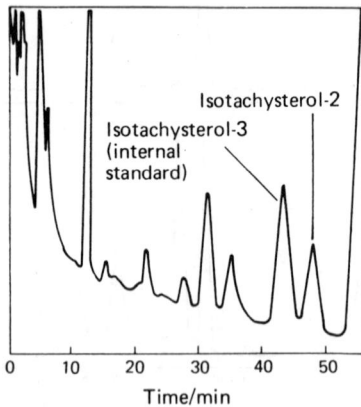

Fig. 30. GLC of isotachysterol derivatives of vitamins D_2 and D_3 obtained from the purified unsaponifiable material of margarine. Column packing, 3% OV-17 on Gas Chrom Q; glass column, 2 m × 4 mm i.d.; oven temp., 235°C; sample size, 100 ng; FID (from Wiggins, 1976).

The formation of the pyro- and isopyro-vitamin D isomers during GLC can be avoided by isomerizing the parent vitamin D_2 or D_3 to its corresponding isovitamin or isotachysterol. Isovitamin D_2 or isovitamin D_3 is formed by reacting the parent vitamin with antimony trichloride reagent (Murray *et al.*, 1966), whilst isotachysterol D_2 or isotachysterol D_3 is formed by reaction with acetyl chloride (Kobayashi, 1965, 1967; Sheppard *et al.*, 1968) (Fig. 26). Isovitamins D_2 and D_3 produce single peaks in the chromatogram that are well separated from each other and from cholesterol (Fig. 29). The separation of isotachysterol D_2 from isotachysterol D_3 is shown in Fig. 30. Conversion of vitamin D to the isotachysterol, rather than to isovitamin D, appears to be the better choice because the former is a more stable isomer (Koshy, 1982).

When vitamin D is determined by GLC it is the potential vitamin D (i.e. the sum of vitamin D and previtamin D) that is measured, as the previtamins are thermally cyclized to the pyro and isopyro isomers or, if reacted with Lewis acids, are isomerized to the isovitamins D or to the isotachysterols (Wiggins, 1976).

The chromatography of the isovitamins D or the isotachysterols is improved if they are converted to their TMS ethers (Jones *et al.*, 1985). Bell & Christie (1974) found the slightly polar OV-17 to be a suitable stationary phase for the chromatography of isovitamin D–TMS ethers (Fig. 31).

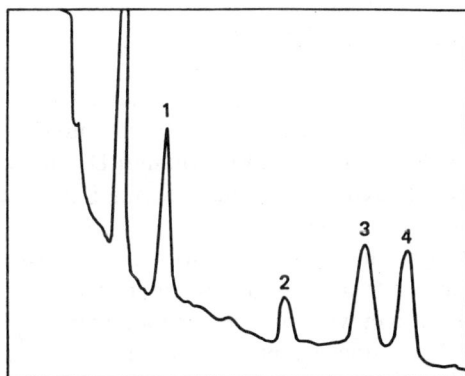

Fig. 31. GLC of TMS ethers of isovitamins D_2 and D_3 obtained from the purified unsaponifiable material of vitamin D_2-fortified full cream dried-milk. Peaks: (1) 5α-cholestane (added as a marker); (2) cholesterol TMS ether; (3) isovitamin D_3 TMS ether (internal standard); (4) isovitamin D_2 TMS ether. Column packing, 3% OV-17 on Gas Chrom Q; glass column, 2·1 m × 3 mm i.d.; oven temp., 235°C; FID (from Bell & Christie, 1974).

As the occurrence of both vitamins D_2 and D_3 in the same sample of food is uncommon, and both compounds remain together in every step preceding GLC, vitamin D_2 can be added as an internal standard at the start of the analysis to account for losses of vitamin D_3 throughout the procedure. Similarly, vitamin D_3 can act as an internal standard in the determination of vitamin D_2. Bell & Christie (1974) showed that this technique is valid for the TMS ethers of isovitamins D_2 and D_3 provided that a correction is made for the slightly different detector response factors for the two vitamin D derivatives. If both vitamins D_2 and D_3 are present in the sample, dihydrotachysterol can be added as an internal standard at the gas chromatographic stage of the analysis. This compound yields a single peak that is well separated from the pyro and isopyro isomers of vitamins D_2 or D_3 and from their corresponding TMS ethers, as well as from isotachysterol derivatives of vitamins D_2 and D_3 and heptafluorobutyrate esters of isotachysterols D_2 and D_3.

The flame ionization detector (FID) has sufficient sensitivity to determine vitamin D in most fortified foods, and those unfortified foods (e.g. fatty fish, dried eggs) that contain relatively large quantities of vitamin D. The sensitivity can be increased by replacing the FID with an electron capture detector (ECD) and preparing an electron-capturing derivative of isotachysterol, such as the heptafluorobutyrate ester (Wilson et al., 1969). Suitable stationary phases for such applications have included 3% OV-17 (Osborne & Voogt, 1978) and 1% FFAP (De Leenheer & Cruyl, 1980). The ECD is capable of reliably determining vitamin D at the $0.1\,\mu g/g$ level in certain foods, such as butter.

In most food samples the vitamin D coexists with relatively large amounts of vitamins A and E, cholesterol, provitamin D and other sterols, which interfere with the GLC assay of vitamin D. The removal of these substances can be achieved by digitonin precipitation of the sterols and/or some form of column chromatography.

Panalaks (1970) used an OV-1 column with an FID to determine vitamin D in fortified non-fat dried milk. Sample preparation involved precipitation of the milk protein with acetone/ethanol, and extraction of the fat with chloroform. The extract was purified on a multi-bore silica gel column, followed by conversion of the vitamin D to isovitamin D, and further purification on two silica micro-columns before GLC analysis. The procedure was as follows.

To a sample of non-fat dried milk, estimated to contain 10–$20\,\mu g$ of vitamin D_2, was added an equal amount of standard vitamin D_3 (or D_2 if the sample contained vitamin D_3). The sample was diluted with water, and an acetone:ethanol mixture (1:1) was used to precipitate the milk protein in the presence of ascorbic acid. The solution, after concentration by rotary evaporation, was extracted with chloroform containing a second antioxidant. The chloroform extract was evaporated to dryness, and the residue was dissolved in hexane for purification by multi-bore silica gel chromatography, using a diethyl ether:petroleum spirit gradient elution programme. The fractions containing the vitamin D were combined, then evaporated to dryness. The residue was treated with antimony trichloride in chloroform to convert the vitamin D to isovitamin D. The reaction was stopped by the addition of tartaric acid, and the reaction mixture was extracted with petroleum spirit. The petroleum extract was successively washed with water, dried, evaporated under nitrogen to 0.5 ml, then applied to a micro-column system consisting of two silica gel-filled Pasteur pipettes clamped one above the other. The micro-columns were eluted with 3.5 ml of chloroform and the first 1.5 ml of eluate was discarded. The next 2.0 ml of eluate was collected, then evaporated under nitrogen to about 0.5 ml and rechromatographed on a pair of newly prepared two-stage micro-columns as before. The 2.0 ml of eluate was evaporated to dryness and the residue was dissolved in 0.1 ml of hexane. A $5\,\mu l$ aliquot of the hexane solution was injected onto a 1.8 m $\times$ 5 mm i.d. GLC column of 3% OV-1 on Gas Chrom Q, and chromatographed with temperature programming. Isovitamins D_2 and D_3 were eluted about 30 min after injection (Fig. 32). An average recovery of 104% of vitamin D_2 was obtained relative to the internal standard (vitamin D_3).

Bell & Christie (1974) used an OV-17 column with FID to determine vitamin D in fortified full cream dried milk. The fat was extracted with ethanol containing a surface-active agent, then saponified. The unsaponifiable extract was purified on a dry column of alumina to yield a fraction containing vitamin D, vitamin A, cholesterol, and other sterols. The fraction was treated with antimony trichloride to convert vitamin D to isovitamin D, and then purified on a second dry column of alumina to remove the sterols and vitamin A. The final extract was treated directly with the silylating reagent for determination of the isovitamin D–TMS ether by GLC. The procedure was as follows.

A sample (at least 100 g) of full cream dried milk was diluted with hot water and mixed to form a creamy paste. The paste was treated with a mixture of ethanol, sodium hexametaphosphate and a surface-active agent (Triton X-100), then extracted with diethyl ether:petroleum spirit (1:1). The organic extract was washed with water, then evaporated to dryness under vacuum before saponification in the presence of vitamin D_3 as the internal

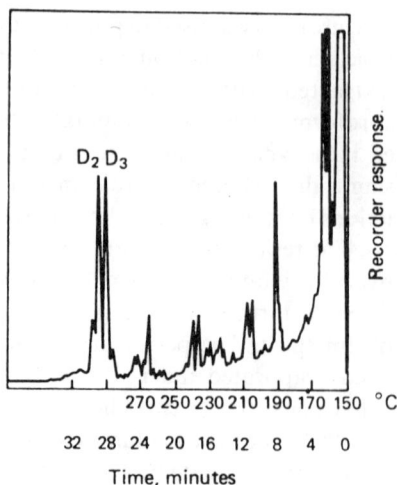

Fig. 32. GLC of isovitamins D_2 and D_3 obtained from a purified lipid extract of vitamin D-fortified non-fat dried milk. Column packing, 3% OV-1 on Gas Chrom Q; glass column, $1·8 \text{ m} \times 5 \text{ mm i.d.}$; oven temp. programme, 150–270°C at 5°C/min then held at 270°C for 15 min; FID (from Panalaks, 1970).

standard. The unsaponifiable fraction was extracted with diethyl ether: petroleum spirit (1:1), and the ether extract was washed with water, then evaporated to dryness. The residue was dissolved in 2 ml of chloroform and adsorbed onto 2 g of deactivated alumina containing a yellow dye; this was done by removing the chloroform on a rotary evaporator. The dried alumina was then poured onto a prepared alumina column (40 cm × 1 cm i.d.), and the column was eluted with chloroform. A fraction containing vitamin D, vitamin A, and sterols was collected, using the band of yellow dye as a marker, and the fraction was evaporated to dryness. The residue was dissolved in 1 ml of chloroform, and treated with antimony trichloride reagent to convert the vitamin D to isovitamin D. The reaction was stopped by the addition of tartaric acid, and the solution was extracted with petroleum spirit. The petroleum layer was washed with water then evaporated to dryness. The residue was dissolved in 2 ml of chloroform, and repurified on a second similar dry column of alumina to remove the vitamin A (as its anhydro derivative) and the sterols. The vitamin D fraction was evaporated to dryness, and the residue was extracted with petroleum spirit, and re-evaporated to dryness in a stream of nitrogen using a dry-block heater set at 50°C. The residue was treated with silylating agent, and the TMS ethers of isovitamin D were subjected to GLC on a $2·1 \text{ m} \times 3 \text{ mm}$

i.d. column packed with 3% OV-17 on Gas Chrom Q (Fig. 31). A recovery factor of 97% of vitamin D_2 was obtained relative to the internal standard (vitamin D_3). Losses of both vitamins were 20–30% when taken through the entire process. The GLC conditions employed were capable of determining $<0.1\,\mu g$ of vitamin D (Bell & Christie, 1973). The above procedure has also been applied to the determination of vitamin D_3 in fatty fish, freeze-dried eggs and margarine (Wiggins, 1978). For the determination of vitamin D in margarine and butter it was found to be necessary to employ preparative TLC on silica gel to further purify the extract after open-column chromatography (Christie, 1975).

7.2.3 Vitamin E

GLC has been more successfully applied to vitamin E in food analysis than it has to vitamins A and D. A review of the early GLC applications for vitamin E analysis has been compiled by Sheppard et al. (1972).

Wilson et al. (1962) established the separation of the four tocopherols and two of the tocotrienols (α- and β-) on packed columns of Celite coated with a stationary phase of SE-30. The unesterified E vitamers were eluted in the following order, with their retention times relative to tocol in parentheses: δ-T (1·13), β-T (1·42), γ-T (1·45), α-T (1·79), β-T3 (1·81) and α-T3 (2·33). The tocopherols and tocotrienols were therefore eluted in accordance with their mono-, di- and trimethyl substitution; the β- and γ-dimethyl tocols were inseparable. α-Tocopheryl acetate was separable between α-tocopherol and α-tocotrienol, but β-tocotrienol coeluted with α-tocopherol. A typical chromatogram of the tocopherols and tocotrienols on a packed column is depicted in Fig. 33. Hall & Laidman (1968) fractionated the unsaponifiable matter of wheat grain and seedlings on an open column of alumina eluted with a petroleum spirit/diethyl ether gradient. Three fractions containing the tri-, di- and monomethyl forms of vitamin E were then individually chromatographed on an SE-30 column to separate the tri-, di- and monomethyl tocopherols from their corresponding tocotrienols. Nair et al. (1966) succeeded in separating the isomeric β- and γ-dimethyl tocols on an SE-52/XE-60 biphase column, after oxidation of the tocopherols to their corresponding para-quinones on a micro-scale using the Emmerie–Engel ferric chloride/2,2'-bipyridyl reagent. The biphase column was also capable of separating α-tocopherol from its oxidation product, α-tocopherylquinone (Nair & Turner, 1963).

In setting up an assay for vitamin E in foods by GLC using packed columns it is usually necessary to purify the sample extract to remove interfering sterols. Cholesterol constitutes the greatest problem as it elutes

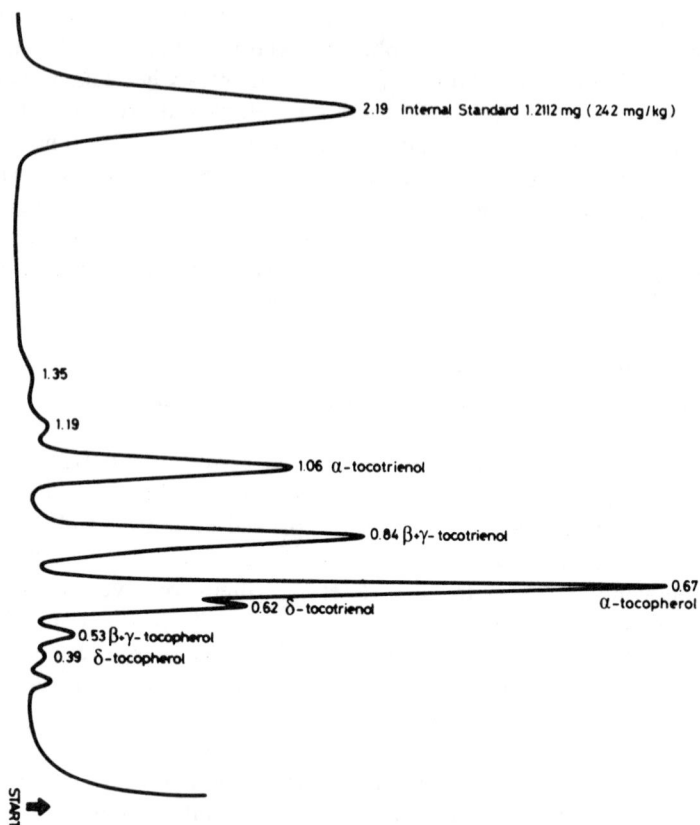

Fig. 33. GLC of E vitamers obtained from the purified unsaponifiable matter of palm oil. (Internal standard = hexadecyl stearate.) Column packing, 2% Silicon oil MS 550/HP on Chromosorb W AW-DMCS; glass column, 1 m × 4 mm i.d.; oven temp., 235°C; FID (from Meijboom & Jongenotter, 1979).

close to α-tocopherol, and packed columns usually lack sufficient resolving power to separate α-tocopherol from an excess of cholesterol (Nelis *et al.*, 1985). The plant sterols campesterol, stigmasterol and β-sitosterol are eluted individually after α-tocopherol (Fig. 34) and, if present, would prevent the estimation of α-tocopheryl acetate and the tocotrienols (Nelson & Milun, 1968). TLC has been used to separate the tocopherols and tocotrienols from the sterols in the unsaponifiable fraction of palm oil. The whole vitamin E band was removed from the TLC plate and subjected to GLC, using hexadecyl stearate as an internal standard (Meijboom &

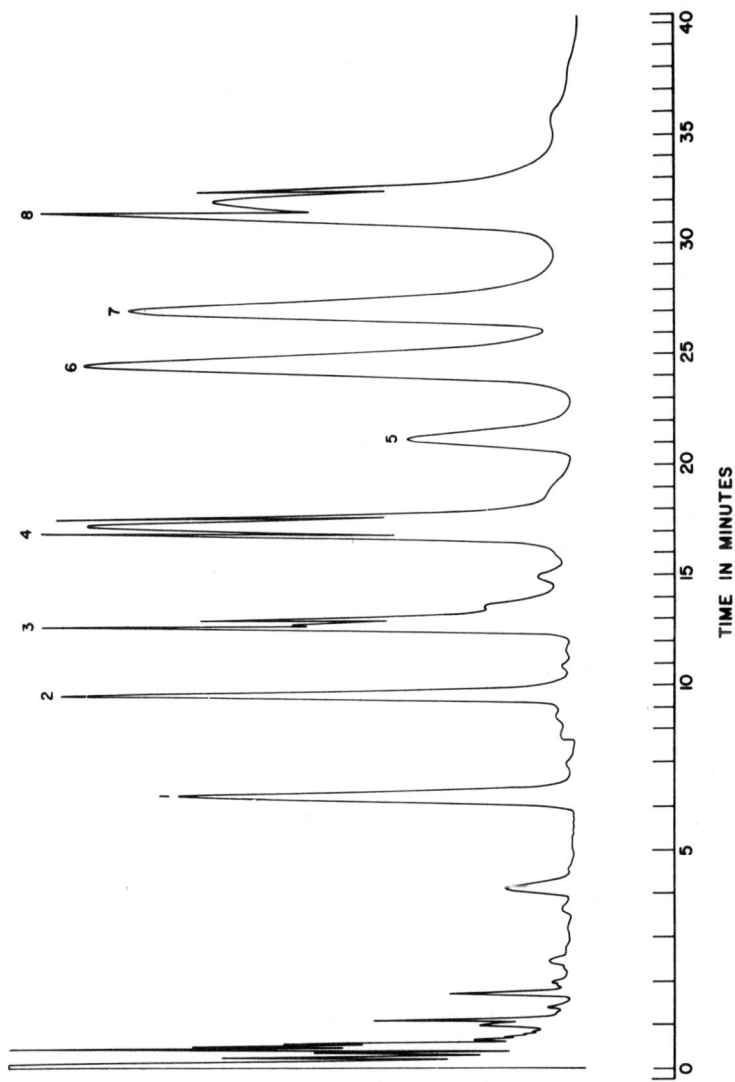

Fig. 34. GLC of E vitamers and plant sterols obtained from the unsaponifiable matter of soy sludge. Peaks: (1) squalene; (2) squalane; (3) δ-tocopherol; (4) $\beta + \gamma$-tocopherol; (5) α-tocopherol; (6) campesterol; (7) stigmasterol; (8) β-sitosterol. Column packing, SE-30 on Gas Chrom Q; glass column, 1·8 m × 3·5 mm i.d.; oven temp., 225°C; FID (from Nelson & Milun, 1968).

Jongenotter, 1979) (Fig. 33). Vitamin A and carotenoids pose no problem as they are eluted rapidly with the solvent; vitamin K is no problem either, as it is eluted much later than the tocopherols (Bunnell, 1967).

Sheppard et al (1971) extracted foods with ethanol containing pyrogallol in a Soxhlet apparatus for 4 h. The ethanol extract was diluted with an equal volume of water, then extracted with hexane in a separating funnel. The hexane extract was reduced in volume under a stream of nitrogen, then purified on an open column of Celite–digitonin to remove sterols, prior to GLC on an SE-30 column. This technique does not involve saponification and therefore permits the estimation of supplemental α-tocopheryl acetate. Cholestane, which is eluted before δ-tocopherol on SE-30 columns, has been used as an internal standard in the GLC of tocopherols (Bunnell, 1967).

Derivatization of the E vitamers to their TMS ethers contributes to reducing retention times and analysis temperatures, whilst also improving peak shape and selectivity (Nelis et al., 1985). The quantitative conversion of the tocopherols to the corresponding silyl derivatives can be confirmed by the absence of the characteristic hydroxy band at $2.7\,\mu m$ in the infrared spectrum (Nair & Machiz, 1967). Slover et al. (1969a) reported that SE-30 is capable of separating the TMS ethers in order of δ-, $\beta + \gamma$-, α-tocopherols and α-tocotrienol. β- and γ-tocotrienols are eluted together between β/γ-tocopherols and α-tocopherol, whilst δ-tocotrienol coelutes with β/γ-tocopherols. Apiezon L high vacuum grease yields a partial separation of β- and γ-tocopherols and permits their individual estimation, provided that the amount of one isomer does not greatly exceed that of the other. The separations obtained with 2% SE-30 and 0.5% Apiezon L stationary phases permitted all four tocopherols, plus α- and β-tocotrienols, to be estimated as their TMS ethers in seeds, fats and oils (Slover et al., 1969a), and in wheat, wheat flour and wheat baked products (Slover et al., 1969b), using didecyl pimelate as an internal standard. The interfering sterols were removed by TLC purification of the unsaponifiable matter. Govind Rao & Perkins (1972) used GC–MS with an SE-30 column to estimate and identify TMS derivatives of tocopherols and tocotrienols in the unsaponifiable fraction of vegetable oils. Preparative two-dimensional TLC of the unsaponifiable matter was employed to isolate the E vitamers in those oils which contained the difficult positional isomers, β- and γ-tocopherol. The combined technique permitted the estimation of seven out of the eight vitamers; the presence or absence of δ-tocotrienol could not be determined as an authentic standard was not available.

Nelson et al. (1970) converted the tocopherols and the plant sterols in soya sludges and residues to their butyrate esters prior to GLC on an SE-30 column with cholesteryl isovalerate as an internal standard. This method was also utilized by Hartman (1977) to determine α-, $\beta + \gamma$- and δ-tocopherols in vegetable oils, but the presence of the plant sterol derivatives in the chromatogram prevented the estimation of the tocotrienols.

Christie *et al.* (1973) used a packed column containing OV-1 as a stationary phase on Gas Chrom Q support to separate the TMS ethers of α-, $\beta + \gamma$- and δ-tocopherols after saponification and removal of the sterols by digitonin precipitation. The internal standard, α-tocopheryl propionate, was satisfactory for the estimation of the tocopherols in the foods studied, but would probably have interfered with the chromatography of α-tocotrienol had this vitamer been present. The procedure was as follows.

Food samples (2–5 g) containing 100–200 μg of tocopherol were saponified in the presence of ascorbic acid as antioxidant, and in an atmosphere of nitrogen. The unsaponifiable matter was extracted with diethyl ether, and the ether extracts were washed with water, then evaporated to dryness under vacuum. The residue was dissolved in 1–2 ml of cyclohexane, and applied to a 250 mm × 10 mm i.d. column of neutral, deactivated alumina. The column was washed with cyclohexane, followed by a 7% solution of diethyl ether in cyclohexane to elute the tocopherols. The eluate was evaporated to dryness and dissolved in ethanol. A standard solution of α-tocopheryl propionate (internal standard) was evaporated to dryness, and an aliquot of the ethanolic extract was added to it. The solution was diluted with water, allowed to stand at about $-15°C$ for 1 h, then centrifuged. The supernatant was added to an ethanolic solution of digitonin, and the digitonides were allowed to precipitate by leaving the solution at about $-15°C$ overnight. The liquid was filtered, extracted with carbon tetrachloride, then evaporated to dryness. The residue was dissolved in 0·5 ml of hexane, and applied to a 120 mm × 10 mm i.d. Celite–digitonin column. The vitamin E fraction was eluted with hexane. The hexane eluate was evaporated to dryness, and the residue was dissolved in cyclohexane, then silylated. The TMS ethers of α-, $\beta + \gamma$-, and δ-tocopherols were separated on a 2·7 m × 4 mm i.d. GLC column packed with 3% OV-1 on Gas Chrom Q. The recoveries of α-tocopherol added to various food samples before saponification ranged from 90 to 98%, depending upon the type of food analysed. The method was reported to be largely unaffected by the carotenoids, and by synthetic antioxidants, such as BHA and BHT.

Erickson *et al.* (1973) used a 2% OV-17 packed column to separate the TMS ethers of α-, $\beta + \gamma$- and δ-tocopherols. The unsaponifiable fraction of cocoa lipids was purified by preparative TLC, and the internal standard, β-

sitosterol, was added prior to derivatization. δ-Tocopherol was absent in the cocoa extracts, and GLC did not suggest the presence of tocotrienols.

Gas chromatography using open-tubular capillary columns was employed for the quantitative determination of the tocopherols and the major phytosterols in the unsaponifiable matter obtained from fats, oils and margarines of vegetable origin (Slover *et al.*, 1983). A synthetic tocopherol that does not occur in nature, 5,7-dimethyltocol, was added to the sample as an internal standard prior to saponification. The TMS ether derivatives of the tocopherols and sterols were chromatographed at about 260°C on a 50 m × 0·25 mm glass capillary column coated with Dexsil 400. This stationary phase permitted the adequate separation of α-tocopherol from cholesterol. A chromatogram of soy bean oil unsaponifiables (Fig. 35) revealed the separation of δ-, γ- and α-tocopherols; a small β-tocopherol peak preceded γ-tocopherol and was partially separated from it. The major sterols (campesterol, stigmasterol and β-sitosterol) were eluted after the tocopherols. In later work, the Dexsil 400 glass capillary column was

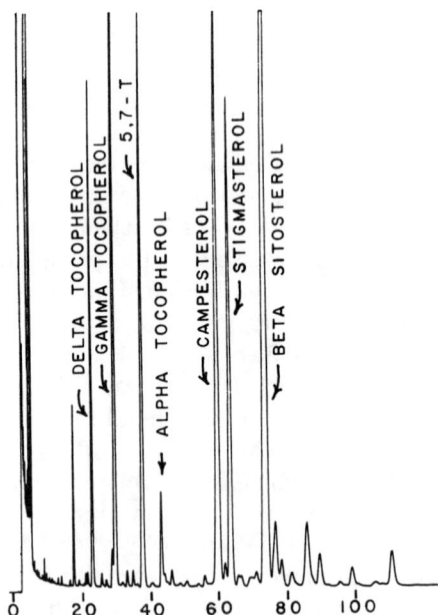

Fig. 35. GLC of TMS ethers of tocopherols and phytosterols obtained from the unsaponifiable material of soy bean oil. Glass capillary column, 50 m × 0·25 mm i.d.; stationary phase, Dexsil 400; oven temp., 260°C; FID (from Slover, 1980).

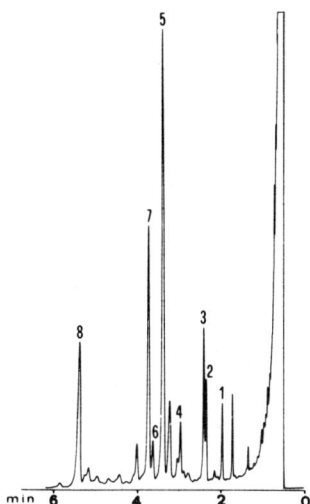

Fig. 36. GLC of TMS ethers of E vitamers obtained from palm oil unsaponifiables after removal of the sterols by TLC. Peaks: (1) δ-T; (2) β-T; (3) γ-T; (4) δ-T3; (5) α-T; (6) β-T3; (7) γ-T3; (8) α-T3. (T = tocopherol: T3 = tocotrienol). Glass capillary column, 15 m × 0·25 mm i.d.; stationary phase, OV-17; oven temp., 240°C; FID (from Lercker & Caboni, 1985).

replaced by a 12 m fused silica capillary column coated with SP 1200 (Slover *et al.*, 1985).

The separation of the eight naturally occurring tocopherols and tocotrienols as their TMS ethers on an OV-17 glass capillary column has been demonstrated (Mordret & Laurent, 1978; Lercker & Caboni, 1985). The E vitamers naturally present in palm oil, after TLC fractionation of the unsaponifiable material to remove the sterols and other interfering compounds, are depicted in Fig. 36; all eight vitamers may be detected. Substitution of OV-17 by SE-30 resulted in the overlapping of γ-tocopherol and δ-tocotrienol (Mordret & Laurent, 1978).

7.2.4 Vitamin K

Phylloquinone (vitamin K_1) and the vitamin K_2 menaquinones (MK-n) exhibit low volatilities, and elute well after the other fat-soluble vitamins in most GLC systems. This results in very long retention times and poor detectabilities. On-column thermal degradation of vitamins K_1 and K_2 to their respective chromenol and chromanol isomers has been reported (Fig. 37), although some authors have attributed the presence of these

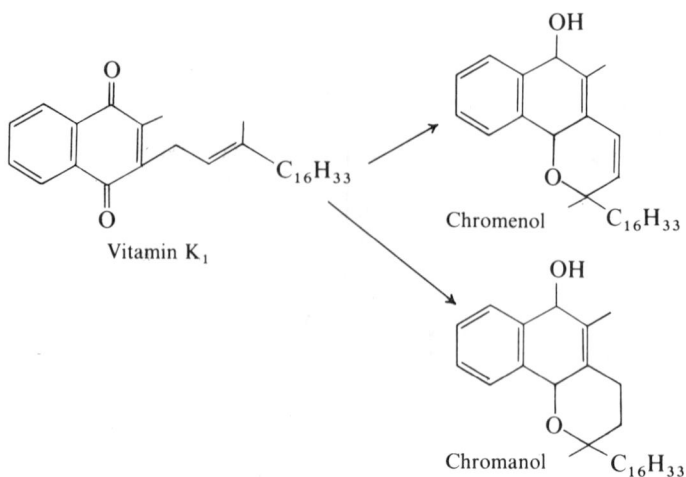

Fig. 37. GLC on-column thermal degradation of vitamin K_1 into its chromenol and chromanol isomers (reprinted from Lefevere *et al.*, 1985, p. 223 by courtesy of Marcel Dekker Inc.).

degradation products in the chromatogram to photodegradation of the original sample (Lefevere *et al.*, 1985).

The majority of gas chromatographic applications have dealt with the separation and quantification of standard mixtures of phylloquinone and the menaquinones; few applications for determining these compounds in biological matrices have been reported. Most GLC determinations have been performed without derivatization using packed columns containing non-polar stationary phases, such as SE-30, Apiezon L or OV-1. Such columns afford a good separation between K_1, K_1-epoxide and low molecular weight menaquinones (MK-1 to MK-7) in the presence of vitamin E. Vitamin K_1, with a predominantly saturated side chain, is eluted well before the menaquinones, which have unsaturated side chains. For menaquinones (MK-n), a linear relationship exists between the number of isoprene units and the log of the retention time. Chromatography on OV-1 separates K_1 from its photodegradation products. To avoid very long retention times, some authors have used columns with low liquid phase loadings (1–2%) and/or high column temperatures (295°C). However, the use of low liquid phase loadings, together with 'bleeding' of the stationary phase at high column temperatures, increases the risk of column deterioration and the formation of artefacts (Lefevere *et al.*, 1985).

Vitamin K_1 and its epoxide metabolite have been determined in blood plasma using the ECD (Bechthold & Jähnchen, 1979), but the FID has been employed in most of the published applications.

Derivatization procedures have been described which overcome the problems of thermolability, whilst improving chromatographic resolution. Conversion of vitamins K_1 and K_2 to their respective dihydroquinones by catalytic reduction with hydrogen gas, and subsequent formation of the

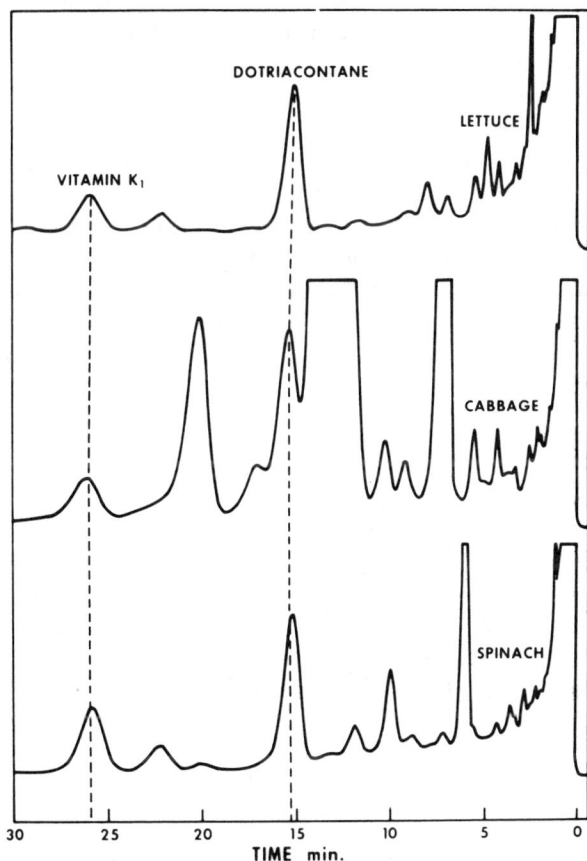

Fig. 38. GLC of vitamin K_1 obtained from the purified lipid extract of lettuce, cabbage and spinach. Dotriacontane is the internal standard. Column packing, 2·5% Dexsil 300 on Chromosorb G AW-DMCS; glass column, 2·1 m × 2 mm i.d.; oven temp., 290°C; FID (Reprinted with permission from Seifert, R. M. (1979). Analysis of vitamin K_1 in some green leafy vegetables by gas chromatography. *J. Agric. Fd Chem.*, **27**, 1301–4). Copyright (1979) American Chemical Society.

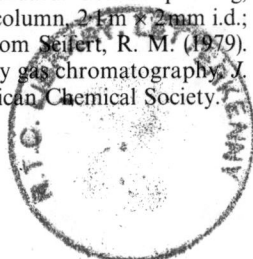

TMS derivatives of the dihydroquinones, afforded the separation of *cis*-
and *trans*-vitamin K_1, as well as vitamin K_2 up to MK-9 (Vetter *et al.*, 1967).
However, TMS–dihydrovitamins K_1 and K_2 are highly susceptible to
hydrolysis and reversion to the original quinones (Dialameh & Olson,
1969). Dihydromethyl esters of vitamin K were found to be more stable
than the TMS ethers (Vecchi *et al.*, 1981). In the opinion of Lefevere *et al.*
(1985), derivatization should not be performed unless it has clearly been
proven to be profitable under the given analytical conditions.

A food chemistry application of GLC was described by Seifert (1979) for
the determination of vitamin K_1 in green leafy vegetables. The leaves were
freeze-dried, extracted with hexane in a Soxhlet extractor, and concentrated by rotary evaporation at 40°C. An aliquot of the concentrated
extract was purified by liquid column chromatography on neutral alumina,
and dotriacontane was added to the concentrated eluate as an internal
standard before injection onto a 2·1 m × 2 mm i.d. Dexsil 300 GLC column
at 290°C. The retention time of vitamin K_1 was approximately 25 min
(Fig. 38), but it took 45 min to elute all peaks. Recovery of standard vitamin
K_1 added to spinach averaged 92%. A fairly high RSD (10·5%) was
obtained for foods containing $0·76 \pm 0·08$ mg of vitamin K_1 per 100 g.

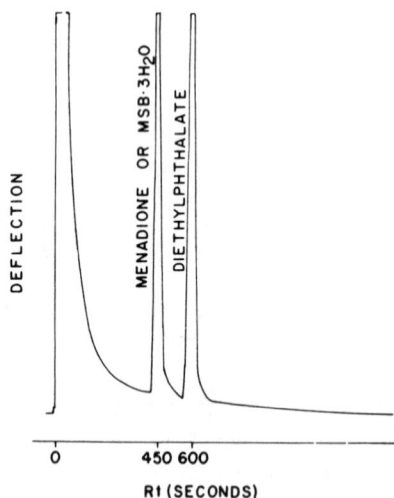

Fig. 39.   GLC of menadione or menadione sodium bisulphite in the methanol
extract of feed premixes using on-column pyrolysis. The diethylphthalate is present
as an internal standard. Column packing, 2% OV-17 on Chromosorb W; glass
column, 6 ft × 1/8 in i.d.; oven temp., 140°C; FID (from Winkler & Yoder, 1972).

Owing to the long retention times, and the possibility of on-column thermal degradation, GLC on packed columns has not attained popularity as a means of determining vitamins K_1 or K_2 in food chemistry. However, the use of open-tubular capillary columns may limit problems of thermal degradation (Lefevere *et al.*, 1985).

Menadione is much more volatile than the natural K vitamins and is not susceptible to on-column degradation. Water-soluble forms of menadione, such as menadione sodium bisulphite (MSB), must be converted to menadione before they can be assayed by GLC. This conversion has been carried out by performing a chloroform extraction of the menadione released by alkaline hydrolysis of the parent compound (Sheppard *et al.*, 1972). However, since menadione decomposes in alkaline solution, this method tends to yield variable results and low recoveries of menadione.

MSB can be assayed directly by GLC using the technique of on-column pyrolysis of the MSB, and subsequent detection of the pyrolysis product, menadione. In the analysis of feed premixes, MSB was extracted with methanol in the presence of diethyl phthalate as internal standard, and the extract was injected directly onto a 3% Dexsil 300 column (Winkler, 1973). A typical chromatogram of menadione and/or the MSB pyrolytic product is shown in Fig. 39. Differential thermal analysis and GC–MS showed that the pyrolysis was quantitative at an injector temperature of 250°C (Winkler & Yoder, 1972). The method of Winkler (1973) has been accepted as Final Action by the Association of Official Analytical Chemists (AOAC, 1984*h*).

Chapter 8

High-Performance Liquid Chromatography (HPLC)

For discussions upon HPLC instrumentation and general chromatographic theory, the reader is referred to standard texts such as (Snyder & Kirkland, 1979; Hamilton & Sewell, 1982; Krstulovic & Brown, 1982; Simpson, 1982; Parris, 1984; Poole & Schuette, 1984; Engelhardt, 1986).

8.1 GENERAL ASPECTS OF HPLC RELEVANT TO FAT-SOLUBLE VITAMIN ASSAYS

8.1.1 Principle of HPLC

HPLC employs closed, reusable columns packed with microparticulate porous silica or derivatized silica, which permit rapid solute distributions between the mobile and stationary phases. A high-pressure pump provides a controlled flow of mobile phase, and a precise sample loading is achieved using either manual syringe injection or automatic injection. Detection of the separated components is achieved by continuous monitoring of the column effluent. HPLC allows hundreds of individual separations to be carried out on a given column, with a far greater speed, efficiency and reproducibility compared with open-column chromatography.

HPLC permits the rapid and non-destructive quantification of the fat-soluble vitamins at room temperature without the need for derivatization, in contrast to GLC which is limited by sample volatility or thermal stability. Separation in HPLC is the result of specific interactions between component molecules and the stationary and mobile phases: in GLC the mobile gas phase plays no part in the separation. Detection in HPLC relies mainly on the UV absorption or fluorescence spectral characteristics of the vitamin, and therefore provides a marked selectivity in addition to the column separation. Accompanying lipids may either be separated from the vitamins or, in most cases, remain undetected, hence extensive sample pretreatment is usually unnecessary.

8.1.2 Column Packings

The particles of silica or derivatized silica prepared for use in HPLC are described as totally porous microparticulate packings, and are available in different sizes within the range of 3–10 μm particle diameter. The majority of published vitamin assays involving HPLC have utilized 5–10 μm silica particles packed into stainless steel columns of 25–30 cm length and internal diameter 4·0–4·6 mm. Particles of 5 μm diameter provide better resolution and efficiency than 10 μm particles, but require a higher pressure to achieve a satisfactory flow rate. Particles of 10 μm diameter represent a good compromise between efficiency, resolution and pressure requirements; they will also accommodate a broader solute polarity range than will 5 μm particles.

Faster separation times with no loss of efficiency can be achieved with 3 μm silica particles packed into shorter columns. However, the use of sub-5 μm particles imposes certain constraints upon the design of the HPLC system (Cooke et al., 1982). To begin with, the column length must be reduced to allow reasonable flow rates, and to maintain an acceptable pressure drop across the column. These changes in particle diameter and column length lead to a corresponding decrease in column volume, thus the band spreading during its elution through the column is small. The resultant smaller peak volumes are susceptible to serious extra-column dilution unless extra-column volumes (e.g. injection loop, connecting tubes and unions, and detector flowcell) are stringently minimized. The response time of the detector and the recorder must also be low in order to maintain chromatographic efficiency (DiCesare et al., 1981).

The microparticulate silica particles may be either irregular or spherical in shape. Spherical packing materials are more difficult to manufacture and hence are more expensive than irregular materials. The surface area of irregular particles is approximately 2·5 times greater than that of spherical particles for a given particle diameter, thus providing a higher loading capacity. It is debatable whether the spherical packings have any major advantages over irregular packings in terms of efficiency and stability, although columns packed with spherical particles are slightly more permeable.

Some assays have utilized stainless steel cartridge columns (typically 10 cm × 4·6 mm i.d.) which fit into specially constructed holders. These columns, by the application of only finger-tight pressure on an end external compression nut, can seal up to 7000 psi, and can be quickly changed or inverted for backflushing.

Radial compression columns produced by Waters Associates have been designed to minimize the 'wall effect', which occurs in conventional HPLC columns, and refers to the greater solute dispersion near the column wall than at the column core. The 'wall effect' is caused by differences between the packing density of particles close to the wall and those at the column centre. This leads to irregular flow patterns across the diameter of the column and results in a lower overall column efficiency. Radial compression columns are prepared from heavy wall polyethylene cartridges (10 cm × 8 mm) that are uniformly radially compressed in a purpose-built hydraulic press. The column wall is forced to deform and mould to the shape of the internal packing structure, thus reducing the number of channels available to the mobile phase at the wall/packing interface. Radial compression columns are packed with conventional packings and are characterized by high permeability, low operating pressures and high efficiency over a wide range of flow rates (Fallick & Rausch, 1979).

The insertion of a short guard column between the injector and analytical column protects the latter against loss of efficiency from sample impurities, strongly retained sample components, and from pump or valve wear particles. To maintain an adequate capacity for sample impurities without introducing excessive peak dispersion the volume ratio of the guard column to that of the analytical column should be in the range 1:15 to 1:25 (Poole & Schuette, 1984). Guard columns have been developed that fit into a special holder which allows the analytical column and guard column to butt against each other. This design reduces the band broadening caused by the presence of connecting tubing and the additional column terminators. The guard column is usually packed with the same stationary phase as the analytical column. Commercially prepared disposable guard columns slurry-packed with particles of the same diameter as used in the analytical column should not increase sample dispersion by more than 5–10%. When a greater loss of column efficiency can be tolerated, guard column modules can be dry-filled at required intervals in the laboratory using microporous or pellicular packings. The latter refer to glass beads coated with silica or derivatized silica, and have a particle size of $> 20 \, \mu m$.

8.1.3 Mobile Phases

Selection of the mobile phase (also referred to as the eluent) is made on the basis of solvent strength and solvent selectivity. Solvent strength is synonymous with polarity for normal-phase LC. Strong solvents are characterized by their ability to dissolve polar solutes and to elute solutes with low capacity factors (k values)† in normal-phase adsorption and partition LC. In reversed-phase LC there is an inverse relationship between polarity and solvent strength. Solvent selectivity has been defined as 'the ability of a given solvent to selectively dissolve one compound as opposed to another, where the polarities of the two compounds are not obviously different' (Snyder, 1974). The general strategy in optimizing a separation is first to adjust the solvent strength to maintain solute k values in the range 1–10 and then, while holding the solvent strength constant, to alter the selectivity of the mobile phase.

Compounds having k values in the optimum range of 1–10 can be separated using isocratic elution, i.e. using a mobile phase whose solvent strength remains constant throughout the separation. Compounds of widely different k values cannot be separated isocratically, since early eluting peaks are insufficiently resolved, and later peaks become broadened to the point of difficult detection. This 'general elution problem' is usually solved by performing gradient elution. In this technique the solvent strength is increased continuously throughout the separation, so that individual components are eluted near their optimum k values. This is achieved using a gradient programmer which changes the mobile phase composition with respect to time. Gradient elution is frequently used with a binary solvent mixture: ternary solvent mixtures allow both solvent strength and solvent selectivity to be altered during the separation.

8.1.4 Detection Systems

Specialized texts on HPLC detectors have been published (Vickrey, 1983; Ryan, 1984; Scott, 1986; Yeung, 1986).

Two types of in-line HPLC detector have been used extensively in food analysis to determine fat-soluble vitamins; namely, absorbance and fluorescence detectors. Electrochemical detection has been applied to the determination of vitamins E and K in biological materials, such as blood and liver, but has not, as yet, been widely adopted in food analysis. Each of these three detectors provides a continuous electrical output that is a function of the concentration of solute in the column effluent passing

† The symbol k (rather than k') is used in this text to denote the capacity factor in accordance with the nomenclature discussed by Ettre (1981).

through the detector flow cell. Since these detectors respond to changes in concentration rather than to changes in mass, they are dependent on solute dilution during chromatography. Thus column size affects the sensitivity of an absorbance detector. For instance, reduction of a column dimension from 250 mm × 4·6 mm to 150 mm × 3·2 mm increased the sensitivity of a UV detector by a factor of approximately two (Nelis *et al.*, 1985).

8.1.4.1 Absorbance detection

Absorbance measurement represents the most widely used detection method employed in HPLC, and may be performed using either a fixed-wavelength photometer or a continuously variable wavelength detector. The latter, which comprise monochromator-type detectors and diode array detectors, permit any wavelength to be selected throughout the UV–visible range of wavelengths (190 nm–900 nm). These detectors, therefore, have the versatility and convenience of allowing operation at the absorption maximum of a solute, or at a wavelength that provides maximum selectivity.

8.1.4.2 Fluorescence detection

Fluorescent compounds can be detected with a high degree of selectivity by means of a fluorescence detector. The sensitivity of a fluorescence detector is higher than that of an absorbance detector, and the linear dynamic range is at least four orders of magnitude (Rhys Williams, 1988; private communication). The sensitivity of fluorescence detection depends, in part, upon the composition of the mobile phase. For example, α-tocopherol and retinol display a five- to six-fold decrease in intensity on changing from hexane to acetonitrile:water (50:50), hence normal phase HPLC provides a greater sensitivity for fluorescence detection compared with reversed-phase systems (Rhys Williams, 1985). The sensitivity may also be affected by coeluting non-fluorescent compounds that have a high absorbance at either the excitation or emission maxima of the fluorescent compound of interest. Such compounds may absorb some of the excitation or emission energy, and therefore reduce the signal generated by the fluorescent compound (DeVries, 1985). To prevent quenching by oxygen, the mobile phase must be degassed and kept under an atmosphere of helium (Rhys Williams, 1980).

Detectors available for fluorescence monitoring in HPLC range in complexity from simple filter fluorometers to dual monochromator spectrofluorometers with scanning capabilities. Cut-off filters, which transmit all light below or above a certain wavelength, generally provide a greater signal than narrow bandpass interference filters or monochromators, but this signal enhancement is obtained at the expense of a loss of selectivity. The bandpass of a monochromator can be altered by changing the slit width. Where excitation and emission maxima are not well separated (e.g. vitamin E, with excitation at 290 nm and emission at 330 nm), a dual monochromator instrument may be necessary (DeVries, 1985). Spectrofluorometers allow the excitation and emission wavelengths to be manually selected or programmed and, with stop-flow scanning, can provide excitation and/or emission spectra.

Of the fat-soluble vitamins, only vitamins A and E possess native fluorescence and can be measured directly by a fluorescence detector. Vitamin K, as such, does not fluoresce, but it can be detected fluorometrically after reduction to its hydroquinone form.

8.1.4.3 Electrochemical detection

The majority of electrochemical detectors used in HPLC are amperometric. In amperometry the working (polarizable) electrode is maintained at a preselected constant potential relative to a reference electrode at or near the limiting current plateau for the electroactive solute. The selected potential is determined from the voltammogram obtained for a stationary sample solution (see Section 6.3). The chromatogram is recorded by measuring the detector cell current as the sample is eluted from the column. The stability of the background current is dependent upon the constancy of the mobile phase flow rate and composition. In flow-through amperometry the mass transfer of the solute to the working electrode occurs by convective diffusion, which results in a thinner diffusion layer at the electrode compared with the thickness of the diffusion layer under stationary conditions. Thus the measured current on an HPLC amperometric detector reaches a higher value than that in a diffusion-controlled voltammetric instrument. The amperometric detector competes in sensitivity and selectivity with the fluorescence detector, and its linear dynamic range is about three orders of magnitude (Scott, 1986).

Electrochemistry in HPLC is dependent upon the column effluent being electrically conductive. Those reversed-phase systems which use semi-aqueous or methanolic mobile phases are compatible with electrochemical detection, since suitable concentrations of an inorganic salt can be added to the mobile phase in the form of a buffer, and this acts as the supporting electrolyte. If the mobile phase is not sufficiently polar to permit the addition of salt, or if the separation process is impaired by the presence of an electrolyte, the electrolyte can be added postcolumn.

Gradient elution is not normally possible with electrochemical detection, as the response of the detector is critically dependent on the constancy of the ionic content of the mobile phase.

Amperometric detection is eminently suitable for the electrooxidation of phenolic compounds and has found application in vitamin E assays. The reversible oxidation–reduction between the quinone and hydroquinone forms of vitamin K has also been exploited in clinical studies by means of amperometry, but has not yet found widespread application in food analysis.

8.1.5 Quantification

Some HPLC methods employ internal standardization, which has been described previously for GLC (see Section 7.1.4). This calibration technique has proved particularly useful in the determination of supplemental vitamin D in foods, where vitamin D_2 can be used as an internal standard for vitamin D_3, and vice versa. Vitamin D assays demand a more extensive sample preparation than the assays of other fat-soluble vitamins, and the addition of an internal standard at the start of the analysis compensates for losses incurred during the procedure. The internal standard also compensates for the thermal isomerization of vitamin D.

For HPLC methods that require a less stringent sample preparation, the external standardization (direct calibration) method is generally preferred. This technique obviates the problem of finding a suitable internal standard and, in common with internal standardization, does not assume that all sample components have been eluted and detected. The external standardization procedure involves preparing a series of standard solutions of the analyte (A). Equal amounts of each standard solution are chromatographed, and a calibration plot is constructed of peak height (h_A) against concentration (W_A). The calibration plot should result in a straight line (within the linear range of the detector) intercepting the origin. The slope of the line is the response factor of the detector to the analyte (K_A). Thus,

$$K_A = \frac{h_A}{W_A}$$

The same volume of sample is injected and the peak height (h'_A) is measured. The concentration of analyte (W'_A) is calculated from the response factor, thus:

$$W'_A = \frac{h'_A}{K_A}$$

Alternatively, the concentration of analyte may be calculated by interpolating the peak height obtained on the calibration plot. Having established that the calibration plot is linear over the working concentration range, a single standard solution may be adequate for calibration. In this case, the external standardization equation becomes simply:

$$\text{Conc. A in sample} = \frac{\text{Conc. A in standard}}{\text{Peak size A in standard}} \times \text{Peak size A in sample}$$

The above procedure applies to peak areas as well as to peak heights.

External standardization involves absolute measurements of peak size, hence the technique depends upon repeatable injection volumes. This, however, can be achieved with an injection valve or autoinjector, both of which facilitate the precise control of injection volume. Peak measurements in external calibration are compared from separate chromatograms, unlike internal standardization where the internal standard peak and analyte peak are present in the same chromatogram. Thus external calibration is more prone to errors arising from changes in the chromatographic conditions (e.g. temperature, flow rate, mobile phase composition). The extent of these changes will depend upon the quality and design of the chromatograph but, in any case, the errors can be minimized by running the samples and calibration standard alternately. Given precise control of injection volume and constant chromatographic conditions, peak size measurement is more precise with external calibration than with internal calibration. This is because the latter technique involves the measurement of two peaks (analyte and internal standard) which increases the precision error by a factor of 1·4 ($\sqrt{2}$). In summary, internal standardization is generally preferred for multi-stage assays where loss of analyte may be a problem; otherwise, external standardization is preferred.

A third calibration method that is advantageous in the analysis of complex mixtures, such as food extracts, is the method of standard additions. This technique compensates for matrix interferences, whereby the presence of other compounds in the sample may affect the retention and/or the peak size of the analyte. In this procedure, three or four successive known amounts of the pure analyte (A) are added to a definite amount of the sample extract, and each mixture is subjected to chromatographic separation. The peak areas or heights are measured and plotted as a function of the added amounts of A. The amount of A in the original sample can then be determined by extrapolating the standard

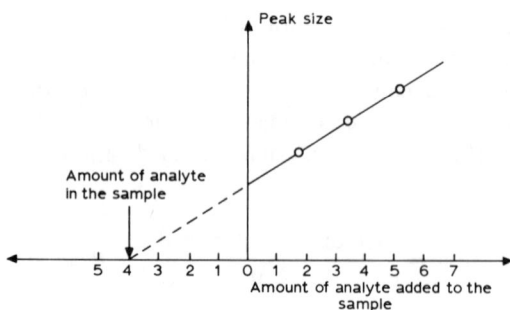

Fig. 40. Standard additions calibration plot.

additions calibration plot to the point of intersection of the concentration axis (see Fig. 40).

If the linearity of the calibration plot has been established, a one-point calibration can be performed. In this procedure, a chromatogram is obtained of the sample, then a known amount of A is added to the sample and a chromatogram of the 'spiked' sample is obtained. The concentration of the analyte can be determined using the calibration factor, R, defined by the following equation.

$$R = \frac{h'_A - h_A}{W_A}$$

where h'_A is the height of A in the 'spiked' sample, h_A is the height of A in the 'unspiked' sample, and W_A is the weight of analyte added. The weight of analyte in the original sample is given by:

$$W_A = \frac{h_A}{R}$$

If a sample can be obtained that is known to be free of the analyte (A) (e.g. an unfortified sample of a foodstuff that is normally fortified), this sample blank can be used as a matrix for preparing standards for normal calibration. That is, various amounts of A are added to the sample blank and a calibration plot is constructed.

8.1.5.1 Preparation of a retinol standard
In vitamin A assays that involve saponification, the instability of retinol, and the unavailability of suitably pure commercial preparations of retinol, prohibit the use of such preparations as reference standards. Thus one

cannot prepare a standard retinol solution by merely weighing a calculated amount of solid retinol.

The Sub-Committee of the Analytical Methods Committee specified the stable all-*trans*-retinyl acetate as the reference material in the HPLC assay for vitamin A in animal feedstuffs (Analytical Methods Committee, 1985). The acetate ester is commercially available in a suitable degree of purity, and provides a means of checking for possible loss of vitamin A during hydrolysis.

The all-*trans*-retinyl acetate is first assayed by direct spectrophotometry (see Section 6.1) and the potency is calculated in IU/g. Another portion of the same retinyl acetate standard is then saponified and extracted alongside the feed samples being assayed; the retinol content of the solution is then calculated spectrophotometrically. If the potency of the saponified extracted standard is less than 93% of the potency of the standard assayed by direct spectrophotometry, the whole process must be repeated for samples and standard.

Hydrolysis of the all-*trans*-retinyl acetate standard is carried out by preparing a solution of the standard in ethanol, so that 1 ml contains approximately 15 000 IU. A 2·5 ml aliquot of this solution is saponified then extracted with petroleum spirit. The combined washed petroleum extracts are diluted to 250 ml, so that the concentration of retinol in this solution is approximately 150 IU/ml. A 5 ml aliquot of the standard retinol solution is pipetted into a 50 ml volumetric flask, and the solvent is removed at ambient temperature with a stream of inert gas. The residue is dissolved in isopropanol, and then diluted to volume with the same solvent. The absorbance of the solution is measured, using isopropanol as a reference, at 310, 325 and 334 nm, and the corrected absorbance at 325 nm is calculated using the Morton and Stubbs equation (see Section 6.1). If the difference between the corrected and uncorrected absorbances exceeds 3% (i.e. if A_{325} (corrected)/A_{325} is less than 0·97), the value of A_{325} (corrected) should be used for the standardization; otherwise A_{325} should be used.

In the HPLC assay, the concentration of the retinol standard solution should be approximately the same as that expected in the sample extract. For example, in the published procedure for determining vitamin A in animal feedstuffs (Analytical Methods Committee, 1985), a retinol concentration of 2·5 IU/ml is expected in the extract for each 1000 IU/kg of vitamin A in the sample. Thus, if a sample with a declared vitamin A concentration of 20 000 IU/kg is to be analysed, a retinol standard solution of 50 IU/ml should be prepared.

To prepare a standard retinol solution for the HPLC assay, an aliquot of the standardized solution is evaporated to dryness at ambient temperature with a stream of inert gas. The residue is dissolved in isopropanol or whatever solvent is used to dissolve the final sample extract. The retinol concentration in the sample extract is calculated by reference to the mean peak size obtained from replicate injections of the retinol standard. Recovery data should not be used to correct the determination, as the losses from the sample and the standard might not be the same.

8.2 HPLC MODES

The HPLC modes encountered in the analysis of fat-soluble vitamins are liquid–solid (adsorption) chromatography and bonded-phase chromatography; a third mode, gel-permeation HPLC, is sometimes employed as a clean-up step.

8.2.1 Liquid–Solid (Adsorption) Chromatography (LSC)

LSC is a form of normal-phase chromatography in which the polar surface of the silica particle constitutes the solid stationary phase. Separations result from the interaction of polar functional groups in the solute molecule with the adsorption sites on the silica surface. The strength of these polar interactions is responsible for the selectivity of the separation. LSC is generally considered to be suitable for the separation of non-ionic molecules which are soluble in organic solvents; such compounds are of moderate polarity, and contain at least one polar functional group. The unique ability of adsorbents to differentiate solutes based on differences in their polar functional groups enables compounds to be separated into classes or groups of similar chemical type. LSC also provides a powerful means of separating *cis/trans* isomers, the separation mechanism being attributed to a steric fitting of solute molecules with the discrete adsorption sites.

The silica particles are characterized by their shape (irregular or spherical), size, and pore structure (mean pore diameter, specific surface area and specific pore volume). Commercial HPLC silica packings used for fat-soluble vitamin assays in foods have surface areas ranging from 170–500 m^2/g; pore diameters range from 60–125 Å. Solute retention (k) in LSC increases with increased surface area and decreased pore diameter. Table 19 lists the various silica packings used in published assays in order of increasing surface area. Solute retention can be expected to be lowest with

Table 19

Underivatized silica packings used in published fat-soluble vitamin assays in foods

Product name	Manufacturer/supplier	Particle size/shape	Specific surface area (m^2/g)	Mean pore diameter ($\mathring{A}$)	Specific pore volume (cm^3/g)
				Pore structure	
Apex Silica	Jones Chromatography	3 or 5 μm (S)	170	100	0·7
Supelcosil LC-Si	Supelco	5 μm (S)	170	100	0·65
Ultrasphere-Si	Altex	5 μm (S)	190	—	—
RESOLVE	Waters Associates	5 μm (S)	200	90	—
μPorasil	Waters Associates	10 μm (I)	300	125	—
Zorbax SIL	DuPont	5 μm (S)	350	75	—
Partisil Silica	Whatman	5 μm (I)	350+	85	0·85
Polygosil 60	Macherey–Nagel	5 μm (I)	450	60	0·75
LiChrosorb Si-60	E. Merck	5 μm (I)	490	60	0·7

S = Spherical.
I = Irregular.

Apex Silica or Supelcosil LC-Si (170 m²/g) and highest with LiChrosorb Si-60 (490 m²/g) under the same conditions and identical column design. A high surface area also permits a high sample loading capacity, which is useful for preparative work. Selectivity (α), on the other hand, is reduced with silica of smaller pore diameter. Hence better separations may be obtained on particles of 100 Å pore diameter than with particles of 60 Å pore diameter. In practice, the mobile phase composition is adjusted to make k more or less the same regardless of surface area (Bristow, 1976).

In LSC the solvent and solute compete for the active sites of the adsorbent, thus the more strongly the mobile phase interacts with the adsorbent, the quicker the solute will elute from the column. The strength of a solvent (for non-electrolytic solvents) is directly related to its polarity in normal-phase chromatography. LSC is frequently carried out using a non-polar solvent (typically hexane) containing a small percentage (usually <5% v/v) of a more polar solvent, such as diethyl ether, amyl alcohol, and isopropanol. The low concentrations of polar additives in the mobile phase have a dramatic effect upon retention and selectivity. These additives, known as moderators or modulators, are preferentially adsorbed from the mobile phase by the hydrogen-bonded silanol groups on the silica surface, and effectively deactivate these strong adsorption sites. The remaining isolated silanol groups are those responsible for the adsorbing properties of the silica. Because the active surface of the silica is now more homogeneous, the modified silica facilitates an improved reproducibility of sample retention and a substantial increase in sample capacity. Higher column efficiency, reduced peak tailing, and a diminished tendency for sample decomposition may also be observed in some cases.

Water, being a very polar solvent, is a very strong moderator. In practice, all systems in LSC are moderated systems because, unless specifically dried, all organic solvents contain an inherent amount of water. The lower the polarity of the mobile phase, the bigger is the influence of small changes in water concentration. With hexane or heptane, a change in water concentration of a few parts per million is sufficient to greatly affect sample retention. It is difficult to standardize the water content of a mobile phase, but a possible alternative is to prepare an isohydric mobile phase, i.e. a mobile phase which corresponds to the same hydration level as the adsorbent. Isohydric mobile phases avoid the long equilibration times usually required with silica columns when changing the eluent, since the eluent is in equilibrium with the adsorbent with respect to water. The mobile phase can be made isohydric with respect to silica by maintaining the water saturation of the mobile phase at about 50% by volume. Mobile phases with approximately 50% water-saturation can be prepared by mixing equal volumes of dry mobile phase with completely water-saturated mobile phase. In the case of a highly non-polar solvent (e.g. hexane or heptane), in which the solubility of water is very low, it is difficult to achieve a complete saturation by simply shaking or stirring the solvent with water. Engelhardt (1977) described a moisture control system as a means of conditioning the mobile phase and the column together.

Gradient elution in LSC is performed by increasing the solvent strength value ($\varepsilon°$) of the mobile phase exponentially during the separation. In practice, it is difficult to ensure that equilibration between the silica adsorbent and the changing mobile phase is occurring sufficiently rapidly. The problem is due to the susceptibility of the silica to water, regardless of whether or not isohydric solvents are used. If both solvents A and B are isohydric at the start of the gradient programme, intermediate compositions of A and B are usually non-isohydric. This leads to the possible uptake of water by the column, resulting in non-reproducible separations and long column regeneration times (Poole & Schuette, 1984). Because of this problem gradient elution is best avoided in LSC for routine applications.

Other potential problems may be encountered in LSC. Column deactivation can occur owing to the strong retention of highly polar compounds present as traces in injected samples or as impurities in the mobile phase; guard columns should be used to reduce this problem. The silica increases the tendency of sample oxidation in the presence of molecular oxygen; deoxygenating the mobile phase with an inert gas such as helium obviates this problem (Snyder & Kirkland, 1979). The mildly acidic nature of the silica surface may cause some decomposition of acid-labile compounds, such as carotenoids.

Temperature is not normally used as a separating variable in LSC as the predominately hydrocarbon mobile phase is of low viscosity and low boiling point at ambient temperature. In any case, selectivity (α) is little affected by changing temperature. Sample retention, however, is very sensitive to temperature change. An increase in column temperature of 1°C results in a 2% decrease in the solute capacity factor (k), therefore column thermostatting at ambient temperature is recommended in LSC, especially where peak height measurements are used in quantitative work.

Column regeneration is periodically required to flush out chemical contaminants that eventually deactivate the adsorbent. Only when the retention of a standard sample becomes constant should the column be used for HPLC separations (Snyder & Kirkland, 1979).

8.2.2 Bonded-Phase Chromatography (BPC)

In BPC the stationary phase is a liquid that is chemically bonded to the silica particle and, unlike liquid–liquid (partition) chromatography, cannot be easily removed during use. Owing to its unique retention mechanism, BPC is considered to be distinct from liquid–liquid chromatography, although many similarities exist.

Most commercially available bonded phases are of the siloxane type (Si—O—Si—R), which are prepared by reacting the surface silanol ($\equiv$Si—OH) groups on the silica support with a chlorosilane or alkoxysilane of the following chemical structure:

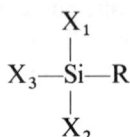

$$X_3\text{—Si—R}$$

with X_1 above and X_2 below the Si.

R is the functional group of interest. In a monofunctional silanizing agent, only one of the substituents X_1, X_2, or X_3 is a reactive group, either chloro or alkoxy (methoxy or ethoxy); the other two substituents are usually methyl groups. Silanizing agents containing two and three reactive groups are referred to as di- and trifunctional. A monofunctional agent such as an organodimethylchlorosilane reacts with the silanol groups on the silica surface to form a monomolecular layer or monomeric phase. Such a phase is also referred to as a 'brush type' or 'bristle structure'. Owing to steric hindrance during the bonding process, not all sites react. Unwanted residual silanols trapped by steric hindrance can be 'end-capped' by reaction with a small monofunctional silane such as trimethylchlorosilane (TMCS), giving a completely hydrophobic surface. Examples of these reactions are illustrated in Fig. 41.

BPC packings can be operated in both normal- and reversed-phase modes. The R group for normal-phase BPC is a polar moiety, such as propylnitrile —$(CH_2)_3CN$ or propylamino —$(CH_2)_3NH_2$. For reversed-phase BPC the functional group is an alkyl moiety, the most common being the octadecyl (C_{18}) hydrocarbon.

The corresponding di- and trifunctional silanizing agents react with surface silanols in a more complicated fashion and, depending on the reaction conditions, can form a monolayer, multilayer or cross-linked polymer of the bonded phase.

Monomeric bonded phases exhibit faster diffusion rates in the stationary phase than do polymeric bonded phases and hence, in theory, provide greater column efficiencies. Monomeric phases also facilitate a more rapid

(a)

$$\equiv Si\!-\!OH + Cl\!-\!\underset{\underset{\displaystyle CH_3}{|}}{\overset{\overset{\displaystyle CH_3}{|}}{Si}}\!-\!R \rightarrow \quad \equiv Si\!-\!O\!-\!\underset{\underset{\displaystyle CH_3}{|}}{\overset{\overset{\displaystyle CH_3}{|}}{Si}}\!-\!R + HCl$$

organodimethylchlorosilane   siloxane bonded phase

(b)

$$\equiv Si\!-\!OH + Cl\!-\!\underset{\underset{\displaystyle CH_3}{|}}{\overset{\overset{\displaystyle CH_3}{|}}{Si}}\!-\!CH_3 \rightarrow \quad \equiv Si\!-\!O\!-\!\underset{\underset{\displaystyle CH_3}{|}}{\overset{\overset{\displaystyle CH_3}{|}}{Si}}\!-\!CH_3$$

TMCS   'end-capped' silanol

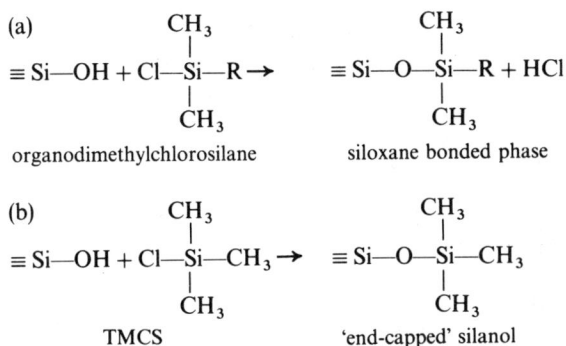

Fig. 41. Reaction between a silanol group on the silica surface and (a) an organodimethylchlorosilane reagent to form a monomeric siloxane bonded phase, (b) TMCS to form an end-capped silanol.

column equilibration after changing the mobile phase composition or after gradient elution. This is not to say, however, that polymeric phases have no useful role in HPLC: their high surface coverage confers a high selectivity for very non-polar solutes, such as polynuclear aromatic hydrocarbons.

Differences in selectivity and chromatographic performance of bonded-phase packings are attributable to particle characteristics (shape and porosity), the chemical nature of the functional group, the amount of organic groups bonded (low versus high carbon load) and their surface configuration, and the percentage of accessible unreacted silanol groups.

Solvents used for mobile phases in BPC may be classified in terms of their strength and selectivity using the empirical scheme proposed by Snyder (1974, 1978). The polarity index P' is a measure of solvent strength. In normal-phase BPC, the higher the solvent P' value, the greater is the solvent strength. In reversed-phase BPC the opposite is true: the lower the solvent P' value, the greater is the solvent strength. Solvent selectivity depends upon the relative ability of the solvent to participate in hydrogen bonding or dipole–dipole interactions. These interactions can be expressed as proton donor (x_d), proton acceptor (x_e) and dipole–dipole (x_n) values. Table 20 lists the P' values and the three selectivity parameters for solvents that are most likely to be used in normal-phase and reversed-phase separations. Solvents of similar selectivity are placed into one of eight solvent groups (I–VIII) based on similarities between their molecular interactions. Thus the polarity index (P') is the variable to alter when adjusting the capacity factor (k), whilst the selectivity (α) is altered by changing the solvent to one from another group.

Table 20
Suggested solvents for HPLC

	P'	x_e	x_d	x_n	Solvent group
Normal-phase					
Diethyl ether	2·8	0·53	0·13	0·34	I
Di-*n*-butyl ether	2·1	0·44	0·18	0·38	I
Chloroform	4·1	0·25	0·41	0·33	VIII
Dichloromethane	3·1	0·29	0·18	0·53	V
Ethyl acetate	4·4	0·34	0·23	0·43	VI
Isopropanol	3·9	0·55	0·19	0·27	II
n-Propanol	4·0	0·54	0·19	0·27	II
Ethanol	4·3	0·52	0·19	0·29	II
Acetonitrile	5·8	0·31	0·27	0·47	VI
Water	10·2	0·37	0·37	0·25	VIII
n-Hexane	0·1				Carrier
Isooctane	0·1				Carrier
Reversed-phase					
Methanol	5·1	0·48	0·22	0·31	II
Tetrahydrofuran	4·0	0·38	0·20	0·42	III
Acetonitrile	5·8	0·31	0·27	0·47	VI
Dioxan	4·8	0·36	0·24	0·40	VI
Dimethylformamide	6·4	0·39	0·21	0·40	III
Methoxyethanol	5·5	0·38	0·24	0·38	III
Water	10·2				Carrier

From Berridge, J. C. (1985). Techniques for the Automated Optimization of HPLC Separations. Reprinted by permission of John Wiley & Sons, Ltd.

A different eluotropic series has been established for reversed-phase separations by measuring the retention of the organic solvents on a reversed-phase column with plain water as the mobile phase. The solvents are listed in order of their retention times relative to that of methanol (see Table 21). The higher the retention value the more the solvent will accelerate the retention of a given solute if the solvent mixed with water is used as the mobile phase (Karch *et al.*, 1976).

8.2.2.1 Normal-phase BPC
Polar bonded-phase packings containing the propylnitrile (cyanopropyl) and alkylamino functional groups, when used with a mobile phase of low polarity, operate as normal-phase systems. That is, non-polar solutes prefer the mobile phase and elute first, whilst polar solutes prefer the stationary

Table 21
Solvent strength on a reversed-phase HPLC column
(according to Karch *et al.*, 1976)

Solvent	Relative retention[a]
Methanol	1·0
Ethanol	3·1
Acetonitrile	3·1
Dimethylformamide	7·6
Isopropanol	8·3
Acetone	8·8
n-Propanol	10·1
Dioxan	11·7

[a] Retention time of solvent relative to that of methanol on
C_{18}-bonded phase with plain water as the mobile phase.

phase and elute later. In general, the polar bonded-phase packings are relatively free from the problems of chemisorption and catalytic activity associated with silica adsorption packings. Polar bonded phases are not usually end-capped, and the presence of some residual silanol groups is desirable to allow 'wetting' of the stationary phase by the mobile phase. The mobile phase consists of a non-polar hydrocarbon solvent (typically hexane) containing small amounts (0·5–1·0% v/v) of a polar modifier, such as isopropanol. The modifier suppresses secondary adsorption effects, which might otherwise cause peak tailing. Polar bonded phases, unlike silica adsorption phases, do not require deactivation, and are not sensitive to the presence of water in the sample or in the solvent. Thus the sample extract can be injected directly onto the column without concern for its water content. Furthermore, BPC columns respond rapidly to changes in solvent polarity, hence can be used in gradient systems.

Nitrile BPC columns are of moderate polarity, and have proved to be a useful alternative to silica adsorption columns. They generally show less solute retention when substituted for silica, but selectivity is similar. The —CN phase provides good selectivity for the separation of geometric isomers and for ring compounds differing in either the position or number of double bonds (Poole & Schuette, 1984). The advantage of nitrile BPC columns over silica adsorption columns is a more rapid equilibration following gradient elution or a change in mobile phase composition. The absence of acidic silanols in nitrile columns overcomes the problem of degeneration of acid-labile solutes, and also produces less tailing with polar solutes. Gillan & Johns (1983) used a nitrile column for the separation of microbial carotenoids to eliminate the effect of underivatized silica on carotenoid degeneration, and to obtain more reproducible retention times. A nitrile column has also been employed to purify the unsaponifiable fraction of vitamin D-fortified milk prior to the determination of the vitamin D by adsorption HPLC (deVries & Borsje, 1982).

Amino BPC columns are of high polarity, and the basic nature of the —NH_2 group imparts a quite different chromatographic selectivity when compared with the acidic surface of silica. An amino column has been employed as a purification step in the determination of vitamin D in fortified low fat milk and infant formulations (Landen, 1985), and also to quantify the vitamin D in fortified instant non-fat dried milk (Cohen & Wakeford, 1980).

A unique type of normal bonded phase is Partisil PAC. This packing contains both amino and nitrile functional groups in a ratio of 2:1 —NH to —CN, and exhibits moderate polarity. The secondary amine may differ in its chromatographic selectivity compared to the primary amine group of most amino bonded phases (Majors, 1980). Partisil PAC columns have been used in HPLC assays to clean up the unsaponifiable fraction of vitamin D-fortified milk (Sertl & Molitor, 1985) and solvent extracts of vitamin D-fortified instant non-fat dried milk (Cohen & Wakeford, 1980). The Partisil PAC packing has also been used in the analytical column for determining the total α-tocopherol in the unsaponifiable fraction of animal feeds (Cohen & Lapointe, 1980a).

Examples of nitrile and amino polar bonded phases used for fat-soluble vitamin assays in foods are listed in Table 22.

8.2.2.2 Reversed-phase BPC

Reversed-phase systems employ bonded-phase packings, in which the silica particle is chemically bonded with a non-polar stationary phase; the mobile phase is a solvent that is more polar than the stationary phase. Solute elution order is the opposite to that observed in normal-phase chromatography: polar solutes prefer the mobile phase and elute first; non-polar solutes prefer the essentially hydrophobic stationary phase, and elute later. The most popular functional group employed in reversed-phase HPLC (RPLC) is an octadecyl (C_{18}) hydrocarbon. The use of a C_{18} alkyl chain permits maximum sample loading and ensures adequate solute retention; the retention time can readily be optimized by adjusting the composition of the mobile phase.

The mechanism governing solute retention in RPLC cannot be adequately

Table 22
Normal-phase BPC packings used in published fat-soluble vitamin assays in foods

Product name	Manufacturer/supplier	Particle size/shape	Specific surface area (m^2/g)	Mean pore diameter $\mathring{A}$	Functional group	Percentage carbon loading (w/w)
Sil-60D-10CN	Perkin–Elmer	10 μm	—	—		—
LiChrosorb-NH$_2$	E. Merck	10 μm (I)	250	100	propylamino	4
μ-Bondapak-NH$_2$	Waters Associates	10 μm (I)	—	125	-amino	9
Partisil PAC	Whatman	5 or 10 μm (I)	—	—	alkyl groups containing amino–nitrile groups in a 2:1 ratio	—

I = Irregular.

explained by simple liquid–liquid partition theory, since the bonded hydrocarbon layer of the stationary phase is only a monolayer thick, and cannot act as a bulk liquid for solubilizing the solutes. In the solvophobic theory of solute retention, the very high cohesive density of the mobile phase, arising from the three-dimensional hydrogen bonding network, provides the driving force. The density forces literally 'squeeze' the less polar solutes out of the mobile phase, enabling them to bind with the hydrocarbon ligands of the stationary phase. The more polar solutes interact with the hydrogen bonding system of the mobile phase in opposition to the solute transfer mechanism. According to the solvophobic theory, therefore, retention in RPLC is a function of sample hydrophobicity, where the selectivity of the separation results almost entirely from specific interactions of the solute with the mobile phase.

McCormick & Karger (1980) pointed out that selectivity based on polar group differences of solute molecules can be very significant in RPLC. This is because the organic component of the mobile phase (e.g. methanol or acetonitrile) is enriched in the stationary phase, and this extracted solvent will interact with solute species. In some reversed-phase packings, solute retention is complicated by interaction of the solute with residual silanol groups on the stationary phase surface.

RPLC is ideally suited to separating non-polar to moderately polar compounds, such as fat-soluble vitamins. The technique is also effective in separating the components of an homologous series, such as α-, $\beta + \gamma$-, and δ-tocopherols or tocotrienols, since hydrophobicity generally increases with the number of carbon atoms in a molecule. Positional isomers, such as β- and γ-tocopherols, cannot be resolved on reversed-phase columns. Saturated compounds are more hydrophobic than the corresponding unsaturated analogues, and hence are retained longer on a reversed-phase column. Compounds of widely different polarity can be separated by gradient elution within a convenient time frame.

RPLC exhibits improved stability and reproducibility compared with normal-phase systems using either silica or polar bonded phases. Interactions between solute and stationary phase on non-polar bonded phases involve weaker forces, thus analyses are rapid and re-equilibration times are short. The latter is particularly useful following solvent compositional changes during method development, and following gradient elution. The weaker forces also minimize the risk of on-column artefact formation. Retention in RPLC is little affected by small variations in the mobile phase composition; for example, no significant effect is seen from slight changes in water content. Hence RPLC is preferable for quantitative work. Since polar compounds are rapidly eluted in an isocratic reversed-phase system, column regeneration is much simpler to carry out compared with normal-phase chromatography.

Differences in selectivity and chromatographic performance between octadecylsilane ODS columns from different manufacturers are attributable to particle characteristics (size, shape and porosity), the coverage of the bonded phase and the surface configuration, and the percentage of accessible unreacted silanol groups.

Microporous materials with pore diameters of 100 Å are more retentive than those of 60 Å. This is because more of the modified surface is accessible to the solute in the larger pore phase (Horváth, 1982).

The amount of ODS ligate bound to the silica surface is commonly expressed as percentage carbon (weight per weight) or simply carbon load, and ranges from 5% to 17%. Table 23 lists the various reversed-phase ODS packings used in published assays in order of increasing percentage carbon loading. High loading ODS bonded phases, such as LiChrosorb RP-18 (17% carbon w/w), are highly retentive, and are particularly useful where solute retention is a problem, such as in the separation of vitamins D_2 and D_3. Such bonded phases require mobile phases with a relatively high proportion of organic component to reduce analysis time. The high carbon load also facilitates a high solute loading capacity, making such a phase useful for preparative HPLC. Packings with low carbon loadings, such as Spherisorb ODS-1 (7% carbon w/w), are less retentive and therefore allow faster analysis times.

Carbon load is not strictly an appropriate term because the percentage of carbon will depend on the surface area of the silica support, and whether or not the silica was fully hydroxylated prior to bonding. A more informative term of surface coverage is carbon content per unit specific surface area, expressed in μmoles/m^2 (Krstulovic & Brown, 1982). The term carbon load is meaningless, for example, when comparing the surface coverage of Vydac TP 201 C_{18} (9% carbon w/w) with μBondapak C_{18}, which has a similar carbon load (10% w/w). As shown in Table 23, the mean pore diameters for the Vydac and μBondapak materials are greatly different (300 Å cf. 125 Å, respectively). A large pore diameter corresponds to a low specific surface area and, in fact, the surface area of the Vydac material (100 m^2/g) is one-third of that of the μBondapak (300 m^2/g). Thus, in terms of carbon content per unit specific surface area, Vydac TP 201 C_{18} has a surface coverage that is three times greater than that of μBondapak C_{18}. This property of the Vydac phase has proved useful in resolving vitamins D_2 and D_3 (Muniz et al., 1982).

Table 23
Reversed-phase BPC packings used in published fat-soluble vitamin assays in foods

Product name	Manufacturer/ supplier	Particle size/shape	Specific surface area (m^2/g)	Mean pore diameter ($\mathring{A}$)	Percentage carbon loading (w/w)	Surface configuration	End-capped or uncapped
Partisil ODS	Whatman	10 μm (I)	—	—	5	Polymeric	Uncapped (50% residual silanols)
Spherisorb ODS-1	Phase Separations	5 or 10 μm (S)	220	80	7	Monomeric	Major silanols capped
Nova-PAK C_{18}	Waters Associates	5 μm (S)[a]	—	60	7	Monomeric	Capped
Hypersil ODS	Shandon	3 or 5 μm (S)	180	—	9	Monomeric	Capped
Vydac TP 201 C_{18}	Separations Group	10 μm (S)	100	300	9	Monomeric	Uncapped
μBondapak C_{18}	Waters Associates	10 μm (I)	300	125	10	Monomeric	Capped
Supelcosil LC-18	Supelco	5 μm (S)	—	100	11	Monomeric	Capped (where necessary)
RESOLVE C_{18}	Waters Associates	5 μm (S)	—	90	12	Monomeric	Uncapped
Ultrasphere ODS	Altex	5 μm (S)	—	—	12	Monomeric	Capped
Nucleosil C_{18}	Macherey–Nagel	5 or 10 μm (S)	—	100	14	Monomeric	Capped
Zorbax ODS	DuPont	5-6 μm (S) or 7-8 μm (S)	—	75	15	Monomeric	Uncapped
LiChrosorb RP-18	E. Merck	10 μm (I)	150	100	17	Monomeric	Uncapped

[a] Present specification quotes 4 μm (Waters Associates, 1985).
S = Spherical.
I = Irregular.

Partisil 10 ODS is a polymeric phase with a low (5%) carbon load and a high (50%) residual silanol content. This packing can be operated either in the normal- or in the reversed-phase mode, according to the mobile phase used.

The eluotropic series listed in Table 20 for solvents used in RPLC is considered by Horváth (1982) to be based on surface tension rather than on polarity. In agreement with the solvophobic theory, water, having the highest surface tension, is the weakest eluent, whereas the organic solvents, having low surface tension, are strong eluents.

The mobile phase used in RPLC is invariably composed of a water–organic solvent mixture where the concentration of the organic component determines the rate of elution of a given compound from the column. Methanol and acetonitrile have been widely used in admixtures with water to effect the separation of compounds which are generally soluble in organic solvents, but insoluble in aqueous solvents. The selectivity of a separation may be conveniently adjusted by changing the type of organic component in the mobile phase. Ternary and quaternary mobile phases allow the fine-tuning of selectivity independently of solvent strength. This versatility is obtained by choosing solvents from different solvent groups (see Table 20) according to their different molecular interactions with a given solute.

Increasing the proportion of water in semi-aqueous mobile phases causes an increased retention of the more hydrophobic solutes relative to the more polar solutes. Increasing the concentration of organic component with time is a convenient way of performing gradient elution in RPLC. The non-polar stationary phase equilibrates rapidly with changes in mobile phase composition, and is therefore well suited for performing gradient elution. Semi-aqueous mobile phases are relatively viscous compared with the predominately hydrocarbon solvents used with polar bonded phases. An improved column efficiency through a higher rate of mass transfer, together with shorter retention times, can be obtained by operating reversed-phase systems at a higher temperature to decrease mobile phase viscosity. An elevated temperature may also cause a change in selectivity (α) for solutes displaying different retention mechanisms (Cox, 1977). A temperature of 50–60°C appears to be convenient if the stability of the sample components allows (Snyder & Kirkland, 1979); a 35°C increase in temperature decreases retention by only a factor of two.

Removal of triglycerides from the sample before injection is essential in reversed-phase HPLC. Triglycerides are insoluble in water, and only sparingly soluble in methanol and acetonitrile. If injected, they may not be completely eluted from the column, and retained material would cause impairment of chromatographic efficiency, peak shape and reproducibility. The use of semi-aqueous mobile phases also poses a solubility problem in the analysis of the non-polar carotenes and the lipophilic vitamin K compounds; the longer chain menaquinones are completely insoluble in pure methanol. Separations at elevated temperatures would obviously improve the solubility of sample components.

Parris (1978) overcame the problem of lipid retention in RPLC by adding a lower polarity solvent (dichloromethane or tetrahydrofuran) to the base solvent (acetonitrile). Tetrahydrofuran, and particularly chlorinated solvents, are very powerful solvents for hydrophobic substances; therefore, to control the elution of lipophilic solutes, a highly retentive column packing (e.g. Zorbax ODS) must be used.

The technique of non-aqueous reversed-phase (NARP) HPLC has been used successfully for the determination of the fat-soluble vitamins. A typical NARP mobile phase consists of a polar basis (usually acetonitrile), a modifier of lower polarity (e.g. dichloromethane, chloroform or tetra-hydrofuran) and, occasionally, a small amount of a third solvent with hydrogen bonding capacity (e.g. methanol). The concentration of the less polar modifier controls retention and, except for tetrahydrofuran, has little effect on selectivity, whilst the third solvent profoundly affects selectivity (Lambert et al., 1985).

The advantage of NARP over semi-aqueous mobile phases used with less retentive column packings is an increased solubility of low polarity compounds in the mobile phase. Thus lipophilic compounds are eluted early and there is a reduced tendency for sterols to precipitate within the HPLC system. The benefit is an improved chromatographic efficiency, solute recovery, and column lifetime. Sample capacity, too, is increased, leading to an improvement of the solute detection limit. Shearer (1983) pointed out that the improved stability of the column bed eluted with non-aqueous mobile phases is influenced by the low viscosity of the solvent, and the correspondingly lower operating pressure required.

Of the several different column packings that have been used in NARP, Zorbax ODS (manufactured by DuPont) possesses the ability to chromatograph, isocratically, compounds of widely divergent polarity. A Zorbax ODS column eluted with acetonitrile:dichloromethane (70:30) gave baseline resolution of the following vitamin standards dissolved in the HPLC mobile phase: retinyl acetate, retinol, α-tocopheryl acetate, vitamins D_2 and D_3 (poorly resolved from one another), β-carotene, and retinyl palmitate. The addition of 0·5 ml of methanol to 1 litre of the mobile phase dramatically improved the resolution of vitamins D_2 and D_3, but retinyl acetate and retinol coeluted (Landen, 1981). Other reversed-phase packings are more selective and require gradient elution to cover such a wide polarity range.

8.2.3 Gel-Permeation Chromatography (GPC)

GPC, using up to four 300 mm × 7·8 mm i.d. μStyragel 100 Å columns connected in series, has been used as an alternative to saponification to remove triglycerides in the analysis of oils and margarine (Landen & Eitenmiller, 1979), breakfast cereals (Landen, 1980), and infant formula foods (Landen, 1982, 1985). μStyragel 100 Å (supplied by Waters Associates) is a semi-rigid gel composed of 10 μm particles of polystyrene cross-linked with divinylbenzene, and has an average pore size of approximately 40 Å (Vivilecchia et al., 1977).

8.3 VITAMIN ASSAYS BY HPLC

Most of the published assays for the fat-soluble vitamins involve the separate determination of each vitamin, often with their respective vitamers. Assay methods for vitamins A, the carotenoids, and vitamins D, E and K that pertain directly to food analysis are summarized in Tables 24–28, respectively. Methods that facilitate the concurrent or simultaneous determination of two or more vitamins are summarized in Tables 29 and 30.

8.3.1 Vitamin A and β-Carotene

Methods for determining vitamin A and, in some cases, β-carotene as well are summarized in Table 24.

Adsorption HPLC on underivatized silica is capable of separating the four isomers of retinol most likely to occur in nature; namely, all-*trans*; 13-*cis*; 9-*cis*; and 9,13-di-*cis*. An example of such a separation is shown in Fig. 42 which depicts a chromatogram of the above four isomers, plus 11-*cis*- and 11,13-di-*cis*-retinol, obtained by photolysis of all-*trans*-retinol. Adsorption HPLC is also capable of separating the retinol and dehydroretinol isomers found in fish liver (Fig. 43). These separations were achieved using a 250 mm × 4 mm i.d. LiChrosorb Si-60 column eluted with hexane containing 0·4% isopropanol at a temperature of 45°C, and monitored by absorbance measurement at 326 nm (Stancher & Zonta,

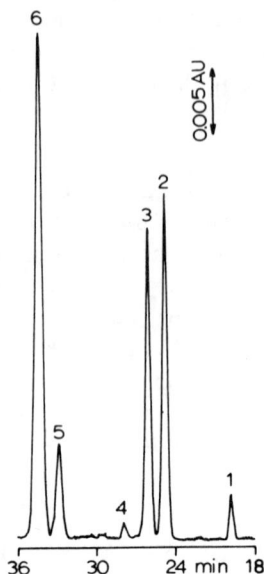

Fig. 42. Adsorption HPLC of retinol isomers in ethanol obtained by photolysis of all-*trans*-retinol. Peaks: (1) 11,13-di-*cis*-retinol; (2) 13-*cis*-retinol; (3) 11-*cis*-retinol; (4) 9,13-di-*cis*-retinol; (5) 9-*cis*-retinol; (6) all-*trans*-retinol. Column, LiChrosorb Si-60; mobile phase, hexane containing 0·4% isopropanol; UV detection, 326 nm, column temp., 45°C (from Stancher & Zonta, 1984).

1984). In foodstuffs, only all-*trans*-retinol and smaller amounts of 13-*cis*-retinol are usually present in significant quantities.

Adsorption HPLC can also separate retinyl acetate from retinyl palmitate, and has been applied to the analysis of margarine and fortified milk. The general procedure entails extracting the whole lipid fraction of the homogeneous sample with a non-aqueous solvent, and removing the polar material. An aliquot of the non-polar lipid extract is then injected directly onto the silica column. Further purification of the lipid fraction is not necessary as silica columns can tolerate relatively heavy loads of triglyceride and other non-polar material. Such material is not strongly adsorbed and can easily be washed from the column with 25% diethyl ether in hexane after the analysis. The amounts of retinyl acetate or retinyl palmitate added to margarine and milk are high enough to dispense with a pre-concentration step. Direct injection of the lipid material onto the HPLC column is possible because the material is dissolved in a non-polar solvent (hexane or heptane) which is compatible with the predominantly hexane (or heptane) mobile phase. An additional advantage of this

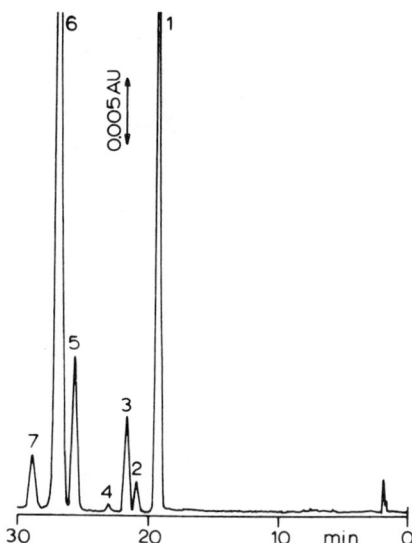

Fig. 43. Adsorption HPLC of isomers of retinol and dehydroretinol obtained from the unsaponifiable matter of cod liver oil. Peaks: (1) 13-*cis*-retinol; (2) 13-*cis*-dehydroretinol; (3) 9,13-di-*cis*-retinol; (4) 9,13-di-*cis*-dehydroretinol (tentative); (5) 9-*cis*-retinol; (6) all-*trans*-retinol; (7) all-*trans*-dehydroretinol. HPLC parameters as in Fig. 42, but different mobile phase flow-rate (from Stancher & Zonta, 1984).

technique is that the vitamin A is maintained in its stable ester form throughout the assay. Adsorption HPLC is particularly appropriate for use with fluorescence detection, as non-polar mobile phases provide a greater sensitivity compared with the polar mobile phases used in reversed-phase HPLC (Rhys Williams, 1985).

Aitzetmüller *et al.* (1979) determined supplemental retinyl palmitate in margarine by dissolving a 120 g sample of margarine in heptane containing 0·05% BHT and 0·02% α-tocopherol, then pouring the resulting emulsion through a 30 cm × 2 cm or 3 cm i.d. glass column filled with 10 g of sodium sulphate (bottom layer) and 20 g of sodium chloride (top layer). The clear non-aqueous eluate was made to a known volume with the heptane containing antioxidant, and an aliquot was injected onto a 5 μm LiChrosorb Si-60 silica column. The mobile phase was heptane:diisopropyl ether (95:5) and the absorbance detection wavelength was 325 nm. The HPLC column was reconditioned after four days of use by pumping a 1:1 mixture of heptane/diethyl ether overnight, followed by prolonged rinsing with the HPLC mobile phase. The average recovery of

Table 24

HPLC methods used for vitamin A compounds and carogene

Analyte	Sample type	Sample preparation	Quantitative HPLC			Reference/ Fig. no.
			Stationary phase	Mobile phase	Detection	
Vitamin A palmitate	Margarine	Heptane extraction, clean-up on Na$_2$SO$_4$/NaCl column	LiChrosorb Si-60	Heptane: diisopropyl ether (95:5)	UV 325 nm	Aitzetmüller et al. (1979)
Vitamin A palmitate	Fortified fluid milk (whole, semi-skimmed, skimmed)	Dispersion in EtOH, partition into hexane	LiChrosorb Si-60	Hexane:diethyl ether (98:2)	UV 325 nm (vitamin A palmitate)	Thompson et al. (1980)
Vitamin A palmitate, carotene	Margarine	Dissolution in hexane, wash with aq. EtOH	LiChrosorb Si-60	Hexane:diethyl ether (98:2)	VIS 453 nm (carotene)	Thompson et al. (1980)
Vitamin A palmitate and acetate	Fortified whole milk powder	Dispersion in non-aq. solvent, partition into hexane	μPorasil	Hexane:CHCl$_3$ (92:8)	UV 313 or 340 nm Fluorescence: excitation 340 nm emission 450 nm	Woollard & Woollard (1981) (Figs 44, 45)
Total retinol	Breakfast cereals, infant formulae, dehydrated whole egg products	Saponification, hexane extraction, evaporation	μPorasil	Hexane:CHCl$_3$ + 1% EtOH (1:1)	UV 313 nm	Dennison & Kirk (1977) (Fig. 46)
Total retinol (all-trans- and 13-cis-)	Breakfast cereals, margarine, butter	Saponification, extraction with hexane:CH$_2$Cl$_2$ (3:1)	Zorbax SIL	Hexane:CH$_2$Cl$_2$: Pr-2-OH (300:200:1·5)	Fluorescence: excitation 365 nm emission 510 nm	Egberg et al. (1977) (Fig. 47)
13-Cis-; 9,13-di-cis-; 9-cis- and all-trans-retinol. Carotene	Cheese	Alkaline digestion (ambient), hexane extraction, evaporation	LiChrosorb Si-60	Hexane: methyl ethyl ketone (90:10)	UV 340 nm (retinoids) VIS 450 nm (carotene)	Stancher & Zonta (1982) (Fig. 48)

Retinol	Milk (unfortified), cheese	Saponification, petroleum spirit extraction, evaporation	Nucleosil C_{18}	MeCN:H_2O (95:5)	UV 328 nm	Bui-Nguyên & Blanc (1980)
Total retinol, β-carotene	Fortified fluid milk (whole, skimmed), infant formulae, margarine	Saponification, hexane extraction, evaporation	LiChrosorb RP-18	MeOH:H_2O (90:10) (retinol) MeOH:H_2O (99:1) (β-carotene)	UV 325 nm (retinol) VIS 453 nm (β-carotene)	Thompson & Maxwell (1977)
Total retinol	Animal feeds	Saponification, 1,2-dichloroethane extraction, evaporation	Spherisorb ODS	MeOH:H_2O (97:3)	UV 325 nm	Lawn et al. (1983) (Figs 49, 50)
Total retinol	Animal feeds	Saponification, petroleum spirit extraction, evaporation	Unspecified ODS	MeOH:H_2O (97:3)	UV 325 nm	Analytical Methods Committee (1985)
Total retinol (all-*trans*- and 13-*cis*-)	Breakfast cereals, margarine, butter	Saponification, precipitation of soaps with acetic acid in MeCN, dilution with H_2O	Vydac TP 201 C_{18}	MeCN:H_2O (65:35)	UV 328 nm	Egberg et al. (1977) (Fig. 51)
Vitamin A palmitate	Fortified non-fat fluid milk	Solvent extraction, formation of methyl esters from triglycerides by alcoholysis, evaporation of hexane extract	Alltech C_{18} (10 μm)	MeOH:H_2O (97:3)	UV 326 nm	Grace & Bernhard (1984)

continued p. 172

Table 24—contd.

| Analyte | Sample type | Sample preparation | Quantitative HPLC | | | Reference/ Fig. No. |
			Stationary phase	Mobile phase	Detection	
Vitamin A palmitate, β-carotene	Margarine	CH$_2$Cl$_2$ extraction, removal of lipid by GP–HPLC on two μStyragel 100 Å columns eluted with CH$_2$Cl$_2$ (UV 340 nm), evaporation of eluate	μBondapak C$_{18}$	MeCN:CH$_2$Cl$_2$ (70:30)	UV 313 nm (vitamin A palmitate) VIS 436 nm (β-carotene)	Landen & Eitenmiller (1979) (Figs 52–54)
Vitamin A palmitate	Breakfast cereals	CH$_2$Cl$_2$ extraction, removal of lipid by GP–HPLC on two μStyragel 100 Å columns eluted with CH$_2$Cl$_2$ (UV 340 nm), evaporation of eluate	μBondapak C$_{18}$	MeCN:CH$_2$Cl$_2$ (70:30)	UV 313 nm (vitamin A palmitate)	Landen 1980 (Figs 55, 56)

MeOH (methanol); EtOH (ethanol); CHCl$_3$ (chloroform); MeCN (acetonitrile); CH$_2$Cl$_2$ (dichloromethane); Pr-2-OH (isopropanol); THF (tetrahydrofuran); EtOAc (ethyl acetate).

retinyl palmitate added to margarine was 97·5%, and the detection limit of the method was 0·27 ppm of retinyl palmitate in the margarine. A similar method could be employed for vitamin A acetate in margarine.

Thompson *et al.* (1980) determined retinyl palmitate and β-carotene in fortified milk (whole, partially skimmed and skimmed) and margarine. Milk (2 ml) was mixed with ethanol, and the lipid was partitioned into hexane. Margarine (5 g) was dissolved in hexane, then shaken with 60% aqueous ethanol to remove polar lipids. An aliquot of the hexane solution was injected onto a 250 mm × 3·2 mm i.d. LiChrosorb Si-60 silica column eluted with 50% water-saturated hexane:diethyl ether (98:2). Retinyl palmitate was determined at an absorption wavelength of 325 nm by combining the peak areas of the 13-*cis* and all-*trans* isomers; β-carotene, which was eluted near the solvent front, was detected at 453 nm. The HPLC column was washed after every twenty samples with 25% diethyl ether in hexane, followed by the mobile phase, until the retention times of vitamin A standards returned to normal. The RSD (ten replicates) for vitamin A in milk was 3%; the RSDs for vitamin A and β-carotene in margarine were 4·5% and 3%, respectively.

Mills (1985) carried out a similar procedure to determine retinyl palmitate in fortified milk, and compared the results with those obtained from the Carr–Price colorimetric method. The variation between the methods was less than 7%, and it was concluded that the procedures were statistically equivalent.

Woollard & Woollard (1981) extracted vitamin A esters from fortified whole milk powder by dispersing the powder in a non-aqueous solvent (dimethylsulphoxide:dimethylformamide:chloroform; 2:2:1 containing ascorbic acid). The lipid fraction was then partitioned into hexane, a portion of which was injected directly onto a μPorasil silica column fitted with a Corasil Type I (Waters Associates) guard column containing pellicular silica, and eluted with hexane:chloroform (92:8). The position of the eluting lipids was revealed by monitoring the absorbance at 280 nm (Fig. 44). Complete resolution of natural retinyl palmitate and supplemental retinyl acetate was obtained with the aid of dual absorbance (340 nm) and fluorescence detection (340 nm excitation; 450 nm emission) (Fig. 45). The fluorometer excitation filter was normally a 12 nm bandpass interference filter, although a high transmittance 320–380 nm filter could be used. The emission filter was a long pass cut-off type. β-Carotene was eluted at the void volume. A wash regime of ethanol (10 ml), followed by chloroform (50 ml), was recommended to return the silica column to its original condition (Woollard, 1987). Recoveries of retinyl acetate and palmitate

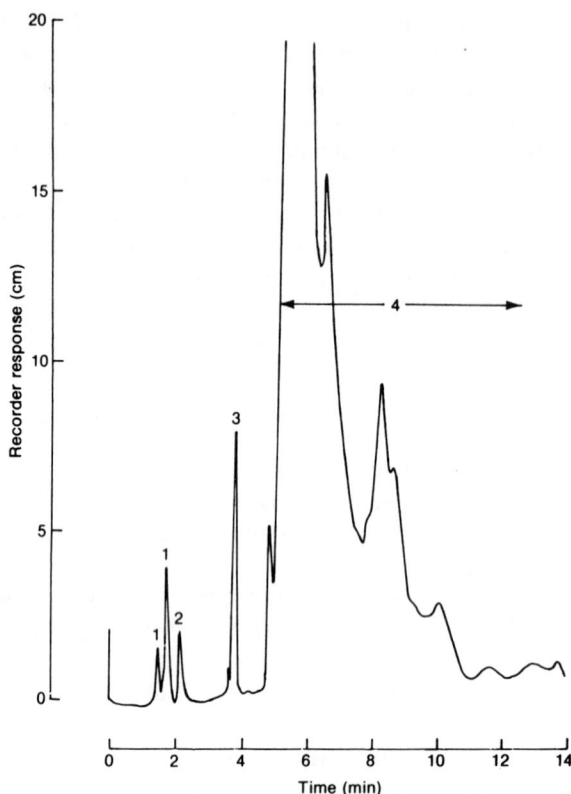

Fig. 44. Adsorption HPLC of purified lipid extract of vitamin A-fortified whole milk powder showing the position of eluting lipids. Peaks: (1) solvent; (2) retinyl palmitate (natural); (3) retinyl acetate (supplemental); (4) co-extracted lipids. Column, μPorasil; mobile phase, hexane:chloroform (92:8); UV detection, 280 nm (from Woollard & Woollard, 1981).

added to unfortified milk powder averaged 98·6% and 99·3%, respectively; the RSD was 5·4%.

Woollard & Fairweather (1985) determined retinyl palmitate and retinyl acetate in UHT-processed milk using a radially compressed 5 μm silica column. Fluorescence detection was employed using an excitation wavelength of 325 nm and a 430 nm cut-off filter to monitor the emission.

Saponification of the sample simplifies the analysis by converting the naturally occurring and supplemental esters of vitamin A to retinol, and allowing a retinol standard to be used in the quantification. The liberation

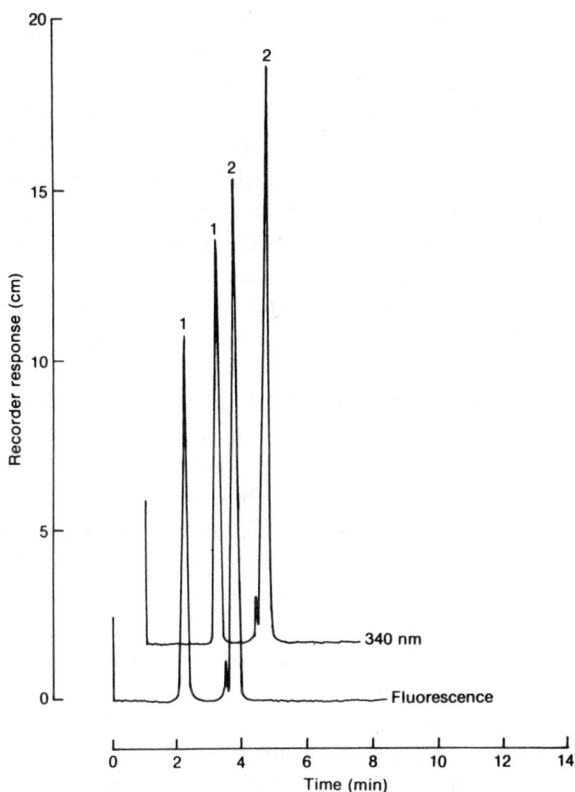

Fig. 45. Adsorption HPLC of vitamin A esters in purified lipid extract of vitamin A-fortified whole milk powder. Peaks: (1) retinyl palmitate (natural); (2) retinyl acetate (supplemental). Column and mobile phase as in Fig. 44; dual detection, UV (340 nm) and fluorescence (340 nm, excitation; 450 nm, emission) (from Woollard & Woollard, 1981).

of the unstable retinol from the relatively stable vitamin A esters during saponification demands protective measures against light and oxygen during the analysis. Subsequent treatment of the unsaponifiable matter depends upon the vitamin potency of the sample and the HPLC mode employed. In methods which use adsorption HPLC, the hexane or heptane solution containing the unsaponifiable matter is compatible with the predominantly hexane (or heptane) mobile phase, thus it is possible to inject an aliquot of the unsaponifiable extract directly onto the silica column. In most reversed-phase methods, the solution containing the unsaponifiable matter must be evaporated to dryness, and the residue redissolved in a solvent that is compatible with the HPLC mobile phase. This step provides the opportunity of concentrating low potency samples.

Adsorption HPLC, using isocratic elution, has been used to determine vitamin A in the unsaponifiable fraction of various food products, including breakfast cereals, milk and cheese. Dennison & Kirk (1977) determined the total vitamin A content of fortified breakfast cereals, infant formula foods, and dehydrated whole egg products after saponification and extraction of the unsaponifiable matter with hexane. The combined hexane extracts were washed with water, filtered over anhydrous sodium sulphate, then evaporated to dryness under vacuum. The residue was dissolved in a portion of the HPLC mobile phase (hexane:chloroform containing 1% ethanol; 1:1), passed through a 0·45 μm fluoropore filter, then analysed on a 300 mm × 4 mm i.d. μPorasil silica column with absorbance detection at 313 nm. Typical chromatograms are depicted in Fig. 46. A standard curve was prepared by dissolving retinol in the mobile phase. The average recovery of vitamin A as retinol in cereal products was 94·3% ± 2·01%. Recovery samples were prepared by adding a known volume of a standard retinyl acetate solution to the samples prior to saponification.

Egberg *et al.* (1977) saponified breakfast cereals and other foods under nitrogen in the presence of ascorbic acid, then extracted the unsaponifiable matter with hexane:dichloromethane (3:1). The organic layer was washed with water to remove residual alkali, and vitamin A oxime was added as an internal standard. An aliquot of the extract was injected, without concentration, onto a 250 mm × 2·1 mm i.d. 5 μm Zorbax SIL silica column eluted with hexane:dichloromethane:isopropanol (300:200:1·5). Complete resolution of 13-*cis*-retinol, all-*trans*-retinol and the internal standard was obtained using a fluorescence detector equipped with a 365 nm interference filter for excitation and a 510 nm cut-off emission filter (Fig. 47).

Stancher & Zonta (1982) used a 250 mm × 4 mm i.d. LiChrosorb Si-60 column eluted with hexane:methyl ethyl ketone (90:10) to determine vitamin A isomers and carotene in cheese. An internal standard mixture of 2-nitrofluorene and azobenzene was added to the hexane extract of the unsaponifiable fraction, which was concentrated by rotary evaporation prior to HPLC. The spectrophotometric detection wavelength was 450 nm for carotene and azobenzene. After the elution of azobenzene, the wavelength was quickly changed to 340 nm in order to detect 2-nitrofluorene and retinol isomers. The technique employed permitted the separation and measurement of the following compounds: carotene; 11,13-

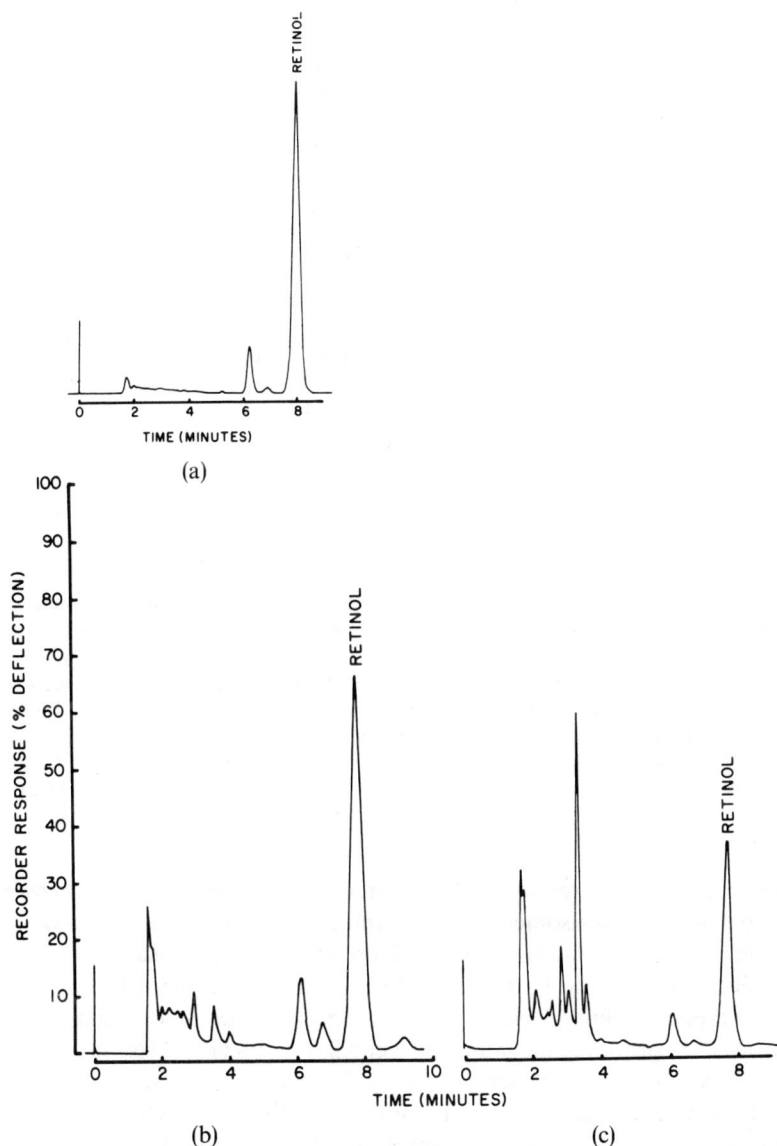

Fig. 46.   Adsorption HPLC of retinol in the unsaponifiable matter from vitamin A-fortified (a) wheat-based breakfast cereal, (b) dehydrated whole egg product, and (c) infant formula. Column, μPorasil; mobile phase, hexane:chloroform (1:1) containing 1% ethanol; UV detection, 313 nm (Reprinted from Dennison & Kirk, 1977. *J. Fd Sci.*, **42**, 1376–9. Copyright © by Institute of Food Technologists).

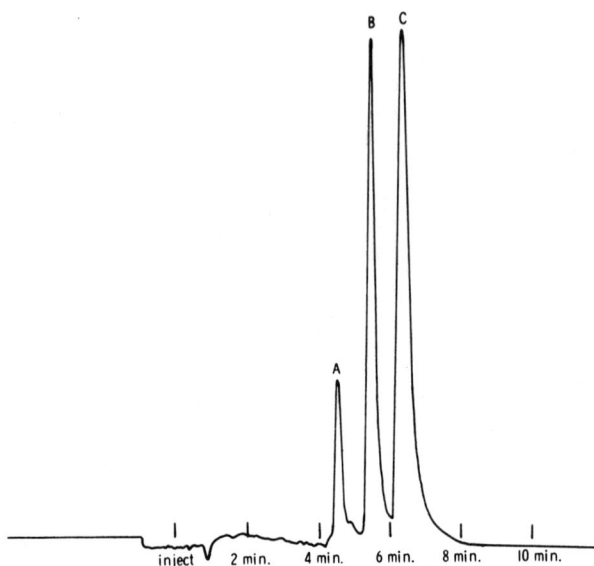

Fig. 47.   Adsorption HPLC of vitamin A in the unsaponifiable matter from cod liver oil. Peaks: (A) 10 ng 13-*cis*-retinol; (B) 21 ng all-*trans*-retinol; (C) 32 ng retinal oxime (internal standard) injected. Column, Zorbax SIL; mobile phase, hexane: dichloromethane:isopropanol (300:200:1·5); fluorescence detection, 365 nm interference filter (excitation) and 510 nm cut-off filter (emission) (Reprinted with permission from Egberg, D. C., Heroff, J. C. & Potter, R. H. (1977). Determination of all-*trans* and 13-*cis* vitamin A in food products by high-pressure liquid chromatography. *J. agric. Fd Chem.*, **25**, 1127–32). Copyright (1977) American Chemical Society.

di-*cis*-retinol; 13-*cis*-retinol; 9,13-di-*cis*-retinol; 9-*cis*-retinol and all-*trans*-retinol (the last two isomers were incompletely resolved) (see Fig. 48).

The removal of the triglycerides from the sample by saponification permits reversed-phase HPLC to be employed. Reversed-phase HPLC with semi-aqueous mobile phases has been utilized to determine vitamin A in various food products, including milk, cheese and breakfast cereals, and in animal feedstuffs. The chromatography yields either a single retinol peak or an all-*trans*-retinol and a 13-*cis*-retinol peak, either of which provides an estimate of the total retinol content. Further separation of *cis* and *trans* isomers of vitamin A is not achieved.

Bui-Nguyên & Blanc (1980) used a 250 mm × 4·6 mm i.d. 10 μm Nucleosil C_{18} column eluted with acetonitrile:water (95:5) with absorbance detection at 328 nm to determine naturally occurring retinol in milk and

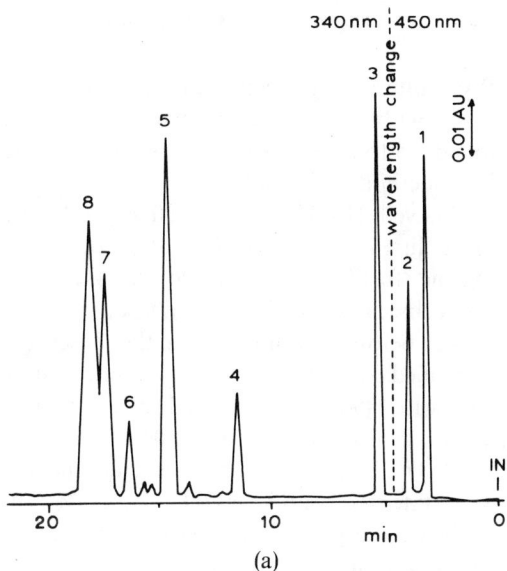

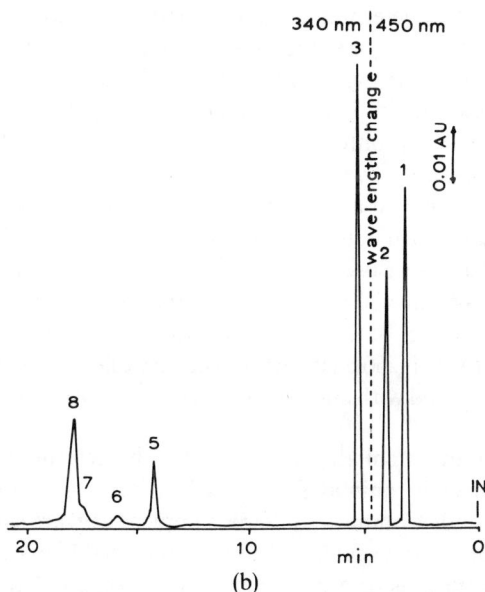

Fig. 48. Adsorption HPLC of vitamin A and carotene. (a) Standard mixture of retinol isomers, carotene and internal standards, (b) unsaponifiable matter from Taleggio cheese. Peaks: (1) carotene; (2) azobenzene (internal standard); (3) 2-nitrofluorene (internal standard); (4) 11,13-di-*cis*-retinol; (5) 13-*cis*-retinol; (6) 9,13-di-*cis*-retinol; (7) 9-*cis*-retinol; (8) all-*trans*-retinol. Column, LiChrosorb Si-60; mobile phase, hexane:methyl ethyl ketone (90:10); UV detection, 450 nm and 340 nm (from Stancher & Zonta, 1982).

cheese. The HPLC column was reconditioned after twenty to thirty analyses by washing with a 95:5 water/acetone solution for 1 h. The recovery of retinol added to cheese before saponification was 93% ± 6%, and the RSD of the method was 4%.

Thompson & Maxwell (1977) used a 250 mm × 3·2 mm i.d. 10 μm LiChrosorb RP-18 column for the determination of vitamin A and β-carotene in margarine, fortified milk (whole and skimmed) and infant formula foods. Margarine (5 g) was dissolved in hexane, then evaporated to dryness under nitrogen before saponification in the presence of pyrogallol; milk (1 ml) was saponified directly. Retinol was determined using a mobile phase of methanol:water (90:10) monitored spectrophotometrically at 325 nm; β-carotene was determined with a mobile phase of methanol:water (99:1) monitored at 453 nm. Recovery of retinol, determined by analysing a solution of retinyl acetate in olive oil, was 99·2% ± 2·3%. The RSDs were 6·8% for twelve replicate analyses of a margarine for retinol, and 5·4% for ten replicate analyses of a margarine for β-carotene.

Lawn et al. (1983) determined the total vitamin A content of feedstuffs by saponification in the presence of ascorbic acid, extraction with 1,2-di-chloroethane, and rotary evaporation of the organic extract to dryness. The residue was dissolved in 5 ml of ethanol, and an aliquot of the filtered solution was injected onto a 250 mm × 4·6 mm i.d. Spherisorb ODS column. The methanol:water (97:3) mobile phase was monitored by absorbance measurement at 325 nm. All-*trans*- and 13-*cis*-retinol were not resolved, although their retention times differed slightly. Therefore, peak area measurements were used to encompass both isomers. Chromatograms of the retinol peak detected by absorbance and by fluorescence are depicted in Fig. 49. The presence of the 13-*cis* and all-*trans* isomers was confirmed by adsorption HPLC (Fig. 50). The mean recovery of eighteen determinations of 'blank' feeds spiked with all-*trans*-retinyl acetate was 102% with an RSD of 10%.

A method based on collaborative tests for the determination of retinol and its derivatives in animal feedstuffs has been recommended by the Analytical Methods Committee (1985). Samples (50 g) are saponified in the presence of sodium ascorbate, and the unsaponifiable matter is extracted with petroleum spirit using a special extraction apparatus that comprises a cylinder and a siphon. The combined petroleum extracts are washed with water, dried, and evaporated under vacuum at 40°C. The residue is dissolved in isopropanol for HPLC on a 250 mm × 5 mm i.d. reversed-phase column (unspecified) eluted with methanol:water (97:3) using spectrophotometric detection at 325 nm.

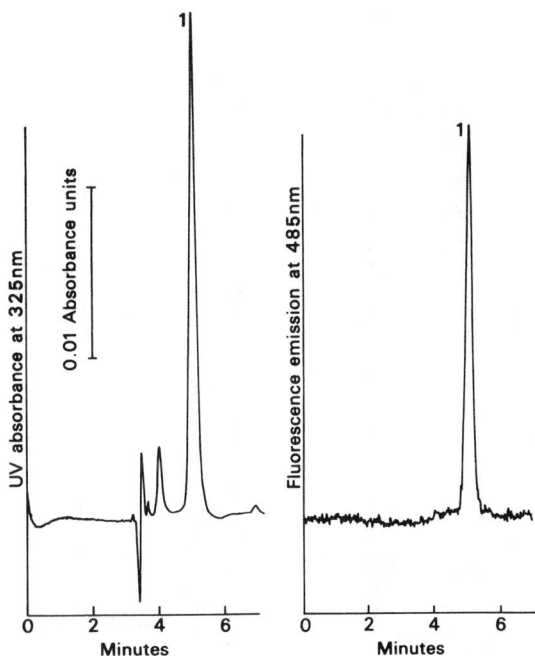

Fig. 49. Reversed-phase HPLC of retinol in the unsaponifiable material from poultry feed. Peak 1 represents total vitamin A (~ 180 ng). Column, Spherisorb ODS; mobile phase, methanol:water (97:3); dual detection, UV (325 nm) and fluorescence (314 nm, excitation; 485 nm, emission) (from Lawn *et al.*, 1983).

In the analysis of breakfast cereals, margarine, butter and other foods, Egberg *et al.* (1977) avoided the time-consuming extraction after saponification by acidifying the unsaponifiable matter with acetic acid in acetonitrile to precipitate the fatty acid salts. The filtered extract was diluted with water, and an aliquot was injected onto a 250 mm $\times$ 3·2 mm i.d. 10 μm Vydac TP 201 C_{18} column eluted with a compatible mobile phase (65% acetonitrile in water) using absorbance detection at 328 nm. Separation of 13-*cis*-retinol and all-*trans*-retinol was obtained which, whilst not as good as that obtained on a silica adsorption column, was sufficient for quantification. Typical chromatograms are depicted in Fig. 51. The reversed-phase technique was adopted as the method of choice because of its ease of operation compared with adsorption chromatography. The average recovery of retinyl acetate added to different food products was

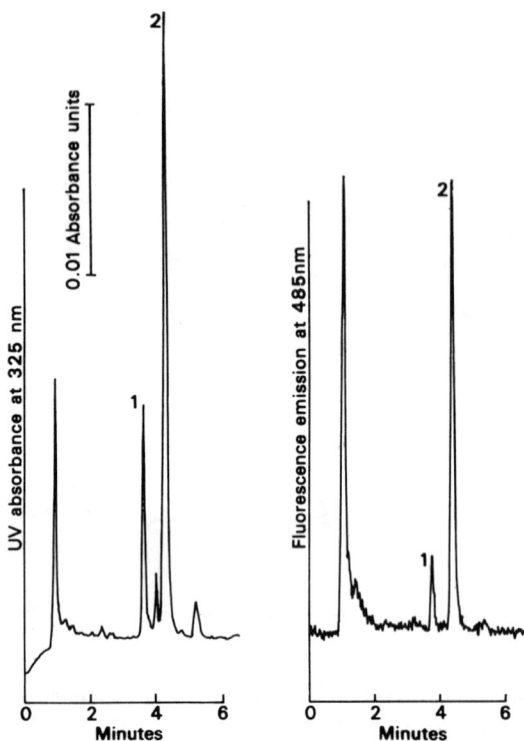

Fig. 50. Adsorption HPLC of vitamin A in the unsaponifiable matter from poultry feed. Peaks: (1) 13-*cis*-retinol (~100 ng); (2) all-*trans*-retinol (~260 ng). Column, Partisil Silica; mobile phase, dichloromethane containing 0·25% ethanol; dual detection as in Fig. 49 (from Lawn *et al.*, 1983).

94·6% ± 6·6%. The pooled RSD was 3·9%. Further details of this method have been published (DeVries *et al.*, 1979).

Grace & Bernhard (1984) avoided saponification in the determination of retinyl palmitate in vitamin A-fortified non-fat milk by converting the reduced amount of triglycerides into their methyl esters by alcoholysis with methanolic KOH solution. Alcoholysis is a milder and more rapid process than saponification, thus there is less potential for destruction of vitamin A. The method entailed extracting a 50 ml sample of milk with a mixture of saturated sodium chloride solution, acidified ethanol, and hexane, plus BHT as an antioxidant. The mixture was centrifuged, and the hexane layer was mixed with methanolic KOH solution. After reaction for 2 min, the mixture was diluted with water, and the hexane layer was evaporated to

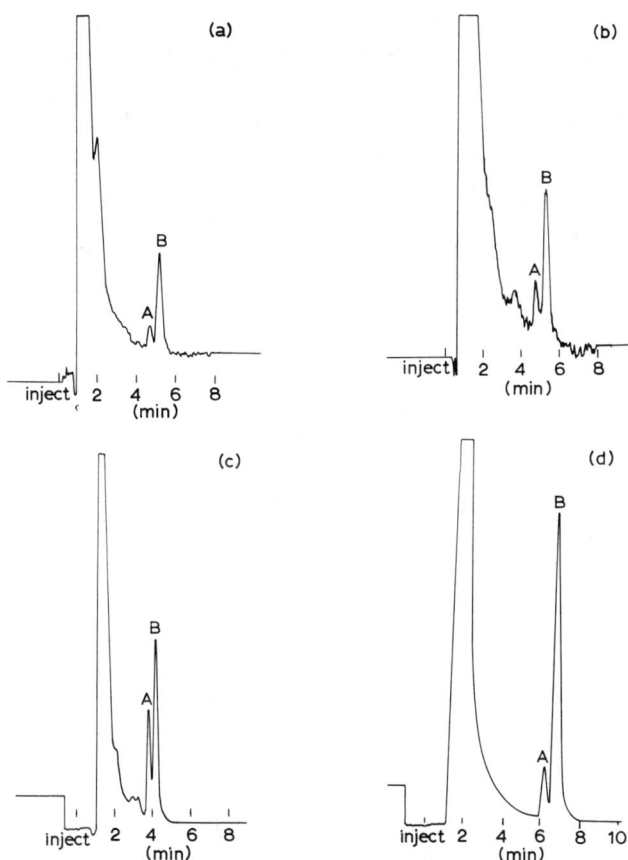

Fig. 51. Reversed-phase HPLC of vitamin A in the unsaponifiable matter from (a) butter, (b) dry cat food, (c) cod liver oil, and (d) fortified breakfast cereal. Peaks: (A) 13-*cis*-retinol; (B) all-*trans*-retinol. Column, Vydac TP 201 C_{18}; mobile phase, acetonitrile:water (65:35); UV detection, 328 nm (Reprinted with permission from Egberg, D. C., Heroff, J. C. & Potter, R. H. (1977). Determination of all-*trans* and 13-*cis* vitamin A in food products by high-pressure liquid chromatography. *J. agric. Fd Chem.*, **25**, 1127–32). Copyright (1977) American Chemical Society.

dryness under vacuum at 60°C. The remaining syrup was diluted with acetone then analysed on a 250 mm × 4·6 mm i.d. 10 μm Alltech C_{18} column using a guard column containing a reversed-phase pellicular packing. The mobile phase of methanol:water (97:3) was monitored by absorbance measurement at 326 nm. Recoveries of retinyl palmitate from spiked samples averaged 99%, with RSDs ranging from 3·2%–10·0%. The small amounts of triglyceride methyl esters present in the final extract did not interfere with the determination of retinyl palmitate, as the bulk of the esters absorb at wavelengths below 326 nm.

Non-aqueous reversed-phase (NARP) HPLC has been used to determine retinyl palmitate and β-carotene in oils and margarine, after dissolution of the sample in dichloromethane, and removal of the triglycerides by gel-permeation HPLC (Landen & Eitenmiller, 1979). The avoidance of saponification in this technique is advantageous in the determination of β-carotene. However, the NARP system is not capable of separating the *cis* and *trans* isomers of vitamin A (Lawn *et al.*, 1983). The procedure was as follows.

Samples of margarine (10 g) were dissolved in dichloromethane containing 0·001% triethylamine and 0·01% BHA, then dried with anhydrous magnesium sulphate and filtered. An aliquot of the filtrate was fractionated by two elution passes through two 300 mm × 7·8 mm i.d. μStyragel 100 Å columns connected in series, with dichloromethane as the mobile phase. A spectrophotometric detector set at 340 nm was used to continuously monitor the column effluent for the vitamin A fraction containing β-carotene, whilst elution of the oil was followed with a refractive index detector. The combined vitamin A/β-carotene fraction was collected manually in a 5 ml vial when the refractive index response approached baseline, and the UV absorption signal indicated the start of a peak.

The eluted fraction was evaporated to dryness in an atmosphere of helium, and the residue was dissolved in a small volume of the mobile phase (acetonitrile:dichloromethane; 70:30) for chromatography on a 300 mm × 7·8 mm i.d. 10 μm μBondapak C_{18} column fitted with a pre-column in-line 2 μm filter. Retinyl palmitate was detected spectrophotometrically at a wavelength of 313 nm, and β-carotene at 436 nm. Recoveries of added β-carotene and retinyl palmitate from vegetable oils were 98·6% ± 2·0% and 95·2% ± 2·6%, respectively, with RSDs of 2·9% for β-carotene and 2·7% for retinyl palmitate. The gel-permeation chromatogram of a standard mixture of retinol, retinyl acetate, retinyl palmitate, and β-carotene is presented in Fig. 52. Retinol and its two esters were resolved, but the elution of β-carotene and retinyl palmitate overlapped. However, by monitoring the column effluent at 436 nm for β-carotene and at 313 nm for retinyl palmitate, elution of both compounds could be followed. Figure 53(a) shows the degree of separation of the oil from the retinyl palmitate and β-carotene fraction during the initial pass of margarine in dichloromethane through μStyragel. In the collected region, the peak response at 340 nm was due primarily to retinyl palmitate.

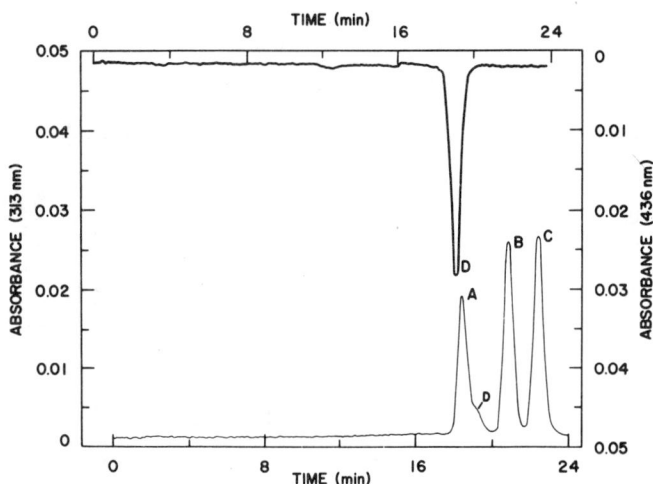

Fig. 52. Gel-permeation HPLC of vitamin A compounds and β-carotene. Standard mixture of 135 ng retinyl palmitate (peak A), 108 ng retinyl acetate (peak B), 100 ng retinol (peak C) and 100 ng β-carotene (peak D). Column, tandem μStyragel 100 Å columns; mobile phase, dichloromethane; dual detection, UV (313 nm) and VIS (436 nm) (from Landen & Eitenmiller, 1979).

Figure 53(b) shows the separation of the oil from the retinyl palmitate and β-carotene fraction during the second pass. The refractive index response indicated virtually complete removal of the oil from the vitamin fraction. The reversed-phase HPLC chromatograms of retinyl palmitate and β-carotene standards, and of the margarine after gel-permeation HPLC fractionation, are depicted in Fig. 54.

A similar method was applied to the determination of retinyl palmitate in fortified dry breakfast cereals (25–35 g samples). The separation of the retinyl palmitate fraction from the lipid in two cereal samples by gel-permeation HPLC is shown in Fig. 55. The reversed-phase separation of retinyl palmitate detected spectrophotometrically at 313 nm, and BHA detected at 280 nm is shown in Fig. 56; supplemental α-tocopheryl acetate present in a wheat base cereal was also detected at 280 nm. Dual wavelength detection facilitated the calculation of the peak response ratio (313/280 nm) as a measure of peak purity for retinyl palmitate. Recovery of added retinyl palmitate in cereal products was 95·4% $\pm$ 4·22% (Landen, 1980).

8.3.2 Carotenoids
There are two essential requirements for the determination of carotenoids in foods; differentiation between α- and β-carotene and, at the same time,

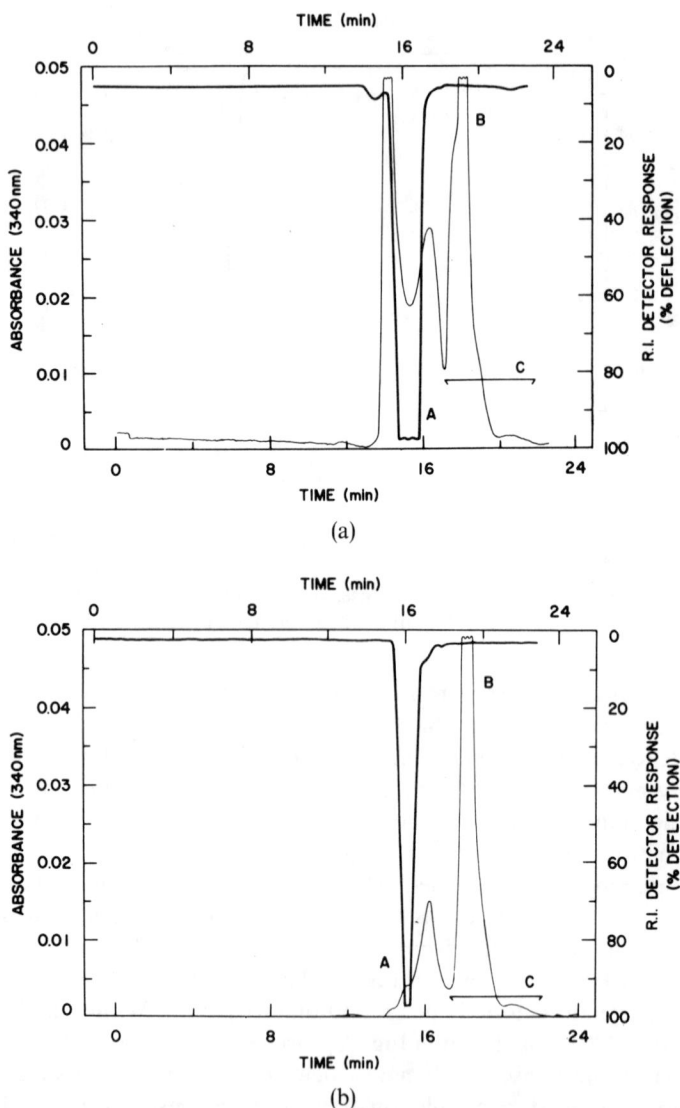

Fig. 53. Gel-permeation HPLC of retinyl palmitate and β-carotene in the lipid portion of margarine. Separation of the lipid (peak A) from the vitamin/carotene fraction (peak B) during (a) the initial pass, and (b) the second pass through μStyragel. Position of the vitamin/carotene fraction collected is indicated by (C). Column and mobile phase as in Fig. 52; dual detection, UV (340 nm) and refractive index (from Landen & Eitenmiller, 1979).

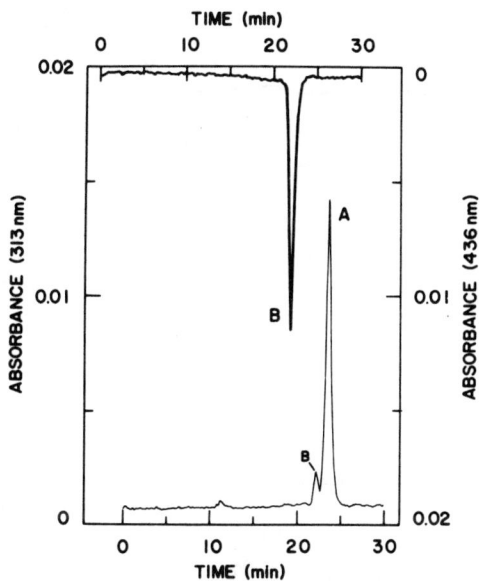

(a)

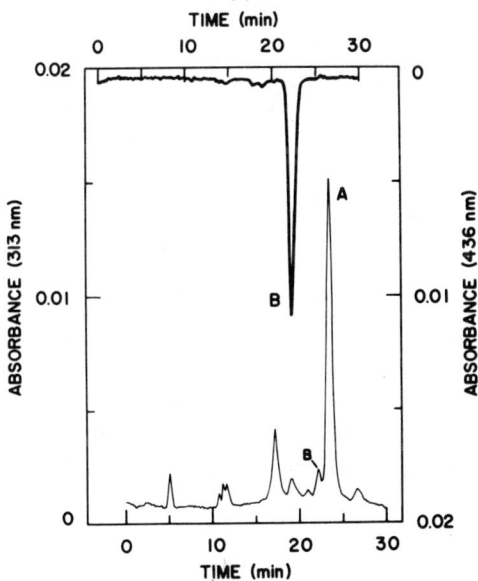

(b)

Fig. 54. Reversed-phase HPLC of retinyl palmitate and β-carotene. (a) Standard mixture of 150 ng retinyl palmitate (peak A) and 60 ng β-carotene (peak B); (b) vitamin/carotene fraction from margarine after two elution passes through μStyragel (see Fig. 53). Column, μBondapak C_{18}; mobile phase, acetonitrile: dichloromethane (70:30); dual detection as in Fig. 52 (from Landen & Eitenmiller, 1979).

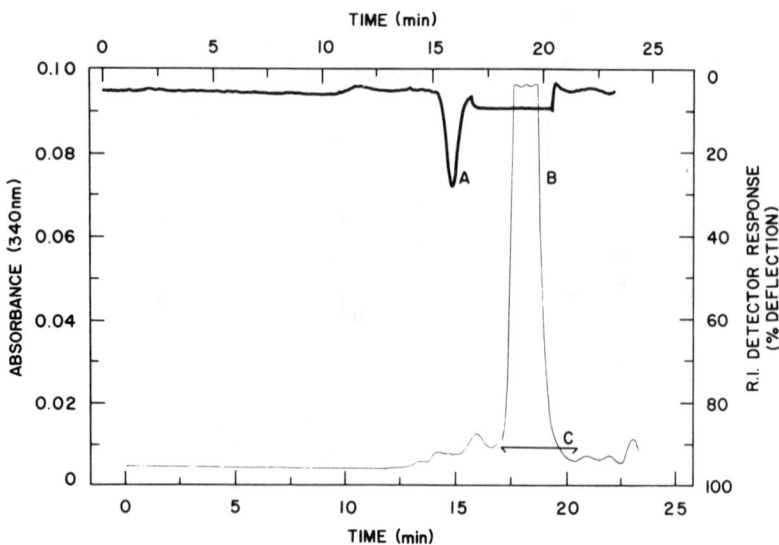

(a)

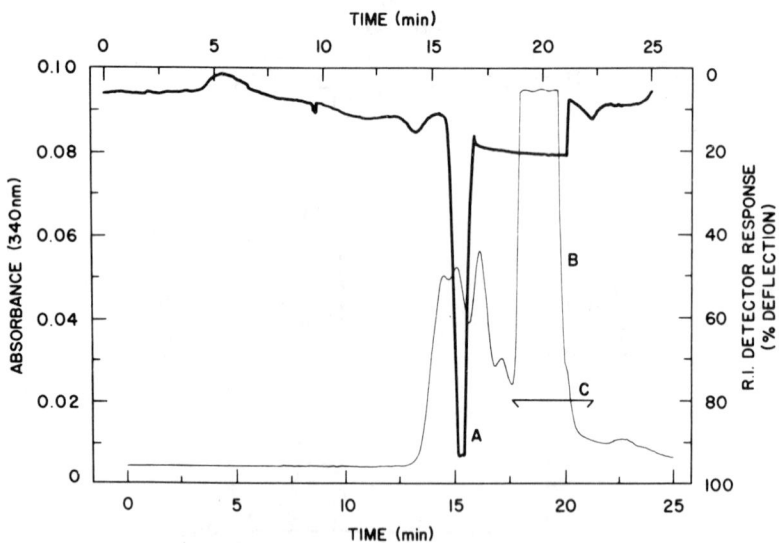

(b)

Fig. 55. Gel-permeation HPLC of retinyl palmitate in the lipid portion of vitamin A-fortified breakfast cereals. Separation of the lipid (peak A) from the vitamin A fraction (peak B) during one pass through μStyragel. (a) Rice-base cereal labelled to contain no fat, (b) wheat-base cereal labelled to contain 1 g fat/1 oz serving (1 oz = 28·4 g). Position of the vitamin A fraction collected is indicated by (C). Column and mobile phase as in Fig. 52; UV detection, 340 nm (from Landen, 1980).

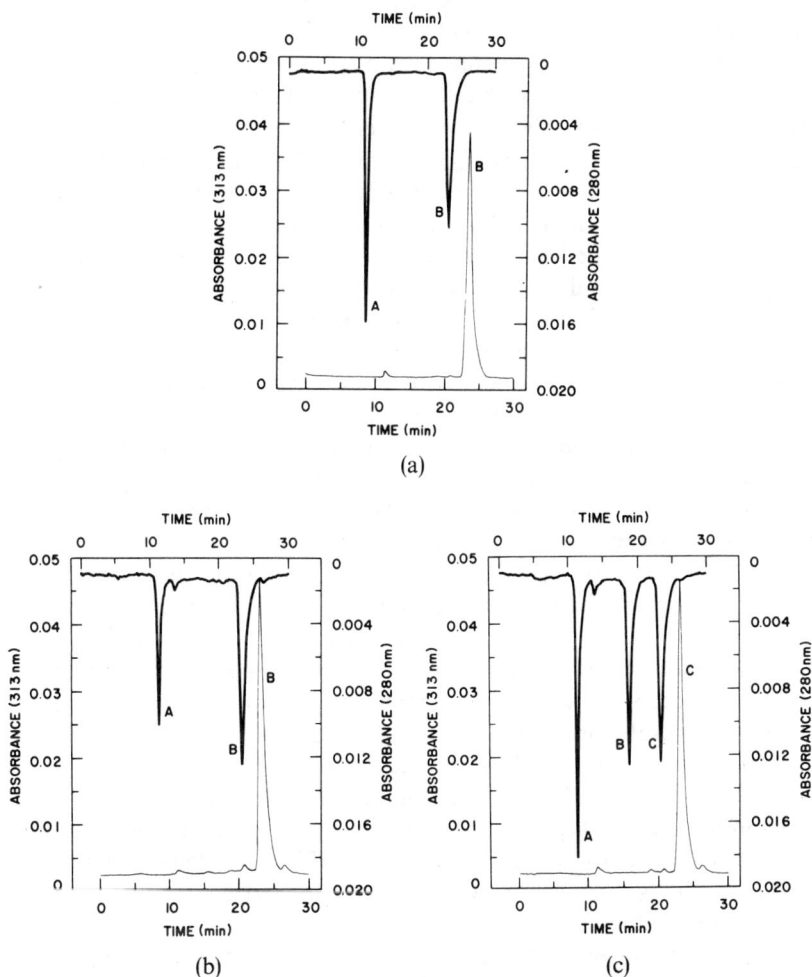

Fig. 56. Reversed-phase HPLC of retinyl palmitate. (a) BHA (peak A) and retinyl palmitate standard (peak B); (b) vitamin fraction from rice-base cereal fortified with vitamin A after gel-permeation HPLC (see Fig. 55). Peak identification as in (a); (c) vitamin fraction from wheat-base cereal fortified with vitamins A and E after gel-permeation HPLC. Peaks: (A) BHA; (B) α-tocopheryl acetate; (C) retinyl palmitate. Column and mobile phase as in Fig. 54; dual UV detection, 313 and 280 nm (from Landen, 1980).

separation of active carotenoids from inactive carotenoids, such as lycopene. If possible, the method should also be capable of resolving *cis* and *trans* isomers of a given carotenoid.

Silica HPLC columns operated with gradient elution facilitate the separation of carotenoids with different functional groups, such as acyclic (e.g. lycopene), monocyclic (e.g. γ-carotene) and bicyclic (e.g. α- and β-carotene) carotenes. *Cis/trans* isomers are also separable on silica, but positional double bond isomers, including α- and β-carotene, are not separable. Quantification of carotenoids by adsorption HPLC on silica columns is unreliable because silica catalyses on-column degradation of carotenoids, presumably due to too strong interactions with active sites (Lambert *et al.*, 1985). The use of nitrile (Gillan & Johns, 1983) or amino (Bushway, 1985) bonded-phase columns overcomes the problem of on-column degradation of carotenoids without affecting selectivity.

In adsorption HPLC using isocratic elution, the carotenoids are eluted as an unresolved group near the solvent front. This technique has been applied to the determination of β-carotene in margarine (Thompson *et al.*, 1980) and in cheese (Stancher & Zonta, 1982) since, in these products, β-carotene is the predominant carotenoid.

Unlike adsorption HPLC, reversed-phase systems are capable of separating positional double bond isomers of carotenoids, such as α- and β-carotene, and there is little risk of on-column carotenoid degeneration on the non-polar bonded phase. Strong mobile phases containing little or no water are necessary to elute carotenoids from reversed-phase columns. NARP is generally preferred for the chromatography of the hydrocarbon carotenoids, such as α- and β-carotene (Fisher & Rouseff, 1986).

Reversed-phase HPLC has been employed to determine β-carotene in milk products and margarine after saponification (Thompson & Maxwell, 1977) and in margarine after gel-permeation HPLC (Landen & Eitenmiller, 1979). Methods for determining naturally occurring carotenoids are presented in Table 25.

Bushway & Wilson (1982) determined the α- and β-carotene contents of fruits and vegetables. Carrots were extracted with a mixture of anhydrous sodium sulphate, magnesium carbonate and tetrahydrofuran (THF). The combined extracts were filtered, concentrated to 75 ml by rotary evaporation at 40°C then diluted to 100 ml with THF for HPLC. Other vegetables and fruit were extracted in a similar manner, and the filtrate was partitioned into petroleum spirit. The combined petroleum fractions were dried, evaporated, then finally dissolved in 0·3 ml of THF for HPLC. The final THF solutions were analysed on a 250 mm × 4·6 mm i.d. Partisil

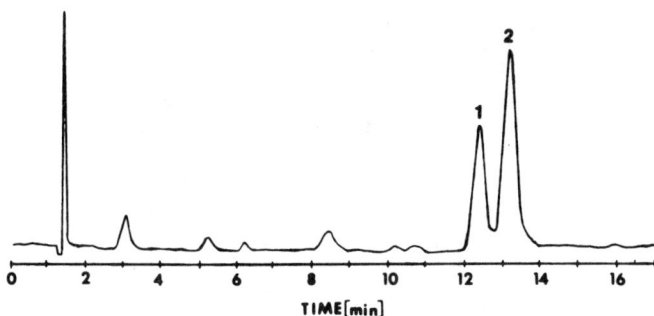

Fig. 57. Reversed-phase HPLC of carotenes in purified extract of carrot. Peaks: (1) α-carotene; (2) β-carotene. Column, Partisil 5 ODS; mobile phase, acetonitrile: tetrahydrofuran:water (85:12·5:2·5); VIS detection, 470 nm (from Bushway & Wilson, 1982).

5 ODS column eluted with acetonitrile:THF:water (85:12·5:2·5) and monitored spectrophotometrically at 470 nm (see Fig. 57). The mean recovery of β-carotene from spiked raw carrots was 100·5%. RSDs of α-carotene and β-carotene for a variety of products ranged from 1·3% to 6·4%.

Speek *et al.* (1986) employed saponification followed by extraction with diisopropyl ether for the determination of β-carotene in vegetables. The HPLC system comprised a 250 mm × 4·6 mm i.d. 3 μm Hypersil ODS column eluted with acetonitrile:methanol:chloroform:water (250:200:90:11) and a spectrophotometric detector set at 445 nm. This system afforded a good separation of α-, β- and γ-carotenes from other carotenoids (Fig. 58). Recoveries of β-carotene added to salad and spinach ranged from 96 to 100%.

Zakaria *et al.* (1979) separated and measured the concentrations of β-carotene and lycopene in tomatoes using NARP. The total pigment content was extracted with acetone, and the non-polar material was partitioned into petroleum spirit. The combined petroleum solutions were washed with water to remove the acetone, and then evaporated to dryness using a rotary evaporator. The residue was subjected to overnight alkaline digestion at ambient temperature, then extracted with petroleum spirit. The petroleum solution was concentrated to 100 ml by rotary evaporation, and kept at −10°C overnight to allow precipitation of the sterols. Aliquots of the filtered petroleum solution were injected onto a 250 mm × 4·6 mm i.d. Partisil ODS column eluted with acetonitrile:chloroform (92:8) and monitored by absorbance measurement at 470 nm. The carotenoids were

Table 25

HPLC methods used for carotenoids

Analyte	Sample type	Sample preparation	Quantitative HPLC			Reference/ Fig. no.
			Stationary phase	Mobile phase	Detection	
α- and β-Carotenes	Fruits, vegetables	Extraction with $THF + Na_2SO_4 + MgCO_3$, filtration, partition into petroleum spirit, evaporation	Partisil ODS	MeCN:THF:H_2O (85:12.5:2.5)	VIS 470 nm	Bushway & Wilson (1982) (Fig. 57)
β-Carotene	Vegetables	Saponification, diisopropyl ether extraction, evaporation	Hypersil ODS (3 μm)	MeCN:MeOH:$CHCl_3$:H_2O (250:200:90:11)	VIS 445 nm	Speek et al. (1986) (Fig. 58)
β-Carotene, lycopene	Tomatoes	Acetone extraction, partition into petroleum spirit, evaporation, alkaline digestion (ambient), petroleum spirit extraction, precipitation of sterols by freezing	Partisil ODS	MeCN:$CHCl_3$ (92:8)	VIS 470 nm	Zakaria et al. (1979) (Fig. 59)

Compound	Sample	Preparation	Column	Mobile phase	Detection	Reference
α- and β-Carotenes	Fruit, vegetables	Extraction with acetone:petroleum spirit (1:1), top layer evaporated	μBondapak C$_{18}$	MeCN:CHCl$_3$ (92:8)	VIS 436 nm	Hsieh & Karel (1983)
Zeinoxanthin, β-Cryptoxanthin, α-Carotene, β-Carotene, cis-β-Carotene	Orange juice	Saponification, hexane extraction, evaporation, magnesia column chromatography, evaporation of eluate	Vydac TP 201 C$_{18}$	MeOH:CHCl$_3$ (94:6)	VIS 475 nm	Quackenbush & Smallidge (1986) (Fig. 61)
α- and β-Carotenes, lycopene	Olive oil	Alkaline digestion (ambient), diethyl ether extraction, evaporation	Supelcosil LC-18	MeCN:Pr-2-OH: 1,2-dichloroethane (92·5:5·0:2·5)	VIS 458 nm	Stancher et al. (1987) (Fig. 62)

Abbreviations: see foot of Table 24.

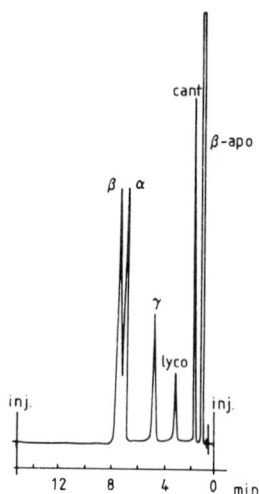

Fig. 58. Reversed-phase HPLC of carotenoid standards. Peaks: (β-apo) β-apo-8'-carotenal; (cant) canthaxanthin; (lyco) lycopene; (γ) γ-carotene; (α) α-carotene; (β) β-carotene. Column, 3 μm Hypersil ODS; mobile phase, acetonitrile:methanol:chloroform:water (250:200:90:11); VIS detection, 445 nm (from Speek *et al.*, 1986).

identified by obtaining stopped-flow spectra of the chromatographic peaks. The HPLC system was capable of separating α-carotene from β-carotene within an elution time of 15 min; lycopene was eluted at about 8 min (see Fig. 59).

Hsieh & Karel (1983) employed a more rapid extraction method, for the determination of α- and β-carotene in fruits and vegetables. Samples were extracted with acetone:petroleum spirit (1:1) until the upper layer became completely colourless. The upper layer was evaporated under vacuum at 30°C, and the residue was dissolved in petroleum spirit before injection onto a 300 mm × 3·9 mm i.d. μBondapak C_{18} column eluted with acetontrile:chloroform (92:8). The detection wavelength was 436 nm. Recoveries of β-carotene added to tomatoes and to dried apricots were 91% and 99% respectively. The RSDs of α-carotene and β-carotene were, respectively, 3·0% and 4·2%.

Bushway (1985) demonstrated the separation of canthaxanthin, β-cryptoxanthin, γ-carotene, α-carotene and β-carotene on a 150 mm × 3·9 mm i.d. Nova-PAK C_{18} column eluted with acetonitrile:methanol:THF (58:35:7) (Fig. 60).

Quackenbush & Smallidge (1986) employed NARP on various 250 mm × 4·6 mm i.d. Vydac C_{18} columns (Vydac TP 201 5 μm or 10 μm; Vydac TP 218) eluted with methanol:chloroform (90:10) and monitored spectrophotometrically at 475 nm to separate carotenes and monohydroxy-carotenoid standards. The system produced baseline separation

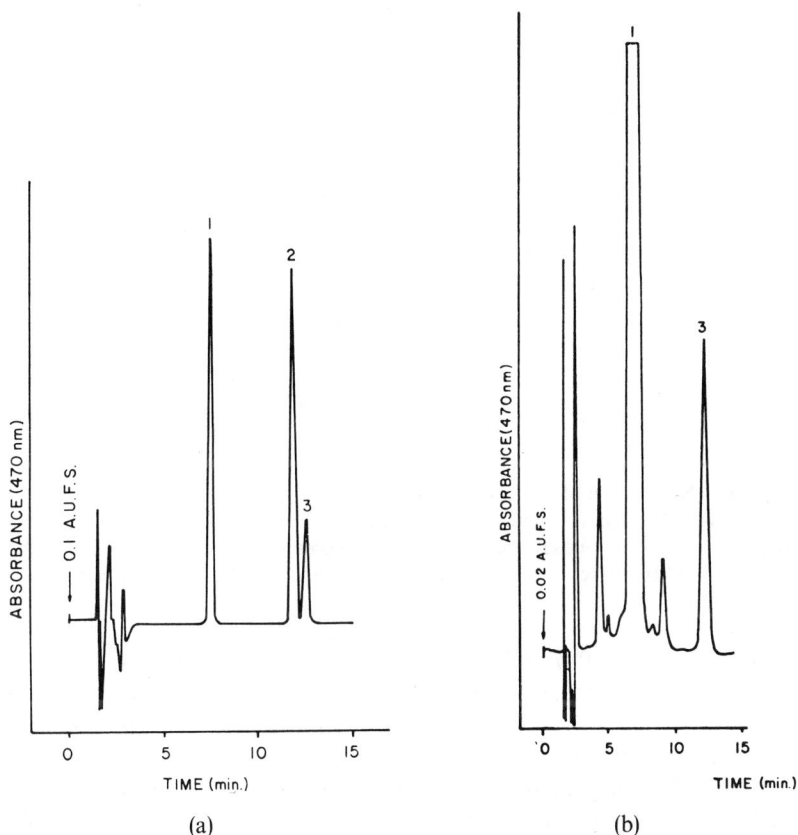

Fig. 59. NARP of carotenes. (a) Carotene standards; (b) purified unsaponifiable material from tomatoes. Peaks: (1) lycopene; (2) α-carotene; (3) β-carotene. Column, Partisil ODS; mobile phase, acetonitrile:chloroform (92:8); VIS detection, 470 nm (from Zakaria *et al.*, 1979).

of β-carotene, α-carotene and β-cryptoxanthin from the biologically inactive zeinoxanthin. The authors proposed that carotenoid esters be saponified, and interfering pigments (residual chlorophylls and xantho-phylls other than cryptoxanthin) removed by open-column chroma-tography on magnesia prior to HPLC. A chromatogram showing the carotenoids present in a purified extract of frozen orange juice, with Sudan I as an internal standard, is depicted in Fig. 61. Vydac columns were also investigated by Bushway (1985).

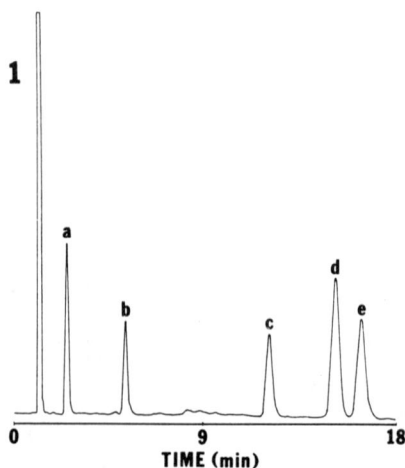

Fig. 60. Separation of carotenoid standards by NARP. Peaks: (a) canthaxanthin; (b) β-cryptoxanthin; (c) γ-carotene; (d) α-carotene; (e) β-carotene. Column, Nova-PAK C_{18}; mobile phase, acetonitrile:methanol:tetrahydrofuran (58:35:7); VIS detection, 470 nm (Reprinted from Bushway, 1985, p. 1541, by courtesy of Marcel Dekker, Inc.).

Stancher *et al.* (1987) utilized NARP for the determination of α-carotene, β-carotene and lycopene in olive oil. Oil samples were subjected to overnight alkaline digestion at ambient temperature; the saponified mixture was extracted with diethyl ether; and the washed ether extract was dried, filtered, then evaporated under vacuum. The remaining oil was dissolved in 1,2-dichloroethane for HPLC using a 150 mm × 4·6 mm i.d. Supelcosil LC-18 column eluted with acetonitrile:isopropanol:1,2-dichloroethane (92·5:5·0:2·5) and a detection wavelength of 458 nm. Lycopene, and α- and β-carotenes, with retention times of approximately 9, 15, and 17 min, respectively, were well separated from three major polar carotenoids, which appeared only partially resolved from one another at about 3 min (see Fig. 62). Spectra of the carotene peaks were recorded by stop-flow scanning. The recovery value obtained with β-carotene was 92%.

Most reversed-phase column packings eluted with non-aqueous mobile phases exhibit too low a retention for the more polar carotenoids. Concomitant chromatography of xanthophylls and carotenes has been carried out using gradient elution, starting from semi-aqueous eluting conditions and finishing with a strong solvent component. However, the use of semi-aqueous mobile phases impairs chromatographic efficiency and peak shape, because of poor sample solubility (Lambert *et al.*, 1985).

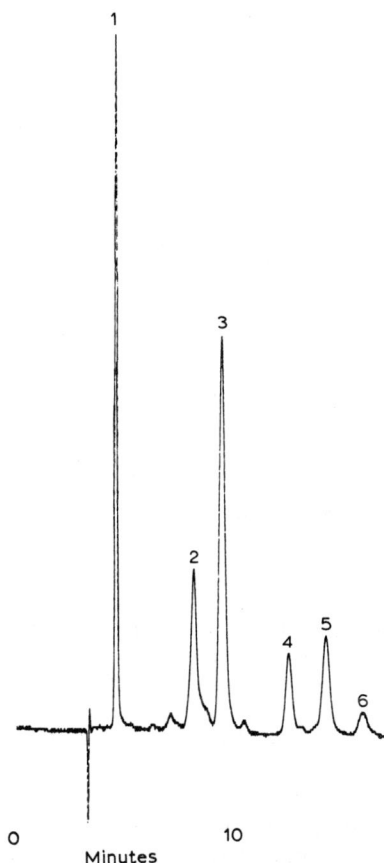

Fig. 61.   NARP of carotenoids in the unsaponifiable matter from frozen orange juice concentrate after magnesia column clean-up. Peaks; (1) Sudan I (internal standard); (2) zeinoxanthin; (3) β-cryptoxanthin; (4) α-carotene; (5) β-carotene; (6) cis-β-carotene. Column, Vydac TP 201 C_{18}; mobile phase, methanol:chloroform (94:6), VIS detection, 475 nm (from Quackenbush & Smallidge, 1986).

To obviate the problem of poor sample solubility associated with semi-aqueous mobile phases, a highly retentive column packing material, such as Zorbax ODS, can be used. Such column packings, operated with non-aqueous mobile phases, separate a wide range of carotenoid standards, without the need for gradient elution. A 250 mm × 4·6 mm i.d. 7 μm Zorbax ODS column eluted with acetonitrile:dichloromethane:methanol (70:20:10) separated nine carotenoid standards, varying from the polar

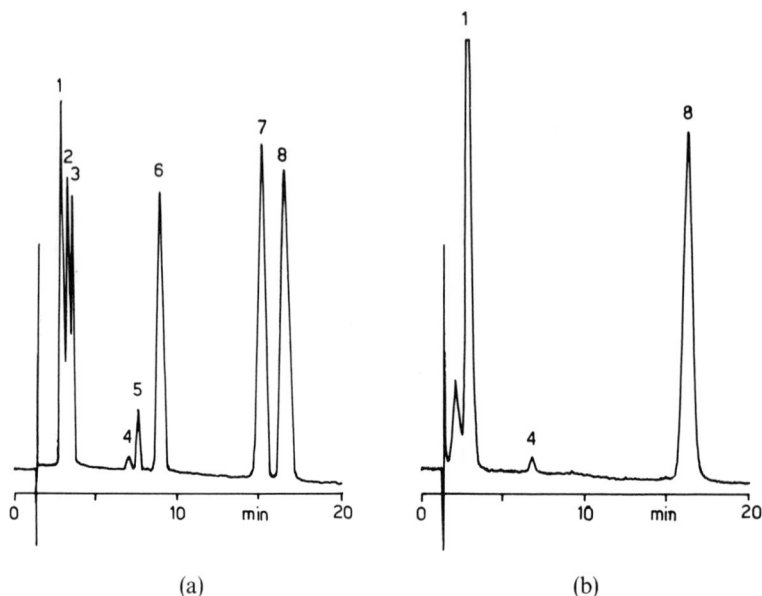

(a)   (b)

Fig. 62. NARP of carotenoids. (a) Carotenoid standards; (b) unsaponifiable matter from olive oil. Peaks: (1) lutein; (2) zeaxanthin; (3) canthaxanthin; (4) β-cryptoxanthin (tentative); (5) β-carotene epoxide; (6) lycopene; (7) α-carotene; (8) β-carotene. Column, Supelcosil LC-18; mobile phase, acetonitrile:isopropanol:1,2-dichloroethane (92·5:5·0:2·5); VIS detection, 458 nm (from Stancher et al., 1987).

xanthophylls to the non-polar carotenes (Nelis & de Leenheer, 1983) (see Fig. 63). The use of n-decanol added at 0·1% by volume as a modifier to a mobile phase of acetonitrile:ethyl acetate (70:30) improved the chromatography of a wide range of carotenoids in terms of stability, enhanced response and greater definition of minor peaks (Lauren et al., 1986).

In the analysis of orange juice, Fisher & Rouseff (1986) modified the isocratic separation of Nelis & de Leenheer (1983) by increasing the solvent strength and flow-rate of the mobile phase to achieve the separation of β-cryptoxanthin, α-carotene and β-carotene in the shortest time possible. The Zorbax ODS column was eluted with acetonitrile:dichloromethane:methanol (65:25:10) and the detection wavelength was 450 nm. The sample preparation entailed extraction of the carotenoids from centrifuged juice solids with methanol; alkaline digestion of the methanol extracts for 1 h at ambient temperature; and clean-up on a 6 ml C_{18} solid-phase extraction column.

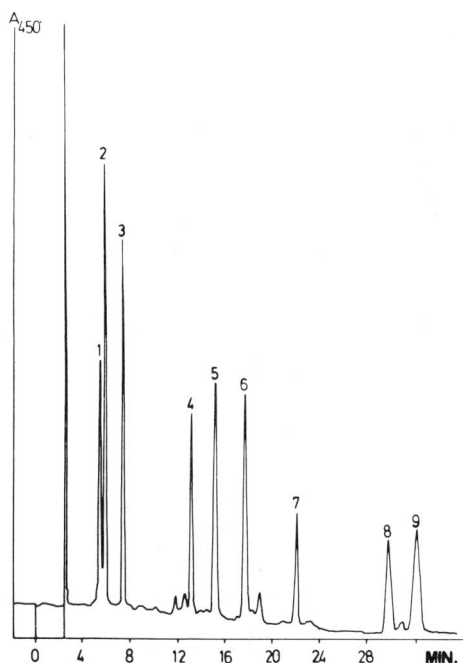

Fig. 63. Separation of carotenoid standards by NARP. Peaks: (1) lutein; (2) zeaxanthin; (3) canthaxanthin; (4) β-cryptoxanthin; (5) echinenone; (6) lycopene; (7) torulene; (8) α-carotene; (9) β-carotene. Column, 7 μm Zorbax ODS; mobile phase, acetonitrile:dichloromethane:methanol (70:20:10); VIS detection, 450 nm (Reprinted with permission from Nelis, H. J. C. F. & de Leenheer, A. P. (1983). Isocratic nonaqueous reversed-phase liquid chromatography of carotenoids. *Analyt. Chem.*, **55**, 270–5). Copyright (1983) American Chemical Society.

8.3.3 Vitamin D

Saponification is the most convenient way of removing the triglycerides from full-fat foods in vitamin D assays. At refluxing temperatures (75–80°C), saponification promotes the thermal isomerization of vitamin D to previtamin D. This poses a problem in the final HPLC analysis as the vitamin D peak in both normal-phase and reversed-phase HPLC is well-separated from the previtamin D peak (de Vries *et al.*, 1979), and it is generally not possible to measure the latter because of interference from coeluting contaminants. To circumvent this problem, the saponification can be performed at ambient temperature overnight. Workers who have

Table 26

HPLC methods used for vitamin D

Analyte	Sample type	Sample preparation	Semi-preparative HPLC	Quantitative HPLC	Reference/ Fig. no.
Vitamin D[a]	Fortified fluid milk (whole)	Alkaline digestion (ambient), diethyl ether extraction, evaporation, hydroxyalkoxypropyl Sephadex column chromatography, evaporation of eluate		LiChrosorb Si-60 50% H_2O-saturated hexane + 0·6% Pr-2-OH UV 265 nm	Thompson et al. (1977) (Fig. 65)
Vitamin D[a]	Fortified milk powder (whole, skimmed)	Saponification, pentane extraction, evaporation, semi-preparative HPLC, evaporation of eluate	Sil-60D-10CN 0·35% amyl alcohol in hexane UV 254 nm	Partisil Silica 0·35% amyl alcohol in hexane UV 254 nm	de Vries & Borsje (1982)
Vitamin D[a]	Animal feeds	Saponification, diethyl ether extraction, evaporation, alumina column chromatography, evaporation of eluate, semi-preparative HPLC, evaporation of eluate	LiChrosorb RP-18 MeCN:MeOH:H_2O (50:50:5) UV 254 nm	Partisil Silica 0·35% amyl alcohol in hexane UV 254 nm	de Vries et al. (1983)
Vitamin D[a]	Fortified fluid milk (whole), infant formulae	Saponification, ether extraction, evaporation, semi-preparative HPLC, evaporation of eluate	Partisil PAC 0·8% amyl alcohol in hexane UV 254 nm	Apex Silica (3 μm) 0·15% amyl alcohol in hexane UV 254 nm	Sertl & Molitor (1985) (Figs 66, 67)
Vitamin D[a]	Fortified whole milk powder	Saponification, benzene extraction, evaporation, semi-preparative HPLC, evaporation of eluate	Nucleosil C_{18} (5 μm) MeOH:MeCN) (1:1) UV 254 nm	Zorbax SIL 0·4% Pr-2-OH in hexane UV 254 nm	Okano et al. (1981) (Figs 68, 69)

Compound	Sample	Procedure	Column 1	Column 2	Reference
Vitamin D[a]	Animal feeds, milk products, liver, fortified foods	Saponification, benzene extraction, evaporation, semi-preparative HPLC, evaporation of eluate	Nucleosil C_{18} (5 μm) MeOH:MeCN (1:1) UV 254 nm	Zorbax SIL 0.4% Pr-2-OH in hexane UV 254 nm	Takeuchi et al. (1984)
Vitamin D_3[a]	Animal feeds	Solvent extraction, evaporation, extraction with MeCN then partition into isooctane, evaporation, silica column chromatography, evaporation of eluate		LiChrosorb-NH_2 Hexane:$CHCl_3$ (70:30) UV 264 nm	Cohen & Lapointe (1979) (Figs 70, 71)
Vitamin D[a]	Fortified non-fat dried milk	CH_2Cl_2 extraction, evaporation, Sep-Pak (silica) clean-up, evaporation of eluate, semi-preparative HPLC, evaporation of eluate	Partisil PAC CH_2Cl_2 UV 254 nm	LiChrosorb-NH_2 CH_2Cl_2:hexane:Pr-2-OH (50:50:2) UV 264 nm	Cohen & Wakeford (1980) (Fig. 72)
Vitamin D_3[a]	Animal feeds	As above, but with Sephadex LH-20 column chromatography after Sep-Pak (silica) clean-up	Partisil PAC CH_2Cl_2 UV 254 nm	LiChrosorb-NH_2 CH_2Cl_2:hexane:Pr-2-OH (50:50:2) UV 264 nm	Cohen & Lapointe (1980b) (Figs 73, 74)
Vitamin D_2 or D_3	Margarine	Vitamin D_2 or D_3 added as internal standard. Saponification, hexane extraction, evaporation, semi-preparative HPLC (two passes), evaporation of eluate	LiChrosorb Si-60 Hexane:CH_2Cl_2 (1:1) UV 295 nm 1st pass; UV 264 nm 2nd pass	Nucleosil C_{18} (5 μm) MeOH:H_2O (95:5) UV 264 nm	van Niekerk & Smit (1980) (Figs 76, 77)

Contd.

Table 26—*contd.*

Analyte	Sample type	Sample preparation	Semi-preparative HPLC	Quantitative HPLC	Reference/ Fig. no.
Vitamin D_3 (naturally occurring)	Eggs, butter, milk, cheese (unfortified)	Eggs, milk concentrated by freeze drying. Vitamin D_2 added as internal standard. Saponification, ether extraction, evaporation, preparation of sterols from a methanolic solution at $0°C$, evaporation of filtrate, preparative TLC, evaporation of extracted vitamin D band		Spherisorb ODS MeOH:H_2O (95:5) UV 265 nm	Jackson et al. (1982)
Vitamin D_2 or D_3	Fortified fluid milk (skimmed), whole milk powder, milk powder with soy bean, chocolate milk powder, diet food	Saponification, petroleum spirit extraction, evaporation, Sep-Pak (silica) clean-up (high fat samples only), evaporation of eluate		Hypersil ODS (two columns) MeOH + 0·5% H_2O UV 265 nm	Bui (1987) (Fig. 78)
Vitamin D_2 or D_3	Fortified fluid milk (whole)	Solvent extraction, formation of methyl esters from triglycerides by alcoholysis, preparative TLC, evaporation of extracted vitamin D band		Ultrasphere ODS MeOH:H_2O (97:3) UV 265 nm	Grace & Bernhard (1984)

Vitamin	Sample	Sample preparation		HPLC conditions	Reference
Vitamin D_2 or D_3	Fortified whole milk powder	Vitamin D_2 or D_3 added as internal standard. Alkaline digestion (ambient), ether extraction, evaporation, precipitation of sterols from a methanolic solution		Two Radial-PAK cartridges containing either RESOLVE C_{18} or Nova-PAK C_{18} MeOH:THF:H_2O (93:2:5) UV 254 and 280 nm (dual)	Indyk & Woollard (1985a) (Figs 79, 80)
Vitamin D_2 or D_3	Infant formulae	Vitamin D_2 or D_3 added as internal standard. Alkaline digestion (ambient), ether extraction, evaporation, silica cartridge clean-up, evaporation of eluate		Column system as above MeOH:THF:H_2O (92:2:6) UV254 and 280 nm (dual)	Indyk & Woollard (1985b) (Fig. 81)
Vitamin D_2 or D_3	Fortified fluid milk (whole, low-fat, skimmed)	Alkaline digestion (ambient), petroleum spirit extraction, evaporation, co-precipitation of sterols with digitonin, petroleum spirit extraction, evaporation, alumina column chromatography, evaporation of eluate		Vydac TP 201 C_{18} MeCN:MeOH (90:10) UV 254 nm	Muniz et al. (1982) (Fig. 82)
Vitamin D_2 or D_3	Fortified fluid milk (whole)	Alkaline digestion (ambient), hexane extraction, evaporation, semi-preparative HPLC, evaporation of eluate	Supelcosil LC-Si 0·5% Pr-2-OH in cyclohexane:hexane (1:1) UV 254 nm	Radial-PAK cartridge containing μBondapak C_{18} or Spherisorb 10 ODS MeCN:MeOH (90:10) UV 254 nm	Thompson et al. (1982) (Fig. 83)

Contd.

Table 26—*contd.*

Analyte	Sample type	Sample preparation	Semi-preparative HPLC	Quantitative HPLC	Reference/ Fig. no.
Vitamin D_2 or D_3	Margarine, infant formulae	As above, but with alumina column chromatography before semi-preparative HPLC	As above, but concentration of Pr-2-OH changed to 0·25%	Radial-PAK cartridge containing μBondapak C_{18} or Spherisorb 10 ODS MeCN:MeOH (90:10) UV 254 nm	Thompson et al. (1982) (Figs 84, 85)
Vitamin D_2 or D_3	Fortified low-fat milk, infant formulae	CH_2Cl_2/Pr-2-OH extraction, evaporation, removal of lipids by GP-HPLC on four μStyragel 100 Å columns eluted with CH_2Cl_2 (UV 280 nm), evaporation of eluate, semi-preparative HPLC, evaporation of eluate	μBondapak-NH_2 CH_2Cl_2:isooctane:Pr-2-OH (600:400:1) UV 280 nm	Zorbax ODS (6 μm) CH_2Cl_2:MeCN:MeOH (300:700:2) UV 254 and 280 nm (dual)	Landen (1985) (Figs 86, 87)

[a]Method unable to distinguish between vitamins D_2 or D_3.
Abbreviations: see foot of Table 24.

saponified at refluxing temperatures have had to compensate for the formation of previtamin D.

Further clean-up to remove sterols, vitamin E vitamers, carotenoids and other interfering material from the unsaponifiable matter is usually necessary in vitamin D assays. This can be achieved in the analysis of fortified foods and animal feeds using one or more of the following techniques; sterol precipitation, open-column chromatography, and semi-preparative HPLC that is different in principle to the final HPLC separation. Sample preparation techniques used in vitamin D assays are summarized in Table 26.

Normal-phase HPLC, using either silica adsorption columns or polar bonded-phase columns, separates previtamin D and vitamin D from all inactive isomers (de Vries *et al.*, 1979). A chromatogram showing the separation of previtamin D_3, *trans*-vitamin D_3, lumisterol$_3$, isotachy-sterol$_3$, *cis*-vitamin D_3 (active form), tachysterol$_3$, 4,6-cholestadienol and 7-dehydrocholesterol (provitamin D_3) is depicted in Fig. 64. A disadvantage of normal-phase HPLC is that it is incapable of resolving vitamins D_2 and

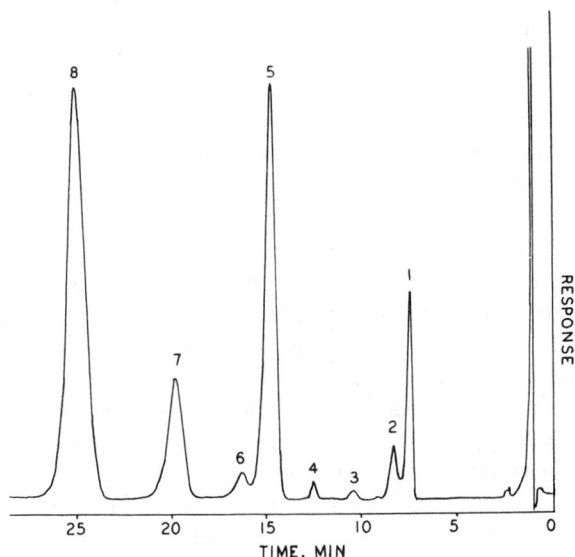

Fig. 64. Adsorption HPLC of vitamin D_3 and its isomers. Peaks: (1) previtamin D_3; (2) *trans*-vitamin D_3; (3) lumisterol$_3$; (4) isotachysterol$_3$; (5) *cis*-vitamin D_3; (6) tachysterol$_3$; (7) 4,6-cholestadienol; (8) 7-dehydrocholesterol (provitamin D_3). Column, LiChrosorb Si-60; mobile phase, hexane containing 0·3% amyl alcohol; UV detection, 254 nm (from de Vries *et al.*, 1979).

D_3 (Fong et al., 1983). In principle, this is not important in the analysis of fortified products, as supplementation is usually carried out with either vitamin D_2 or D_3, and any naturally occurring vitamin D that may be present is usually below the limit of detection. However, in practice, this lack of separation precludes adding vitamin D_2 to the sample at the start of the analytical procedure to act as an internal standard for the quantification of vitamin D_3 (or vice versa). Internal standardization is desirable, in view of the multi-step procedure, to compensate for any losses of vitamin D that may be incurred, including any conversion of vitamin D to previtamin D by thermal isomerization.

Thompson et al. (1977) used low-pressure column chromatography on hydroxyalkoxypropyl Sephadex (HAPS) to purify the unsaponifiable fraction of fortified whole fluid milk prior to the determination of vitamin D on a silica HPLC column. Milk samples (50 g) were subjected to alkaline digestion at ambient temperature overnight in the presence of pyrogallol. The unsaponifiable matter was extracted with diethyl ether and finally with hexane, and the combined extracts were washed with water and evaporated to dryness under vacuum at 60°C. The residue was dissolved in 0·3–0·5 ml of hexane and applied to a 60 cm × 1 cm glass column packed with HAPS. The column was connected to a low-pressure pump and the absorbance of the effluent was monitored at 254 nm. Most of the UV-absorbing material eluted during the first 50 min of chromatography; the bulk of the unsaponifiable matter was held on the column for at least 95 min. The vitamin D fraction was collected between 65 min and 90 min, and evaporated to dryness in a stream of nitrogen. The residue was dissolved in 0·2 ml of hexane, and chromatographed on a 250 mm × 3·2 mm i.d. LiChrosorb Si-60 column eluted with 50% water-saturated hexane containing 0·6% isopropanol and monitored at 265 nm (see Fig. 65). The mean recovery of vitamin D from spiked samples of milk was 97·9%. The high percentage recovery indicated that the cold saponification procedure resulted in negligible isomerization of vitamin D to previtamin D.

de Vries & Borsje (1982) employed normal-phase HPLC on a polar bonded-phase column to purify the unsaponifiable fraction of vitamin D-fortified milk powder (skimmed and whole milk) prior to measurement of the vitamin D peak on a silica HPLC column. Samples (50 g) of milk powder were saponified for 45 min at 80°C on a steam bath in the presence of sodium ascorbate, and the unsaponifiable matter was extracted with pentane. The combined pentane extracts were washed with alcoholic KOH solution, and then washed with water to neutral pH. The pentane extract was dried by adding filter paper strips, and then evaporated to dryness

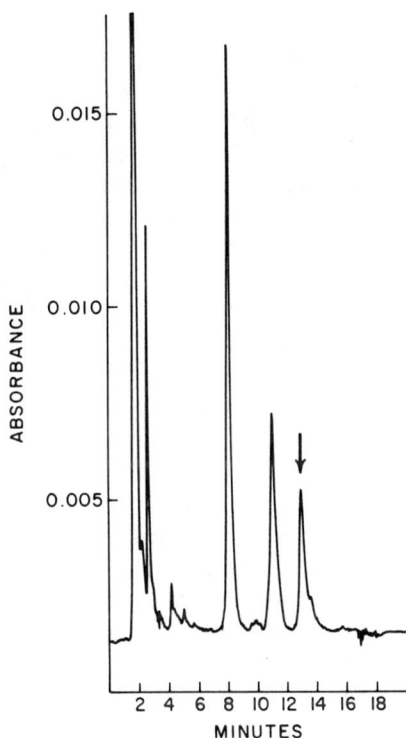

Fig. 65. Adsorption HPLC of vitamin D in the unsaponifiable matter from vitamin D-fortified whole fluid milk after hydroxyalkoxypropyl Sephadex (HAPS) column clean-up. Arrow denotes vitamin D peak. Column, LiChrosorb Si-60; mobile phase, 50% water-saturated hexane containing 0·6% isopropanol; UV detection, 265 nm (from Thompson *et al.*, 1977).

under vacuum at $< 40°C$ in the presence of BHT. The residue was dissolved in 2·0 ml of hexane:toluene (95:5), and a 200 μl aliquot of this solution was analysed on a 250 mm × 4·6 mm i.d. nitrile bonded-phase column of Sil-60D-10CN. Elution of the preparative HPLC column was effected with hexane containing 0·35% amyl alcohol, and the absorbance of the effluent was monitored at 254 nm. The vitamin D fraction (collected in a 10 ml volumetric flask) was evaporated to dryness under nitrogen, in the presence of added BHT, and the residue was dissolved in 2·0 ml of hexane:toluene (95:5). A 500 μl aliquot of this purified extract was injected onto a 250 mm × 4·6 mm i.d. 5 μm Partisil Silica column eluted with 0·35% amyl alcohol in hexane, and monitored at 254 nm. This method, which was subjected to a collaborative study, has been adopted as Official First Action by the AOAC (AOAC, 1984*i*). The saponification conditions employed (45 min at 80°C) result in a constant ratio of previtamin D/vitamin D, and a vitamin D_3 standard subjected to the entire analytical procedure gave 80% vitamin D_3 on analysis. Therefore, results of the HPLC method were multiplied by the factor 1·25 to allow for the formation of previtamin D during refluxing for saponification (Borsje *et al.*, 1982).

For the determination of vitamin D in animal feeds and pet foods (de Vries *et al.*, 1983), the unsaponifiable matter was subjected to open-column chromatography on alumina to remove vitamin E and carotenes, and then to semi-preparative HPLC on a reversed-phase column for further clean-up. The quantification was performed using adsorption HPLC. The procedure was as follows.

Samples were saponified in the presence of sodium ascorbate and EDTA (ethylenediaminetetraacetic acid, disodium salt). The unsaponifiable matter was extracted with diethyl ether, and the combined ether layer was washed with KOH solution followed by water until neutral to phenolphthalein. Petroleum spirit was added, and the dried ether layer was evaporated under vacuum at 40°C in the presence of BHT. The residue was dissolved in 5 ml of hexane, and the hexane solution was quantitatively transferred, with the aid of additional hexane, to a glass column packed with neutral alumina deactivated with petroleum spirit. The hexane eluate, which contained the carotenes, was discarded, after which vitamin E and the antioxidant ethoxyquin (if present) were removed by elution with hexane:diethyl ether (92:8). The column was then eluted with hexane:diethyl ether (60:40), discarding the first 20–25 ml of eluate. The eluate, containing vitamins A and D, was collected when the front of the fluorescent vitamin A band (located by means of a portable UV lamp) reached 3 cm from the bottom of the column. The eluate was evaporated under vacuum, transferred to a centrifuge tube with diethyl ether, re-evaporated, and dissolved in 1·0 ml of methanol with warming. Acetonitrile (1·0 ml) was added, and the clear supernatant was injected onto a 250 mm × 4·6 mm i.d. LiChrosorb RP-18 column eluted with acetonitrile:methanol:water (50:50:5). The vitamin D fraction, detected photometrically at 254 nm, was collected and evaporated under nitrogen in the presence of BHT. The residue was dissolved in 2·0 ml of the next HPLC mobile phase:toluene (95:5) and analysed on a 250 mm × 4·6 mm i.d. 5 μm Partisil silica column. The mobile phase of hexane containing 0·35% amyl alcohol was monitored at 254 nm. The correction factor of 1·25 was applied to account for the thermal isomerization of vitamin D. The method has been adopted as the AOAC Official Final Action (AOAC, 1984*j*).

Sertl & Molitor (1985) used a similar procedure to that described by de Vries & Borsje (1982) for the analysis of vitamin D-fortified milk and infant formula foods, but with simplified extraction and clean-up steps. Milk samples (15 ml) were saponified for 30 min in a 75°C water bath in the presence of ascorbic acid. The unsaponifiable matter was extracted with a mixture of petroleum spirit and diethyl ether. The ether layer was washed successively with water and ethanol, then evaporated to dryness under vacuum. The residue was dissolved in acetone and evaporated to dryness again. The extract was reconstituted with diethyl ether, transferred to a centrifuge tube, and evaporated to dryness with nitrogen. The residue was dissolved in hexane, and applied to a 250 mm × 4·6 mm i.d. amino-nitrile bonded-phase column of 5 μm Partisil PAC preceded by a guard column (30 mm × 4·6 mm i.d.) packed with Spheri-5-Amino (Brownlee Laboratories). Elution of the clean-up column was carried out with 0·8% amyl alcohol in hexane, using absorbance detection at 254 nm. The vitamin D fraction of milk and infant formulae from the semi-preparative column (see Fig. 66) was collected in a 12 ml vial and evaporated to dryness with nitrogen. The residue was dissolved in hexane for quantitative chromatography on a 150 mm × 4·5 mm i.d. 3 μm Apex Silica column with photometric monitoring at 254 nm. The mobile phase was hexane containing 0·15% amyl alcohol. The chromatograms of the vitamin D fractions obtained by semi-preparative HPLC on the analytical HPLC column are displayed in Fig. 67. The chromatography did not separate vitamins D_2 and D_3. The mean recovery of added vitamin D from milk was 97%. Within-day precision was 4·5% RSD, whilst the overall method RSD (reflecting technician-to-technician, day-to-day, and within-day variability) was 7·7%. A 30 min saponification at 75°C was calculated to produce a constant ratio mixture of 14% previtamin D : 86% vitamin D based on the rate constants published by Keverling Buisman et al. (1968). Hence, a factor of 1·16 was used to obtain the potential vitamin D content.

Okano et al. (1981) used a reversed-phase HPLC column to clean up the unsaponifiable fraction of vitamin D-fortified whole milk powder prior to measurement of the vitamin D peak on a silica column. Samples (1 g) of fortified dried milk were saponified by refluxing for 30 min at 80°C in the presence of pyrogallol in an atmosphere of argon. The unsaponifiable matter was extracted with benzene, and the benzene extract was washed successively with aqueous KOH solution and water. The benzene extract was filtered and evaporated to dryness under vacuum below 40°C. The residue was dissolved in 500 μl of the mobile phase (methanol:acetonitrile; 1:1) and the vitamin D_2 fraction was isolated on a 300 mm × 7·5 mm i.d.

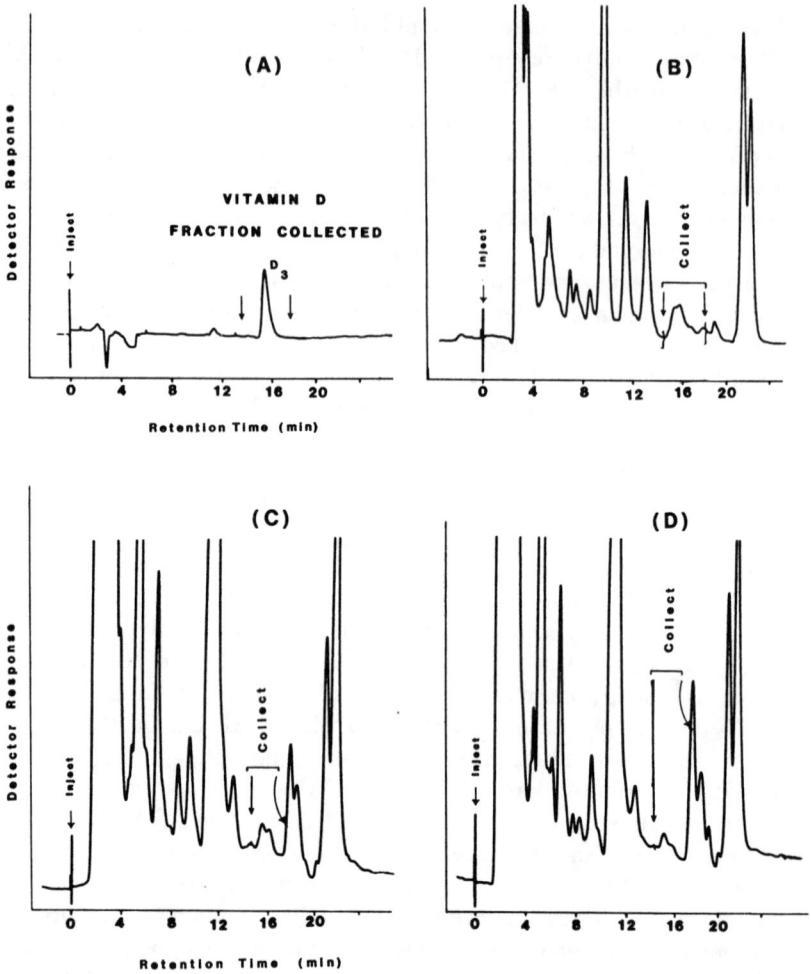

Fig. 66. Semi-preparative normal-phase HPLC of vitamin D in the unsaponifiable matter from vitamin D-fortified (B) whole milk, (C) milk-based infant formula, and (D) soy-based infant formula; (A) vitamin D standard. Position of vitamin D fraction collected is indicated by arrows. Column, Partisil PAC; mobile phase, hexane containing 0·8% amyl alcohol; UV detection, 254 nm (from Sertl & Molitor, 1985).

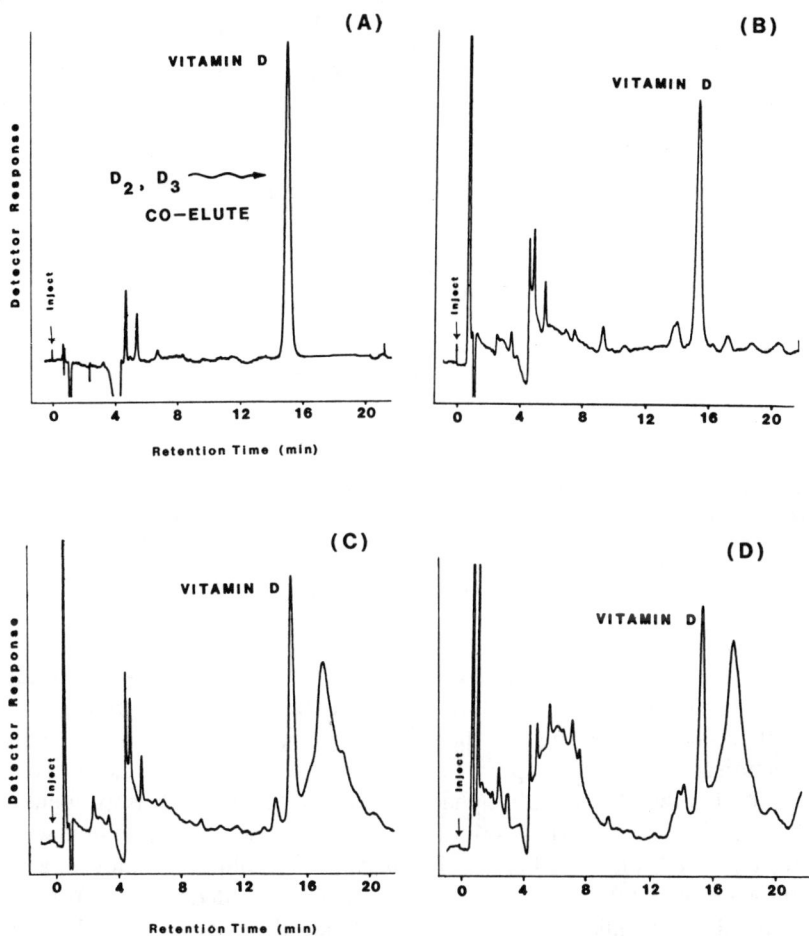

Fig. 67. Adsorption HPLC of the vitamin D fraction isolated by semi-preparative HPLC (Fig. 66) from vitamin D-fortified (B) whole milk, (C) milk-based infant formula, and (D) soy-based infant formula; (A) vitamin D standard. Column, 3 μm Apex Silica; mobile phase, hexane containing 0·15% amyl alcohol; UV detection, 254 nm (from Sertl & Molitor, 1985).

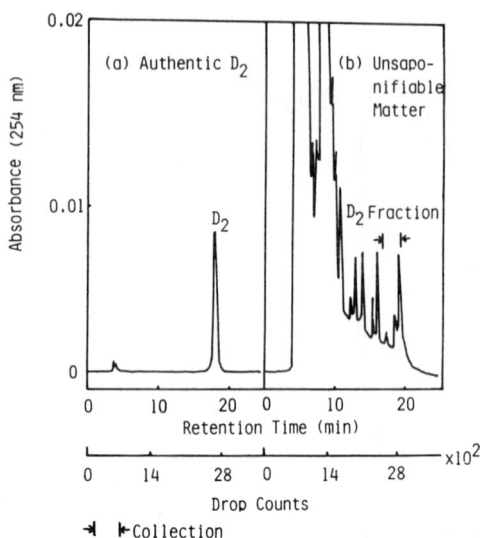

Fig. 68. Semi-preparative reversed-phase HPLC of (a) authentic vitamin D_2 and (b) vitamin D in the unsaponifiable matter from vitamin D_2-fortified whole milk powder. Position of vitamin D fraction collected is indicated by arrows. Column, Nucleosil C_{18}; mobile phase, methanol:acetonitrile (1:1); UV detection, 254 nm (from Okano *et al.*, 1981).

Nucleosil $5C_{18}$ reversed-phase HPLC column using a 254 nm fixed-wavelength absorbance detector. A chromatogram of the semi-preparative HPLC is depicted in Fig. 68. The vitamin D_2 fraction (collected in a mini-fraction collector) was evaporated to dryness, and the residue was dissolved in 200 μl of the second mobile phase (hexane containing 0·4% isopropanol) for analysis on a 250 mm × 4·6 mm i.d. Zorbax SIL silica column with detection at 254 nm (see Fig. 69). The silica HPLC column was not capable of separating vitamins D_2 and D_3. The recovery of added vitamin D_2 from fortified dried milk was 94·3% with a standard deviation of 2·3%. The 254 nm fixed-wavelength detector, which was capable of operating at 0·001 AUFS, enabled a relatively small (1 g) sample size to be taken. The reduced amount of contaminating lipophilic material in the sample obviated the need for cumbersome clean-up procedures, such as open-column chromatography or preparative TLC. In routine assays the whole procedure was applied to the sample and a standard solution of vitamin D_2 simultaneously, so that the assayed value of the sample was exactly corrected for thermal isomerization by comparing the peak height with that

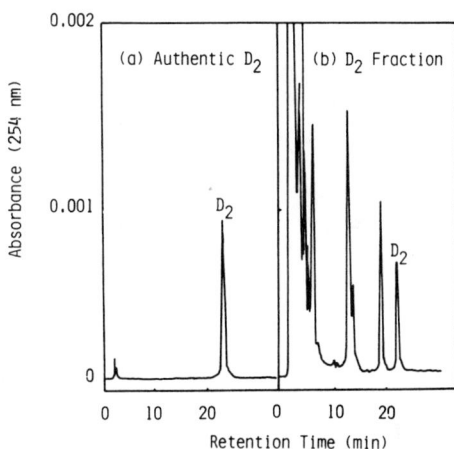

Fig. 69.   Adsorption HPLC of (a) authentic vitamin D_2 and (b) the vitamin D fraction isolated by semi-preparative HPLC (Fig. 68) of vitamin D_2-fortified whole milk powder. Column, Zorbax SIL; mobile phase, hexane containing 0·4% isopropanol; UV detection, 254 nm (from Okano *et al.*, 1981).

obtained from the vitamin D_2 standard solution. The procedure described was also applied to the determination of vitamin D in animal feeds, milk products, liver and fortified foods (Takeuchi *et al.*, 1984).

Cohen & Lapointe (1979) determined the vitamin D_3 content of animal feeds using a liquid partition step as a preliminary clean-up after extraction, then further clean-up on an open column of silica before final analysis by normal-phase HPLC. Feed samples were extracted with a mixture of isooctane:dioxan (80:20), filtered, then shaken with 0·3 ml of tetraethylenepentamine to render the chlorophyll partly insoluble before evaporation to near dryness under vacuum. The residue was extracted with acetonitrile, and the filtered extracts were evaporated to 60–80 ml. The acetonitrile solution was extracted with isooctane, and the isooctane solution was shaken with sodium phosphate tribasic to precipitate inorganic salts, and to remove any traces of amine. After filtration and evaporation to dryness, the residue was dissolved in benzene and transferred to a glass column containing 10 g of silica gel. The column was washed with benzene to remove any oily compounds and most of the carotenoid pigments, and the fat-soluble vitamins were then eluted with benzene containing 1% ethyl acetate. The vitamin fraction was evaporated to dryness, and the residue was dissolved in chloroform for analysis on a 250 mm × 4·2 mm i.d. LiChrosorb-NH_2 column. The mobile phase was

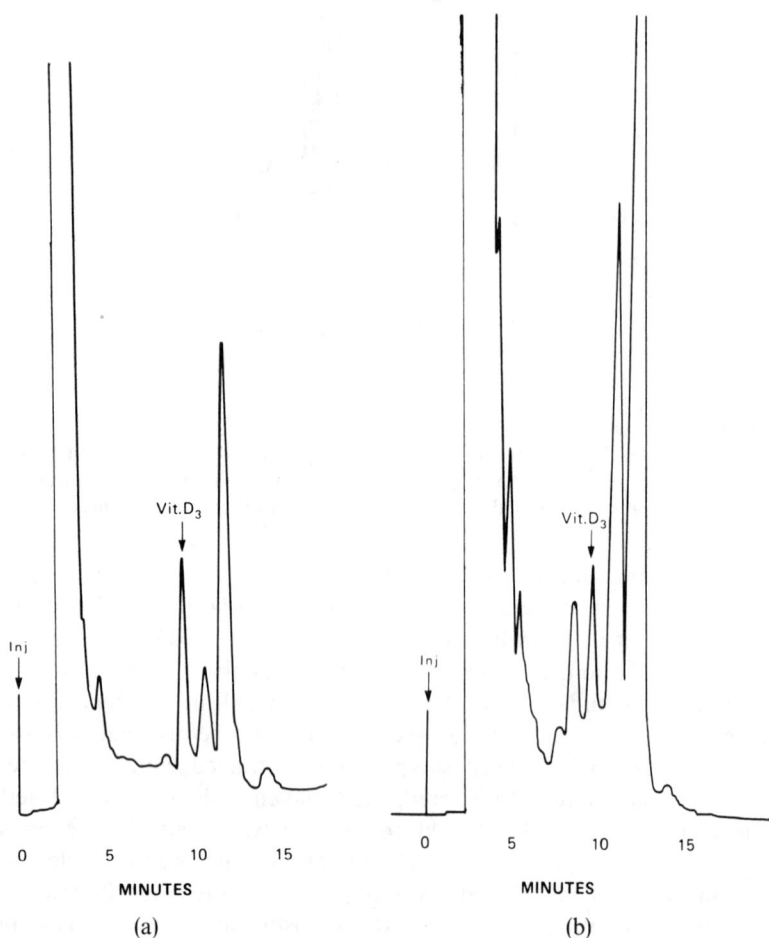

Fig. 70. Normal-phase HPLC of vitamin D from (a) beef supplement fortified at a level of 10 000 IU (250 μg) of vitamin D_3/kg, and (b) cattle supplement fortified at a level of 2000 IU (50 μg) of vitamin D_3/kg, following solvent extraction, liquid–liquid partition, and silica column clean-up. Column, LiChrosorb-NH_2; mobile phase, hexane:chloroform (70:30); UV detection, 264 nm (from Cohen & Lapointe, 1979. Reproduced from the *Journal of Chromatographic Science* by permission of Preston Publications, a Division of Preston Industries, Inc.).

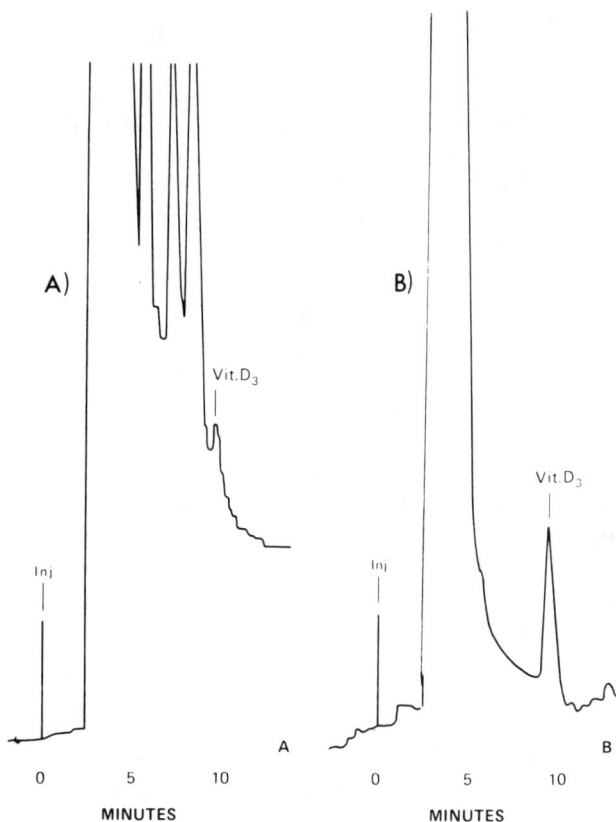

Fig. 71. Normal-phase HPLC of vitamin D from turkey starter fortified at a level of 330 000 IU (8250 μg) of vitamin D_3/kg (A) before, and (B) after silica column clean-up, following solvent extraction and liquid–liquid partition. HPLC parameters as in Fig. 70 (from Cohen & Lapointe, 1979. Reproduced from the *Journal of Chromatographic Science* by permission of Preston Publications, a Division of Preston Industries, Inc.).

hexane:chloroform (70:30) and the absorbance detector was set at 264 nm. Chromatograms of a vitamin D_3 standard, and purified extracts from beef and cattle supplements, are shown in Fig. 70. The effect of the silica clean-up column upon the resolution of vitamin D_3 found in a turkey starter is illustrated in Fig. 71. The overall percentage recovery of vitamin D_3 in feeds was $94\cdot4 \pm 2\cdot4\%$. The minimum detectable amount of vitamin D_3 in animal feeds was found to be in the region of 200 IU (50 μg) per kg.

Cohen & Wakeford (1980) used a Sep-Pak silica cartridge, followed by

HPLC on a polar bonded-phase column to clean up the lipid fraction of vitamin D_3-fortified instant non-fat dried milk. Dried milk samples (10 g) were extracted with dichloromethane containing sodium phosphate tribasic solution and BHT. After evaporation to near dryness under vacuum at 50°C, the residue was dissolved in isooctane:dioxan (95:5) and passed through a Sep-Pak (Waters Associates) silica cartridge by means of a glass syringe. The purified solution was evaporated to dryness under vacuum at 50°C, washed with dichloromethane, and re-evaporated in a stream of nitrogen. The residue was dissolved in dichloromethane and injected onto a 250 mm × 4 mm i.d. column of 10 μm Partisil PAC. The column was eluted with dichloromethane, and the fraction containing the vitamin D was evaporated to dryness in a stream of nitrogen. The residue was dissolved in 1 ml of the HPLC mobile phase (dichloromethane: hexane:isopropanol; 50:50:0·2) and an aliquot of this extract was analysed on a 250 mm × 4 mm i.d. polar bonded-phase column with alkylamine functionality (10 μm LiChrosorb-NH₂). Both preparative and analytical HPLC columns were fitted with guard columns (100 mm × 2 mm i.d.) containing pellicular Co:Pell PAC (Whatman), which consists of amino and nitrile groups bonded to 25–37 μm silica particles. The absorbance detection wavelength of both columns was 264 nm. Chromatograms showing the resolution of vitamin D_3 in a sample of non-fat dried milk before and after semi-preparative HPLC are depicted in Fig. 72. Recoveries of vitamin D_3 added to unfortified instant non-fat dried milk at three different fortification levels were (with standard deviations) 97·1% (4·7%), 100·3% (3·9%) and 95·8% (2·8%). The lower limit of detection was 5 ng of vitamin D_3 injected.

Cohen & Lapointe (1980*b*) developed a procedure for determining low concentrations of vitamin D_3 (4000 IU (100 μg) down to 500 IU (12·5 μg) per kg) from a variety of animal feeds. The overall procedure entailed initial extraction with dichloromethane, followed by Sep-Pak filtration, and further purification using a Sephadex LH-20 column. The vitamin D fraction was then subjected to semi-preparative HPLC on a Partisil PAC column and final analysis on a LiChrosorb-NH₂ column. The initial extraction and two-stage normal-phase HPLC procedures have been described above (Cohen & Wakeford, 1980). The intermediate purification steps were carried out as follows.

The evaporated dichloromethane extract was dissolved in benzene and passed through a Sep-Pak silica cartridge. The vitamin D fraction was eluted from the cartridge with 1% ethyl acetate in benzene, and the eluate was evaporated to dryness under vacuum. The residue was dissolved in 1 ml

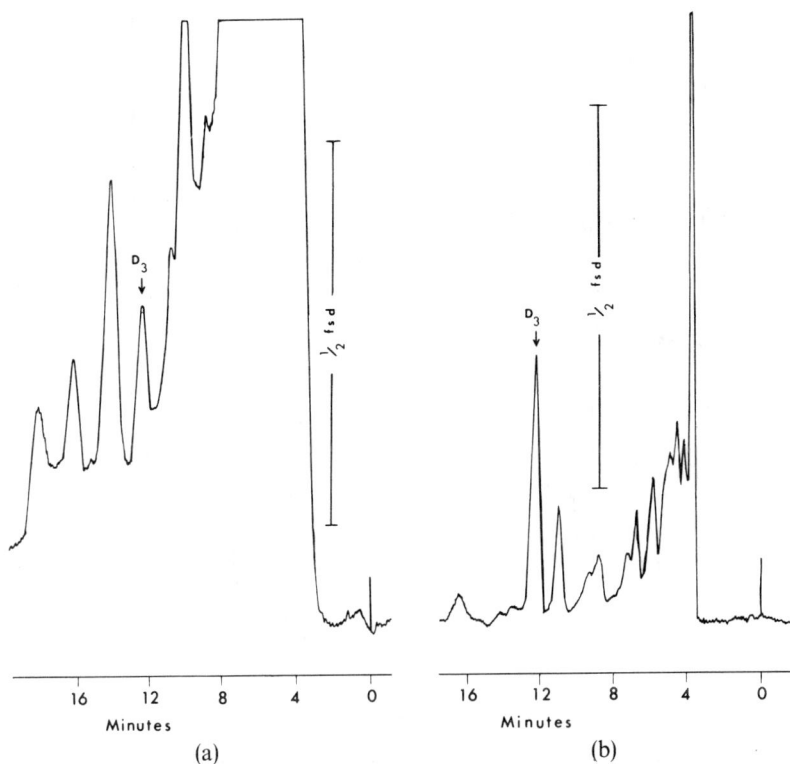

Fig. 72. Normal-phase HPLC of vitamin D from vitamin D_3-fortified non-fat dried milk (a) before, and (b) after semi-preparative HPLC on Partisil PAC, following solvent extraction and Sep-Pak filtration. Column, LiChrosorb-NH$_2$; mobile phase, dichloromethane:hexane:isopropanol (50:50:0·2); UV detection, 264 nm (from Cohen & Wakeford, 1980).

of chloroform:isooctane (98:2) and purified on a column of Sephadex LH-20 packed and eluted with the same solvent. A 254 nm fixed-wavelength absorbance detector was used to monitor the effluent. The eluted vitamin D fraction was evaporated to dryness under vacuum, redissolved in dichloromethane, then re-evaporated to 0·5 ml under nitrogen on a 50°C water bath. An aliquot of this solution was injected onto the semi-preparative Partisil PAC column, and the analysis was continued as described for non-fat dried milk (Cohen & Wakeford, 1980). Chromatograms showing the resolution of vitamin D_3 in horse feed, pig grower and sow breeder are given in Figs 73 and 74. The average percentage recovery of vitamin D_3 in the animal feeds tested was 94·2 ± 5·2%.

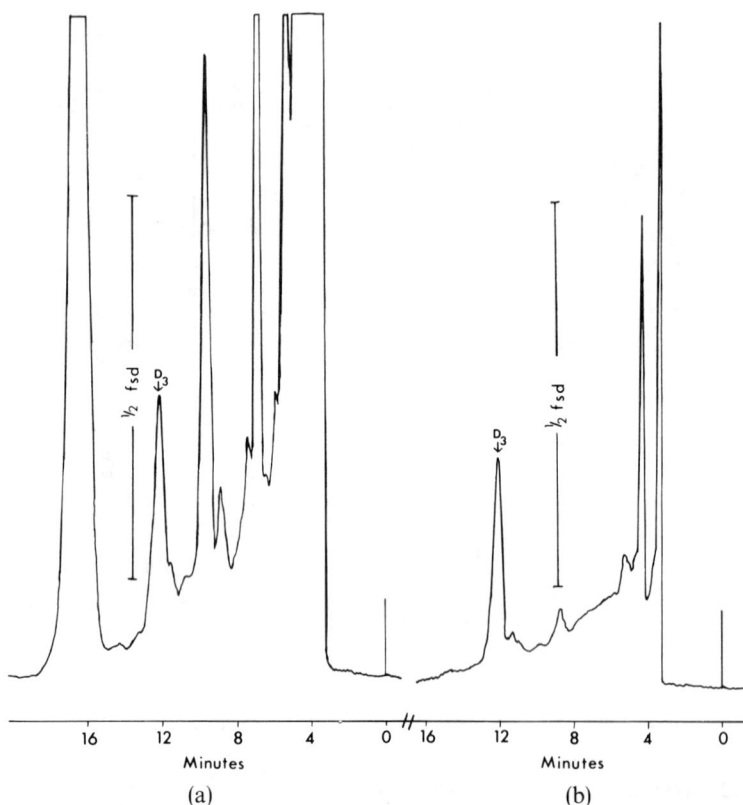

Fig. 73. Normal-phase HPLC of vitamin D from horse feed fortified at a level of 2840 IU (71 μg) of vitamin D_3/kg (a) before, and (b) after semi-preparative HPLC on Partisil PAC, following solvent extraction, Sep-Pak filtration and Sephadex LH-20 column clean-up. HPLC parameters as in Fig. 72 (from Cohen & Lapointe, 1980*b*).

Reversed-phase HPLC, as in the normal-phase mode, affords the isocratic separation of vitamin D from previtamin D and inactive isomers (Fig. 75), hence compensation must be made for the thermal isomerization of vitamin D if a heat treatment such as saponification is employed. In contrast to normal-phase HPLC, the reversed-phase mode, using certain stationary phases, can separate vitamin D_2 from D_3, allowing one of the two vitamins to be used as an internal standard for the other. The internal standard, if added to the sample at the start of the analytical procedure, compensates for any conversion of vitamin D to previtamin D as the isomerization rates of vitamins D_2 and D_3 are virtually equal. The internal

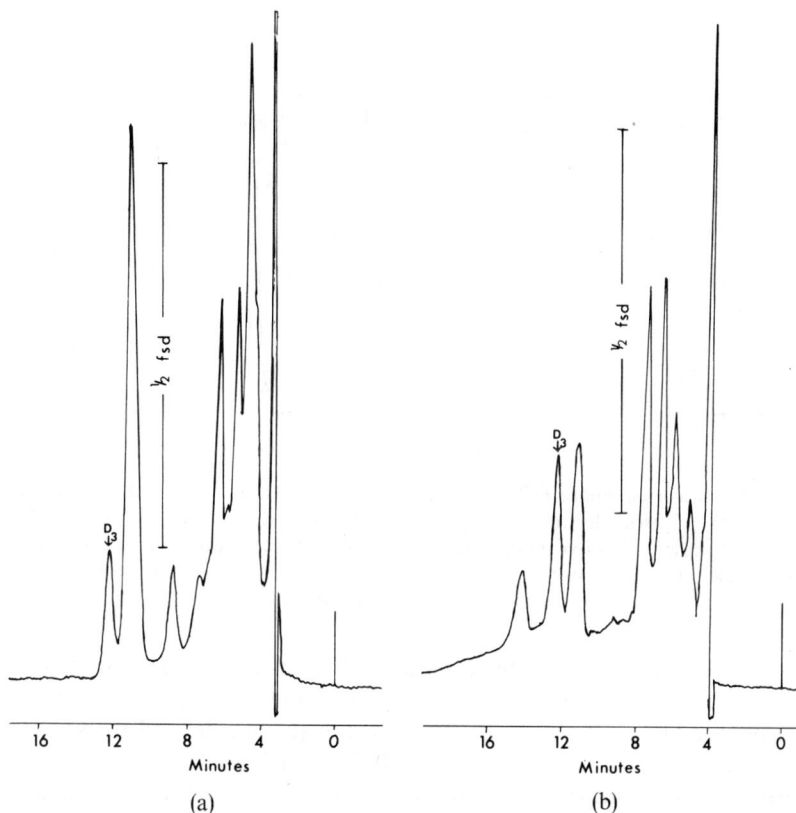

Fig. 74. Normal-phase HPLC of the vitamin D fraction isolated by semi-preparative HPLC on Partisil PAC of (a) pig grower fortified at a level of 500 IU (12·5 μg) of vitamin D_3/kg, and (b) sow breeder at a level of 1268 IU (31·7 μg) of vitamin D_3/kg, following solvent extraction, Sep-Pak filtration, and Sephadex LH-20 column clean-up. HPLC parameters as in Fig. 72 (from Cohen & Lapointe, 1980*b*).

standard also compensates for losses of vitamin D incurred during the extraction procedure.

van Niekerk & Smit (1980) applied the above principle to the determination of vitamin D in margarine using semi-preparative HPLC on a silica column as a clean-up step. Margarine (10 g) samples were saponified by refluxing for 30 min in the presence of α-tocopherol as antioxidant, and vitamin D_2 or D_3 as internal standard. The unsaponifiable matter was extracted with hexane, and the combined hexane extracts were washed with

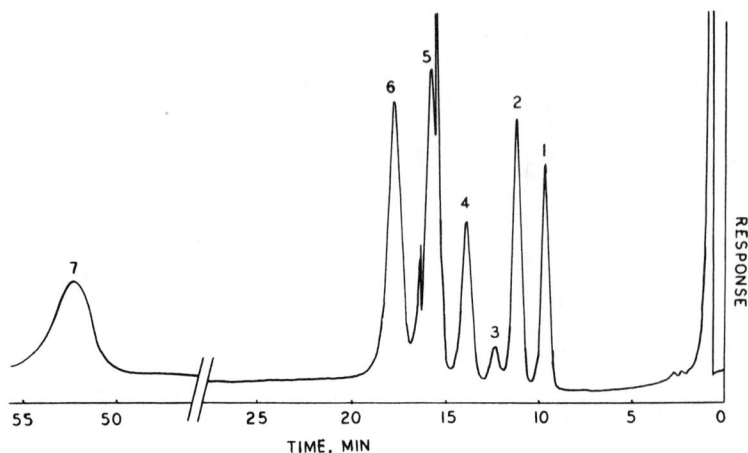

Fig. 75. Reversed-phase HPLC of vitamin D_3 and its isomers. Peaks: (1) *trans*-vitamin D_3; (2) isotachysterol$_3$; (3) previtamin D_3; (4) tachysterol$_3$; (5) vitamin D_3; (6) lumisterol$_3$; (7) 7-dehydrocholesterol (provitamin D_3). Column, LiChrosorb RP-18; mobile phase, acetonitrile:propionitrile:water (79:15:6); UV detection, 254 nm (from de Vries *et al.*, 1979).

water then dried with sodium sulphate. The dried hexane extract was concentrated to 1 ml by rotary evaporation, and filtered through a 0·6 μm membrane filter. γ-Tocopherol was added to the filtrate, and the solvent was evaporated by heating on a 40–50°C water bath under a stream of nitrogen. The residue was dissolved in chloroform, and an aliquot was purified on a 250 mm × 4 mm i.d. 5 μm LiChrosorb Si-60 silica column eluted with hexane:chloroform (1:1); the absorbance detector was set at 295 nm. The vitamin D fraction was collected, using the γ-tocopherol as a tracer to determine its exact elution time, and evaporated to dryness in a stream of nitrogen. The residue was dissolved in chloroform and reinjected on the same system with the detector set at 264 nm. Chromatograms from the silica HPLC column of the unsaponifiable material and of the isolated vitamin D fraction rechromatographed on the same column are depicted in Fig. 76. The vitamin D fraction was evaporated to dryness in a stream of nitrogen, and dissolved in methanol for quantitative reversed-phase HPLC on a 250 mm × 4 mm i.d. 5 μm Nucleosil C_{18} column eluted with methanol:water (95:5) and monitored at 264 nm. The separation of vitamins D_2 and D_3 was incomplete, but was considered sufficient to permit one of the vitamins to be used as an internal standard for the other. A chromatogram showing the resolution of vitamins D_2 and D_3 obtained

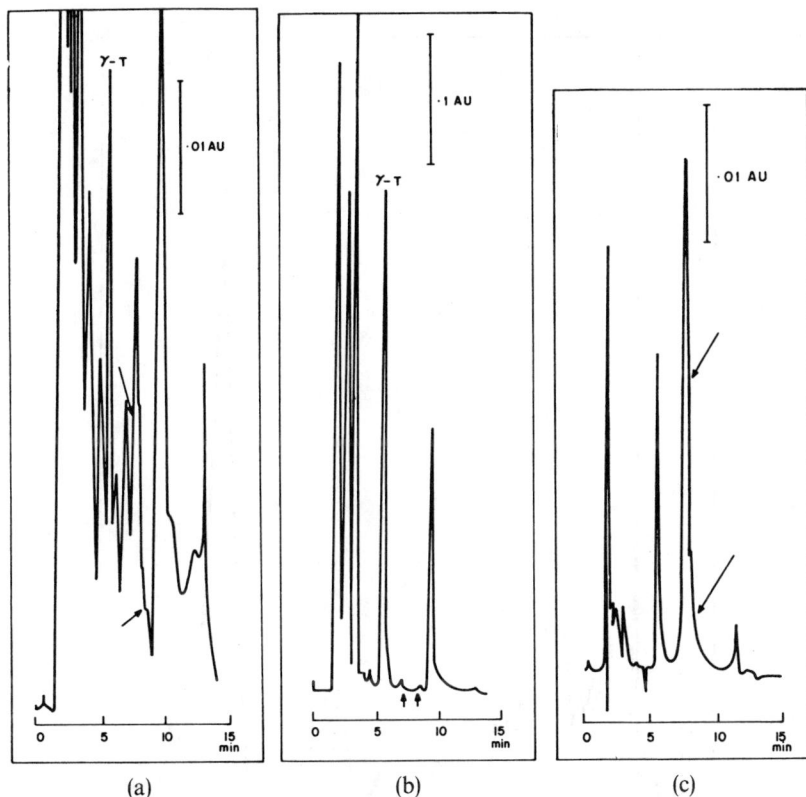

Fig. 76. Semi-preparative adsorption HPLC of vitamin D in the unsaponifiable matter from margarine monitored during the first pass at (a) 264 nm, and (b) 295 nm. The isolated vitamin D fraction was re-chromatographed on the same column with UV detection at 264 nm (c). Position of vitamin D fraction collected is indicated by arrows; γ-T is the γ-tocopherol marker peak. Column, LiChrosorb Si-60; mobile phase, hexane:chloroform (1:1) (from van Niekerk & Smit, 1980).

with the reversed-phase analytical column is given in Fig. 77. The mean recovery of added vitamin D_3 to an unfortified margarine mix was 100·1% (RSD 13·2% for twelve replicates) as calculated from the ratio of D_2 and D_3 peak areas. The detection limit was 1 ng of vitamin D_3 injected.

Jackson *et al.* (1982) determined naturally occurring vitamin D_3 in eggs, butter, milk and cheese. Eggs and milk were concentrated by freeze-drying before analysis. Samples (50 g) were saponified in the presence of vitamin D_2 as internal standard and ascorbic acid as antioxidant. The unsaponifiable matter was extracted with petroleum spirit:diethyl ether (1:1) and the

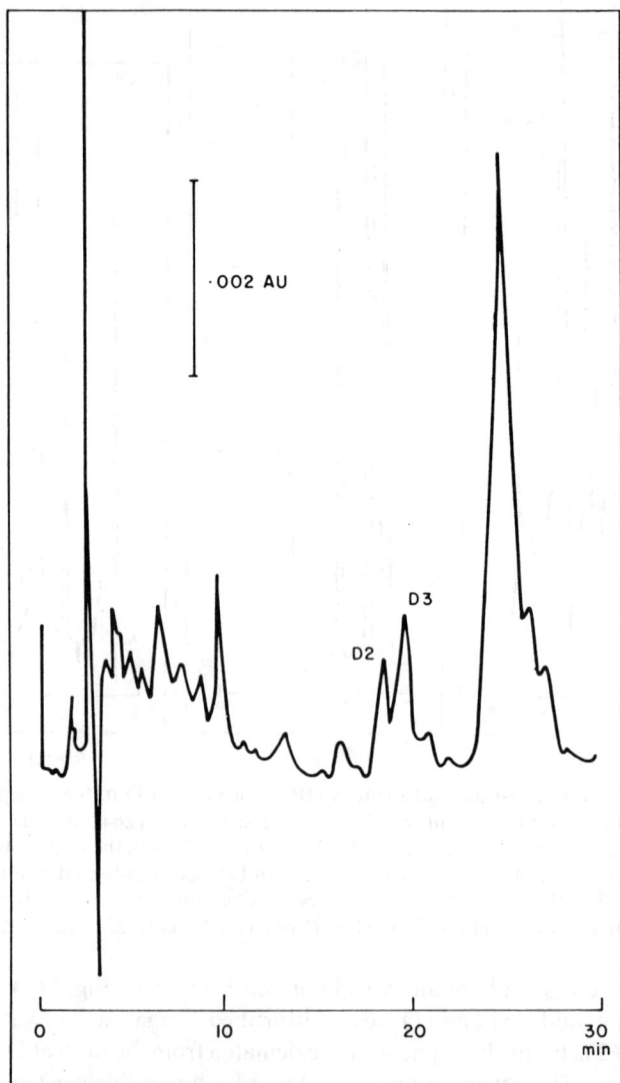

Fig. 77. Reversed-phase HPLC of the vitamin D fraction isolated by semi-preparative HPLC (Fig. 76) of margarine. Column, 5 μm Nucleosil C_{18}, mobile phase, methanol:water (95:5); UV detection, 264 nm (from van Niekerk & Smit, 1980).

combined washed extracts were evaporated to dryness under vacuum. The sterols were removed by precipitation from an ice-cold methanol:water (90:10) mixture, and the filtrate was evaporated to dryness under vacuum. The residue was subjected to preparative TLC on a silica plate developed with hexane:ethyl methyl ketone:dibutyl ether (34:7:6) containing 0·5% BHA. The vitamin D band was removed, the silica was extracted with methanol, and the combined extracts were evaporated to dryness. The residue was transferred to a small specimen tube with petroleum spirit and the solvent was evaporated at 40°C under a stream of nitrogen. The extract was dissolved in 200 μl of methanol containing 0·1% BHA, then injected onto a Spherisorb ODS column eluted with methanol:water (95:5) and monitored spectrophotometrically at 265 nm. The separation of vitamins D_2 and D_3, although not baseline-resolved, was adequate to permit quantification.

Bui (1987) employed saponification in the determination of vitamin D_3 in a variety of fortified food products (homogenized skimmed milk, milk powder, milk powder with soy bean, chocolate drink powder, diet food). Samples containing starch were digested with the enzyme takadiastase before saponification so as to avoid the formation of lumps in solution. High fat samples were subjected to clean-up on a silica Sep-Pak cartridge. This entailed dissolving the unsaponifiable matter in 3 ml of hexane, and loading 2 ml of this solution onto the cartridge. Interfering compounds were removed by washing with 3 ml of hexane:ethyl acetate (85:15) before elution of the vitamin D with 5 ml of hexane:ethyl acetate (80:20). The vitamin D eluate was evaporated to dryness in a stream of nitrogen, and the residue was dissolved in 500 μl of 1% THF in methanol. An aliquot of this solution was injected onto two 120 mm × 4 mm i.d. 5 μm Hypersil ODS columns connected in series. The mobile phase was methanol containing 0·5% water, and the absorbance detector wavelength was 265 nm. Chromatograms of skimmed milk, milk powder and milk powder containing soy bean are depicted in Fig. 78. Quantification was performed using vitamin D_3 as an external standard. The mean recovery of vitamin D_3 added to unfortified skimmed milk was 98%, and the limit of detection was 10 ng of vitamin D_3 injected. No mention was made of the reversible thermal isomerization of vitamin D to previtamin D.

Grace & Bernhard (1984) avoided saponification by subjecting hexane extracts of vitamin D-fortified whole milk to alcoholysis, then separating the triglyceride esters from the vitamin D esters by means of preparative TLC. Removal of the triglyceride esters was necessary as the esters absorb strongly at the detection wavelength (265 nm) used in the subsequent

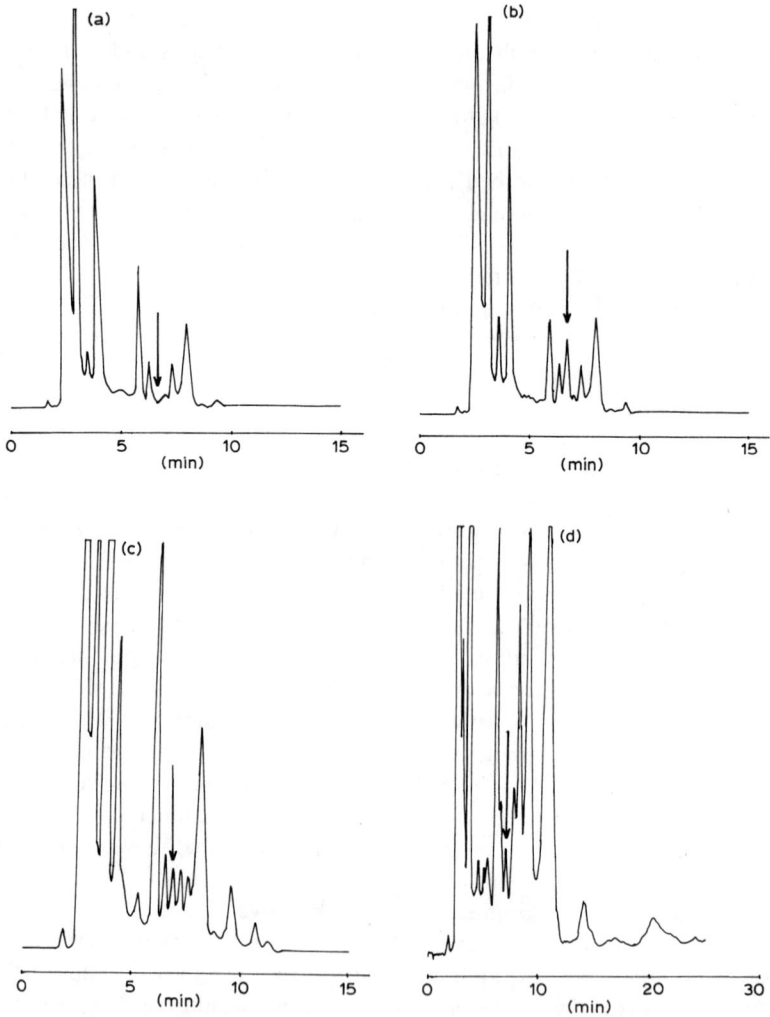

Fig. 78. Reversed-phase HPLC of the unsaponifiable matter from (a) unfortified skimmed milk, (b) vitamin D_3-fortified skimmed milk, (c) fortified milk powder, and (d) fortified milk powder with added soy bean after clean-up on a silica Sep-Pak cartridge. Arrow indicates position of vitamin D. Column, tandem $5 \mu m$ Hypersil ODS; mobile phase, methanol containing 0·5% water, UV detection, 265 nm (from Bui, 1987).

HPLC step. The method entailed extracting a 50 ml sample of whole milk with a mixture of saturated sodium chloride solution, acidified ethanol and hexane. The milk solution was centrifuged, and the triglycerides were converted into their methyl esters by alcoholysis with methanolic KOH solution. After reaction for 2 min, the mixture was diluted with water, and the hexane layer was evaporated to dryness under vacuum at 60°C. The remaining syrup was diluted with hexane, then applied to a silica preparative TLC plate containing an indicator with an activation peak of 254 nm for visualization. The plate was developed initially with hexane:ethyl acetate (80:20) followed by hexane:isopropanol (85:15). The vitamin D band was scraped from the plate and extracted with ethyl acetate. The filtered extract was evaporated to dryness under nitrogen using a 47°C water bath, and the residue was dissolved in 0·5 ml of methanol. The methanolic solution was filtered through a membrane filter, diluted to 1·0 ml with methanol, then refrigerated to allow precipitation of a slightly soluble lipid material. The clear solution was analysed on a 250 mm × 4·6 mm i.d. 5 μm Ultrasphere ODS column eluted with methanol:water (97:3) and detected at 265 nm. Because a maximum of only 82% recovery of vitamin D from the TLC plate was obtained, results were multiplied by the correction factor of 1·22.

Indyk & Woollard (1985a) found that removal of the cholesterol from the unsaponifiable fraction of whole milk powder by precipitation in methanol constituted a sufficient clean-up procedure for the determination of supplemental vitamin D_3. This simplified procedure was attributable to the tandem column HPLC system employed, which adequately separated vitamins D_2 and D_3 from each other, and from vitamins A and E, and thus obviated the need for preliminary chromatographic clean-up. Residual sterols were not detected at the absorption wavelength employed for the quantification (280 nm), hence did not interfere with the analysis. The procedure was as follows.

Samples (10 g) of fortified whole milk powder were subjected to alkaline digestion overnight at ambient temperature in a sealed, nitrogen-flushed flask with the inclusion of pyrogallol as antioxidant, and vitamin D_2 as internal standard. The unsaponifiable matter was extracted with petroleum spirit:diethyl ether (90:10), then washed with water and evaporated to dryness under vacuum at <40°C. The residue was dissolved in methanol to precipitate the sterols, which were removed by filtration through a 0·45 μm membrane filter. An aliquot of the clear filtrate was injected into the HPLC system, which comprised two RCM-100 radial compression units (Waters Associates) connected in series, each unit being equipped with a

10 cm × 8 mm i.d. Radial-PAK cartridge containing 5 μm spherical C_{18}-bonded silica (either RESOLVE C_{18} or Nova-PAK C_{18}). The mobile phase was methanol:tetrahydrofuran:water (93:2:5) and was monitored photometrically by dual wavelength detection at 254 nm and 280 nm. The chromatography of the sample extract was completed within approximately 40 min, after which time late-eluting substances (mainly carotenoids) were removed at an elevated flow rate with 100% methanol. The approximate retention times of the separated vitamin A, vitamin D and vitamin E components were: vitamin A (combined *trans*- and *cis*-retinols) (8 min), vitamin D_2 (26·5 min), vitamin D_3 (28·5 min), γ-tocopherol (33 min) and α-tocopherol (38·5 min). Dual wavelength chromatograms of unfortified and fortified whole milk powder extracts are shown in Fig. 79. The large peak that coeluted with the vitamin D_2 peak at 254 nm was presumed to be a sterol; this peak was not detected at 280 nm. Quantification was performed by the internal standardization method at the 280 nm wavelength. Confirmation of peak identity was routinely achieved by monitoring the spectral ratio (as peak heights) at 254 nm and 280 nm, and comparing the ratio with that of pure vitamin D_3. Recoveries of >95% were obtained when authentic vitamin D standards were added at different levels to unfortified whole milk powder. The RSD of the method (mean of five samples) was 6·0%. The approximate limit of detection was 0·75 μg of vitamin D_3 per 100 g of milk powder.

With simple sensitivity attenuation, it was feasible to simultaneously determine the concentrations of vitamins A and E with vitamin D by the above method. There was no interference from sterols at the detection wavelength of 280 nm, but at 254 nm a large interfering peak was detected. (Absorption of vitamin D at 280 nm is 75% of that at the λ_{max} of 265 nm.) The Nova-PAK system yielded a greater sensitivity compared with the RESOLVE system. This was considered to be a probable consequence of the Nova-PAK packing material being end-capped: the RESOLVE material is not end-capped, and thus permits some degree of 'mixed mode' chromatography. The ability to employ internal standardization without sample clean-up depends upon the use of a semi-aqueous mobile phase. The presence of water causes a delayed retention of the more hydrophobic E vitamers relative to the more polar calciferols. The tetrahydrofuran component was found to assist in reducing overall solute retention without sacrificing resolution. When NARP was employed in an otherwise similar analysis (Indyk & Woollard, 1984), endogenous γ-tocopherol interfered with the vitamin D peaks, thus preventing the use of internal standardization without prior removal of vitamin E.

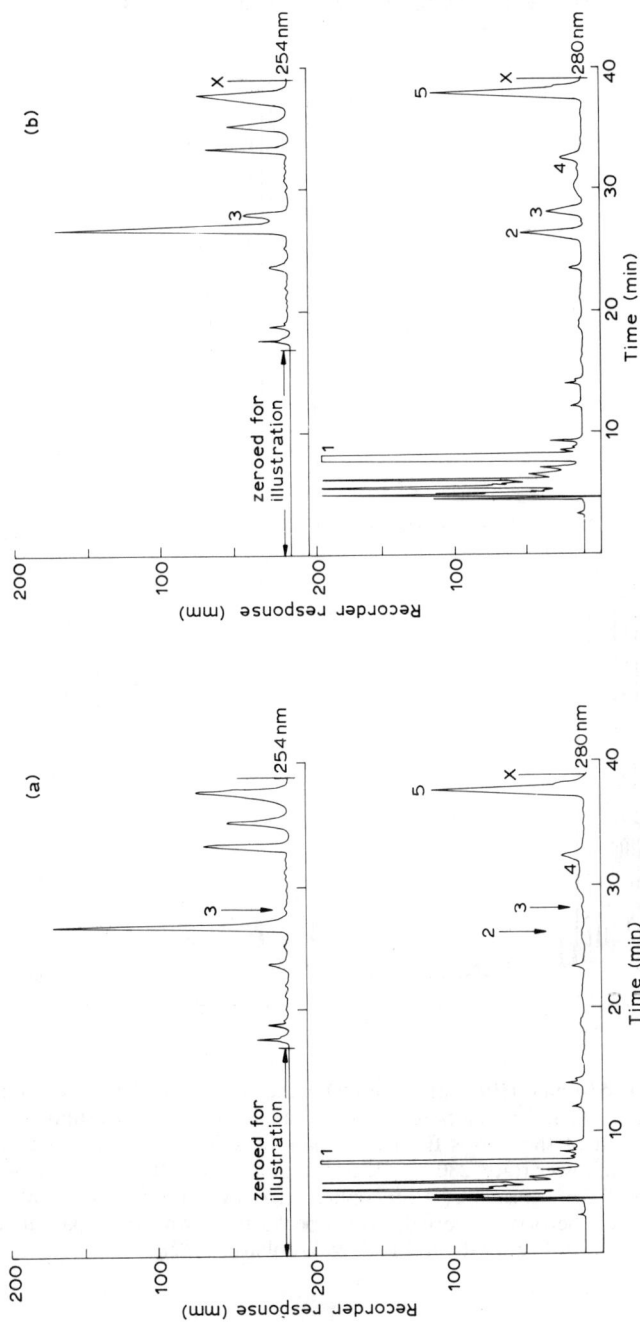

Fig. 79. Reversed-phase HPLC of vitamin D in the unsaponifiable matter from (a) unfortified whole milk powder, (b) vitamin D$_3$-fortified whole milk powder, after precipitation of the sterols from a methanolic solution. Upper trace: UV detection, 254 nm; lower trace, 280 nm. Peaks: (1) vitamin A (*trans*- and *cis*-retinols); (2) vitamin D$_2$ (internal standard); (3) vitamin D$_3$; (4) γ-tocopherol (endogenous); (5) α-tocopherol (endogenous); other peaks unknown. Column, tandem Rad-PAK, 5 μm, C$_{18}$ cartridges; mobile phase, methanol:tetrahydrofuran:water (93:2:5) (from Indyk & Woollard, 1985a).

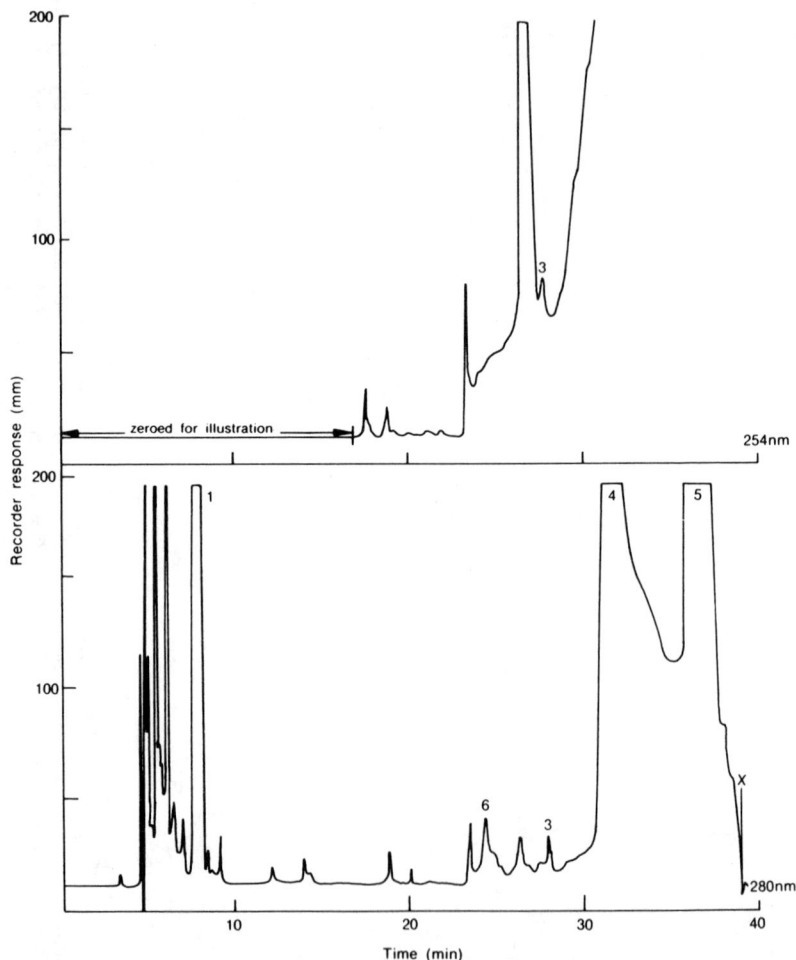

Fig. 80.   Reversed-phase HPLC of vitamin D in the unsaponifiable matter from a fully vitaminized infant formula powder containing 5% w/w corn oil supplement, after precipitation of the sterols from a methanolic solution. Upper trace: UV detection, 254 nm; lower trace, 280 nm. Peaks: (1) vitamin A; (3) vitamin D_3; (4) γ- and β-tocopherol (from corn oil); (5) α-tocopherol (from vitamin E supplement and corn oil); (6) δ-tocopherol (from corn oil); other peaks unknown. HPLC parameters as in Fig. 79 (from Indyk & Woollard, 1985a).

Neither semi-aqueous nor non-aqueous reversed-phase techniques could be used without a clean-up procedure for the analysis of infant formula foods, owing to the large amounts of supplemental and endogenous vitamin E that interfere with the HPLC. The increased background from E vitamers in infant formulations is illustrated in Fig. 80. Indyk & Woollard (1985b) modified the procedure of Indyk & Woollard (1985a) by removing the vitamin E from milk powders and infant formula foods by chromatographic clean-up. The unsaponifiable fraction of the sample was dissolved in 1 ml of hexane and applied to a dry-packed silica cartridge contained in a specially-designed manifold. Elution to waste with hexane: chloroform (21·5:78·5) removed the vitamin E, whilst the vitamin D fraction was obtained by elution with 100% methanol. The chromatography following silica clean-up for fully vitaminized infant formula powders containing (a) 5% w/w corn oil and (b) 30% w/w oil blend is compared in Fig. 81.

The problems of incomplete solute solubility ascribed to semi-aqueous mobile phases did not arise in the assays described by Indyk & Woollard

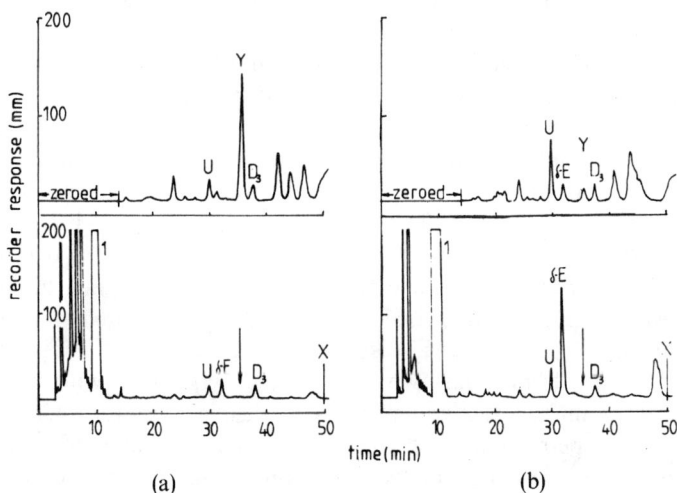

(a)   (b)

Fig. 81. Reversed-phase HPLC of vitamin D in the unsaponifiable matter from fully vitaminized infant formula powder, after silica column clean-up. Formulae contain (a) 5% w/w corn oil, and (b) 30% w/w oil blend. Peak identity: (1) vitamin A; (U) α-tocopherylquinone (tentative); (Y) unknown; (D_3) vitamin D_3; (δ-E) δ-tocopherol. The arrow denotes the elution position of the internal standard, vitamin D_2. Column, tandem Rad-PAK, 5 μm C_{18}; mobile phase, methanol:tetrahydrofuran:water (92:2:6). UV detection, 254 nm (upper trace) and 280 nm (lower trace) (from Indyk & Woollard, 1985b).

1984, 1985*a*, *b*). In the milk powders and infant formula foods analysed, complete solute solubility up to at least 15% water in methanol was reported. The only notable disadvantage inherent in employing an aqueous mobile phase was a reduced sensitivity as compared to a non-aqueous system. This is largely a consequence of greater solute retention and the requirement for an elevated operational flow-rate.

The resolution of vitamins D_2 and D_3 using NARP depends upon the type of reversed-phase packing material and the composition of the mobile phase. For instance, a μBondapak C_{18} column eluted with acetonitrile: dichloromethane (70:30), that was used successfully to determine vitamin A in margarine and fortified breakfast cereals (Landen & Eitenmiller, 1979; Landen, 1980), failed to adequately resolve vitamins D_2 and D_3 (Landen, 1981).

The complete separation of vitamins D_2 and D_3 by NARP has been achieved on a Vydac TP 201 C_{18} column (Muniz *et al.*, 1982), a radially compressed Radial-PAK A C_{18} cartridge (Thompson *et al.*, 1982) and a 6 μm Zorbax ODS column (Landen, 1985). These systems, which are described below, have been employed in the analysis of vitamin D-fortified milk, infant formulations and margarine.

Muniz *et al.* (1982) subjected 100 ml samples of milk (whole, low-fat or skimmed) to overnight alkaline digestion at ambient temperature with constant shaking in the dark. The unsaponifiable matter was extracted with petroleum spirit, and the combined petroleum extracts were washed with aqueous KOH solution followed by water, then evaporated to dryness on a steam bath under nitrogen. The residue was immediately dissolved in digitonin solution, diluted with methanol, and stored at $-20°C$ overnight to precipitate the cholesterol. The mixture was centrifuged, and the supernatant was extracted with petroleum spirit then evaporated to dryness under nitrogen. The residue was dissolved in petroleum spirit, and applied to a 300 mm × 10 mm i.d. glass column dry-packed with neutral deactivated alumina. The column was washed successively with 15% diethyl ether in petroleum spirit, 100% petroleum spirit, and 15% acetone in hexane. The 15% acetone fraction containing the vitamin D was evaporated to dryness under nitrogen, and the residue was immediately dissolved in acetonitrile. An aliquot of the acetonitrile extract was chromatographed on a reversed-phase 10 μm Vydac TP 201 C_{18} column (250 mm × 3·2 mm i.d.) fitted with a guard column (150 mm × 4 mm i.d.) packed with Bondapak C_{18}/Corasil (Waters Associates) or Mikro Pak MCH-5 (Varian). The mobile phase was acetonitrile: methanol (90:10) and the absorbance detection wavelength was 265 nm. This system completely separated vitamins D_2 and D_3 with elution times between 6 and 8 min. Chromatograms of unfortified and fortified low-fat and skimmed milks are given in Fig. 82. The recovery of added vitamin D_2 from fluid milk varied from 85·2% to 99·7%; vitamin D_3 recoveries varied from 85·9% to 98·8%. The RSD was 3·4%. The minimum detectable quantity of vitamin D in milk was 0·4 ng/ml.

Thompson *et al.* (1982) subjected 15 ml samples of whole milk to overnight alkaline digestion at ambient temperature in the presence of pyrogallol as antioxidant. The unsaponifiable matter was extracted with hexane, and the combined extracts were washed consecutively with 5% aqueous KOH, water, and 55% aqueous ethanol to remove interfering polar constituents. The hexane solution was evaporated to dryness under vacuum at 50°C, and the residue was dissolved in the HPLC mobile phase (0·5% isopropanol in cyclohexane:hexane; 1:1) for purification on a 150 mm × 4·6 mm i.d. column of 5 μm silica (Supelcosil LC-Si) with photometric detection at 254 nm. The fraction containing the vitamin D was collected (see Fig. 83) and evaporated to dryness under nitrogen. The residue was dissolved in the next mobile phase (methanol) for injection onto a 10 cm × 8 mm i.d. radially compressed Radial-PAK cartridge containing μBondapak C_{18} with photometric detection at 254 nm.

Margarine samples (50 g) and diluted infant formula foods were treated in a similar manner to that described for milk except that, before semi-preparative adsorption HPLC, the residue from the hexane extract was dissolved in hexane:isopropanol (99:1) and passed through 5 cm of neutral deactivated alumina dry-packed in a Pasteur pipette. For the semi-preparative HPLC on the silica column, the concentration of isopropanol in cyclohexane:hexane (1:1) was changed from 0·5% to 0·25% to improve the separation of vitamin D from other absorbing lipids. Chromatograms from the semi-preparative silica and quantitative reversed-phase HPLC columns are depicted in Figs 84 and 85, respectively. Recovery of vitamin D added to unfortified milk just before saponification was 96–99%. The RSDs for milk and margarine were, respectively, 3% and 9%.

Landen (1985) avoided thermal isomerization of vitamin D in the analysis of fortified milk and infant formula foods by extracting the total lipid fraction with a solvent mixture. The samples (6·5 g of liquid or reconstituted powdered milk) were homogenized in isopropanol/dichloro-methane with magnesium sulphate added to remove water, and BHT as antioxidant. The extract was evaporated to dryness under vacuum below 30°C; dissolved in isooctane; filtered through a 0·5 μm filter; re-evaporated; and dissolved in 1 ml of dichloromethane. This solution was fractionated

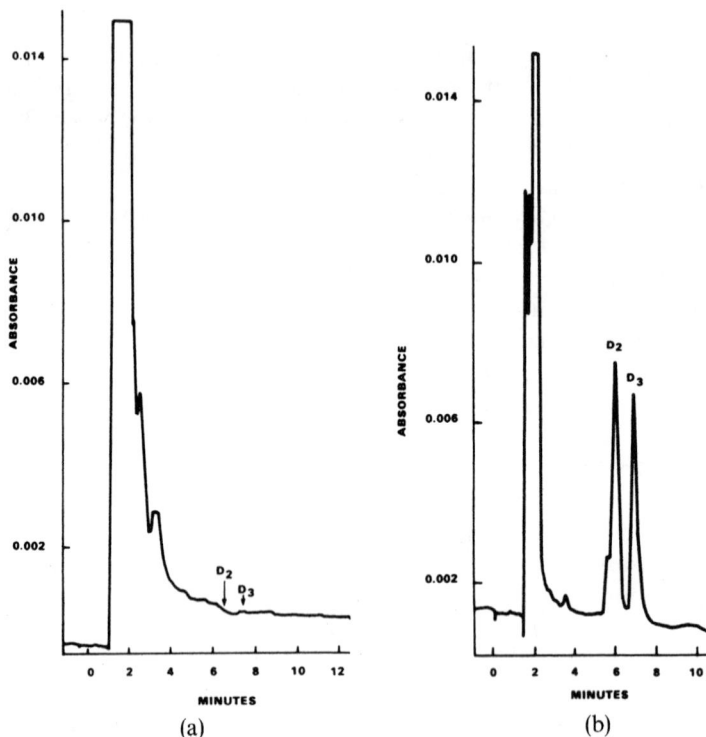

Fig. 82. NARP of vitamin D in the unsaponifiable matter from vitamin D-fortified milk, after co-precipitation of the cholesterol with digitonin and alumina column clean-up. (a) Unfortified 3·8% low-fat milk, (b) low-fat milk fortified with vitamins D_2 and D_3.

on four μStyragel 100 Å columns (300 mm × 7·8 mm i.d.) connected in series, using a mobile phase of dichloromethane containing 0·001% triethylamine. The column effluent was continuously monitored with refractive index and absorbance detectors. After elution of the oil fraction, as monitored by refractive index, the vitamin D fraction, detected at 280 nm, was collected. The injection and collection were repeated twice to collect sufficient vitamin D for quantification.

The combined fractions, plus added BHT, were evaporated to dryness under vacuum below 30°C, then immediately dissolved in 150 μl of the next HPLC mobile phase (dichloromethane:isooctane:isopropanol; 600:400:1) for further purification on a 300 mm × 7·8 mm i.d. μBondapak-NH$_2$ polar bonded-phase column. Cholesterol was monitored by refractive index, and

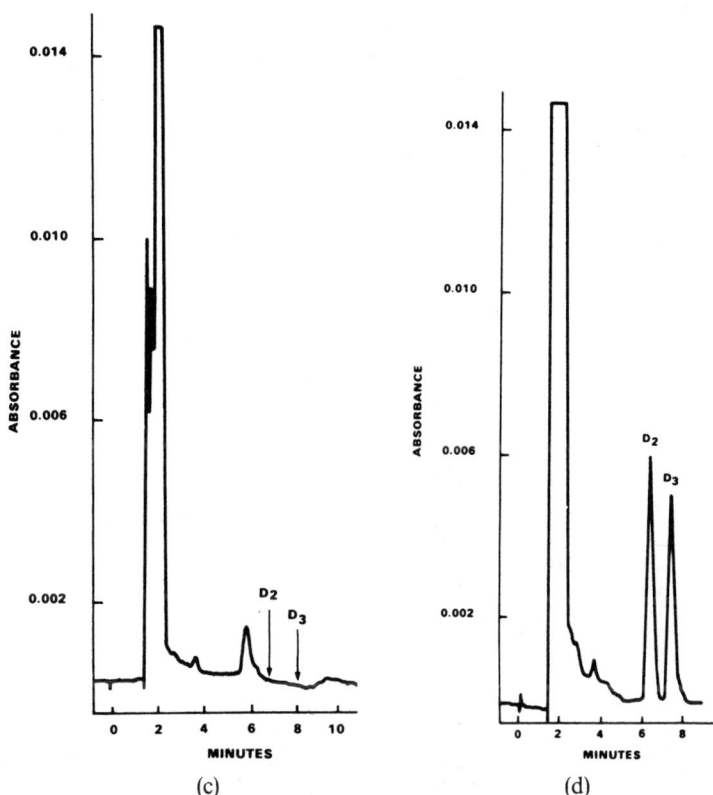

Fig. 82—*contd.*   (c) Unfortified skimmed milk ($<0.5\%$ fat), and (d) skimmed milk fortified with vitamins D_2 and D_3. Column, Vydac TP 201 C_{18}; mobile phase, acetonitrile:methanol (90:10); UV detection, 265 nm (from Muniz *et al.*, 1982).

the vitamin D fraction, detected at 280 nm (see Fig. 86), was collected in a 5 ml vial. The fraction, plus added BHT, was evaporated to dryness under reduced pressure in an atmosphere of helium below 30°C, and the residue was dissolved in 250 μl of the third mobile phase (acetonitrile:dichloromethane:methanol; 700:300:2) for quantification of the vitamin D on a 250 mm × 4·6 mm i.d. column of 6 μm Zorbax ODS with absorbance detection at 280 nm (see Fig. 87). Determination of peak purity was obtained by comparing the ratio of the sample peak response at 254 nm to the response at 280 nm with that ratio obtained from a standard vitamin preparation. The mean recovery of added vitamin D_3 from an infant formulation was $89·6\% \pm 6·7\%$. The RSD was $7·5\%$.

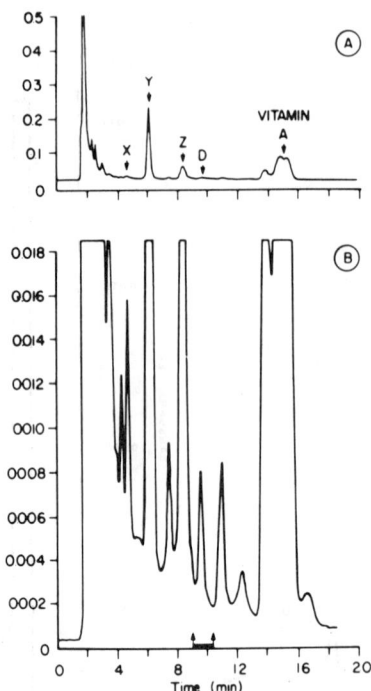

Fig. 83.   Semi-preparative adsorption HPLC of vitamin D in the unsaponifiable matter of vitamin D-fortified whole milk at (A) low, and (B) high sensitivity. Position of elution of vitamin D is indicated by D in (A), and position of vitamin D fraction collected is indicated by arrows in (B). Peaks Y and Z are characteristic of milk. Column, Supelcosil LC-Si; mobile phase, cyclohexane:hexane (1:1) containing 0·5% isopropanol; UV detection, 254 nm (from Thompson *et al.*, 1982).

8.3.4 Vitamin E

HPLC methods for estimating vitamin E in foods and feeds are summarized in Table 27.

Normal-phase HPLC is capable of separating isocratically all of the eight E vitamers, and is the most suitable technique for studying the natural vitamin E content of a particular food. The vitamers are eluted in the following order: α-T, α-T3, β-T, γ-T, β-T$_3$, γ-T$_3$, δ-T and δ-T3 (see Fig. 88). Supplemental α-tocopheryl acetate, if present, would elute in front of α-tocopherol under the above conditions; retinol would elute after the E vitamers. The use of a short (100 mm × 4·6 mm i.d.) column packed with 3 μm Spherisorb substantially reduced the analysis time needed for the

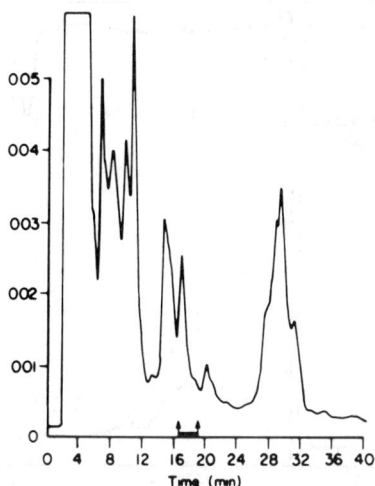

Fig. 84. Semi-preparative adsorption HPLC of vitamin D in the unsaponifiable matter of margarine, after alumina column clean-up. Position of vitamin D fraction collected is indicated by arrows. HPLC parameters as in Fig. 83, except that isopropanol component of mobile phase is changed to 0·25% (from Thompson *et al.*, 1982).

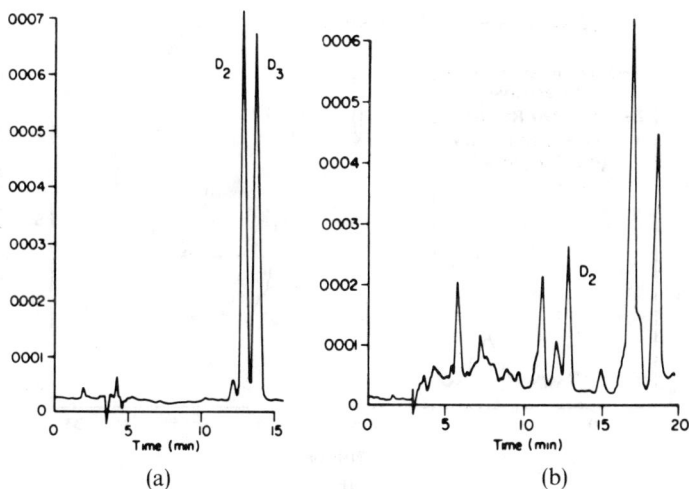

(a)   (b)

Fig. 85. NARP of (a) vitamin D standards, and (b) the vitamin D fraction isolated by semi-preparative HPLC (Fig. 84) of margarine. Column, 5 μm Rad-PAK A C_{18} cartridge; mobile phase, methanol; UV detection, 254 nm (from Thompson *et al.*, 1982).

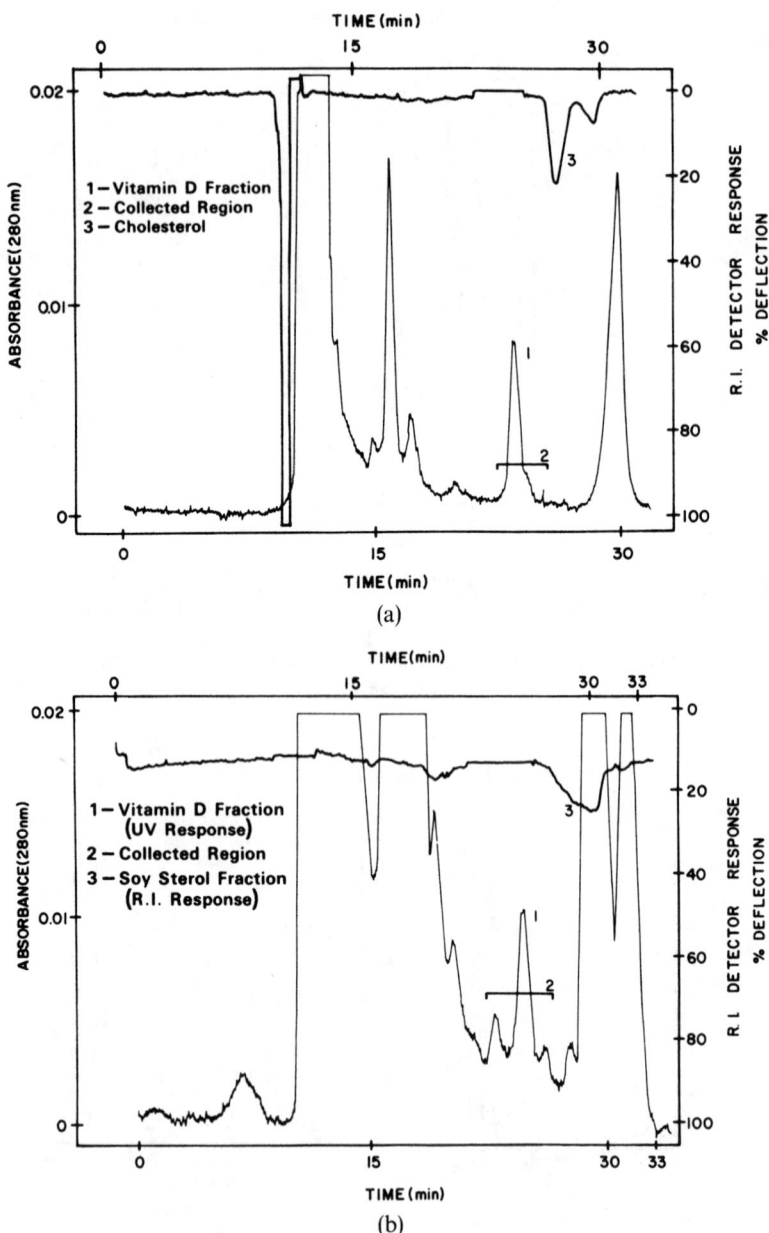

Fig. 86. Semi-preparative normal-phase HPLC of the vitamin D fraction isolated by gel-permeation HPLC from solvent extract of vitamin D-fortified (a) 2% low-fat milk and (b) infant formula. Column, μBondapak-NH$_2$; mobile phase, dichloromethane:isooctane:isopropanol (600:400:1); dual detection, UV (280 nm) and refractive index (from Landen, 1985).

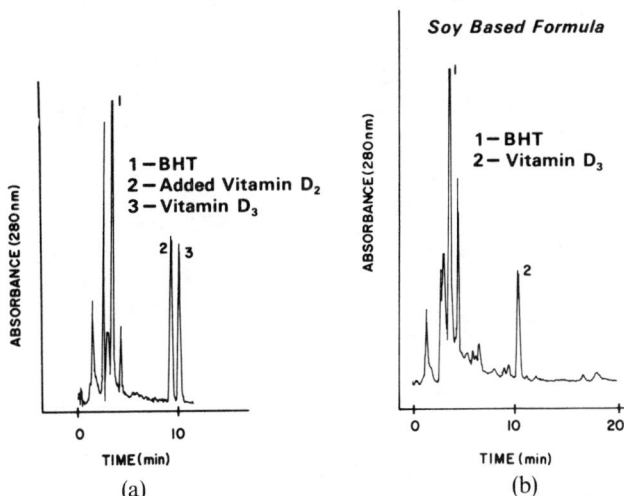

Fig. 87. NARP of the vitamin D fraction isolated by semi-preparative HPLC (Fig. 86) of vitamin D-fortified (a) 2% low-fat milk, and (b) infant formula after gel-permeation HPLC. Column, 6 μm Zorbax ODS; mobile phase, acetonitrile: dichloromethane:methanol (700:300:2); UV detection, 280 nm (from Landen, 1985).

baseline separation of tocopherols when compared to columns of 300 mm or 250 mm length packed with either 10 μm or 5 μm silica particles (Shen & Sheppard, 1986).

Detection of the E vitamers is usually performed by absorbance or fluorescence measurement. Absorbance measurement permits the quantification of α-tocopherol at concentrations down to 0·6 μg/ml, with a minimum detectable amount of pure α-tocopherol at 60 ng (Nelis et al., 1985). According to Thompson & Hatina (1979) the sensitivity of a fluorescence detector with the E vitamers under normal-phase conditions is at least ten times superior to that of a spectrophotometric detector, and is also more selective. The relative sensitivity is illustrated in Fig. 89, which displays chromatograms of E vitamers obtained by passing the column effluent first through a fluorescence detector and then through a spectro-photometric detector; both detectors were set at the optimum wavelengths for vitamin E. The fluorescence excitation and emission wavelengths differ by only 40 nm, thus creating potential problems of spectral overlap. If a filter-type fluorescence detector is employed, the emission filter must be designed to avoid spectral overlap with the light source. Spectral overlap does not occur when instruments with narrow-band monochromators are

Table 27

HPLC methods used for vitamin E compounds

| Analyte | Sample type | Sample preparation | Quantitative HPLC | | | Reference/ Fig. no. |
			Stationary phase	Mobile phase	Detection	
α-, β-, γ-, δ-T α-, γ-, δ-T3	Seed oils	Dissolution in hexane	Partisil Silica	50% H_2O-saturated hexane: dibutyl ether (90:10) + 0·05% Pr-2-OH	UV 292 nm or fluorescence: excitation 290 nm emission 330 nm	Taylor & Barnes (1981) (Fig. 90)
α-, β-, γ-, δ-T α-, β-, γ-, δ-T3	Oils, foods (unfortified)	Dissolution in hexane (oils); diethyl ether extraction (foods)	LiChrosorb Si-60	Isooctane:tert-butyl methyl ether (98:2)	Fluorescence: excitation 295 nm emission 330 nm	Gertz & Herrmann (1982)
α-, β-, γ-, δ-T α-, β-, γ-, δ-T3	Seed oils, margarine, butter	Dissolution in hexane	LiChrosorb Si-60 (column temperature 45°C for separation of all E vitamers)	Diisopropyl ether gradient of 8% to 17·6% in hexane	Fluorescence: excitation 290 nm emission 325 nm	Syväoja et al. (1986)
α-, β-, γ-, δ-T, α-T3	Seed oils	Dissolution in hexane	Polygosil 60	Hexane: diisopropyl ether (90:10)	Fluorescence: excitation 296 nm emission 320 nm	Speek et al. (1985)
α-, β-, γ-, δ-T α-, β-, γ-, δ-T3	Seed oils	Dissolution in hexane	Partisil PAC	Hexane:THF (94:6)	Fluorescence: excitation 210 nm emission 325 nm	Rammell & Hoogenboom (1985)
α-, β-, γ-, δ-T α-, β-T3	Wheat germ oil	Hexane extraction in Soxhlet apparatus	LiChrosorb Si-60	50% H_2O-saturated hexane: diethyl ether (95:5)	Fluorescence: excitation 290 nm emission 330 nm	Barnes & Taylor (1980)
α-, β-, γ-, δ-T α-, β-, γ-, δ-T3	Wheat flour, wheat germ	Hexane extraction in Soxhlet apparatus, evaporation	LiChrosorb Si-60	Hexane: diisopropyl ether (97:3)	Fluorescence: excitation 290 nm emission 330 nm	Håkansson et al. (1987)

Compounds	Sample	Extraction	Column	Mobile phase	Detection	Reference
α-, β-, γ-, δ-T α-, β-, γ-T3	Cereals, flour foods (unfortified)	Extraction with boiling Pr-2-OH, re-extraction with acetone, partition into hexane, evaporation	LiChrosorb Si-60	50% H_2O-saturated hexane + 0.2% Pr-2-OH or 5% diethyl ether	Fluorescence: excitation 290 nm emission 330 nm	Thompson & Hatina (1979)
Total α-T β-, γ-, δ-T α-, β-, γ-T3	Infant formulae (fortified)	Saponification, diethyl ether extraction, evaporation	LiChrosorb Si-60	50% H_2O-saturated hexane + 0.2% Pr-2-OH or 5% diethyl ether	Fluorescence: excitation 290 nm emission 330 nm	Thompson & Hatina (1979)
Vitamin E acetate	Infant formulae (fortified)	Dispersion in non-aq. solvent mixture, partition into hexane	Radial-PAK cartridge containing RESOLVE silica	Hexane + 0.08% Pr-2-OH	UV 280 nm	Woollard & Blott (1986) (Figs 91–93)
Vitamin E acetate	Animal feeds	Dispersion in non-aq. solvent mixture, partition into hexane	Radial-PAK cartridge containing RESOLVE silica	Hexane + 0.08% Pr-2-OH	UV 280 nm	Blott & Woollard (1986)
Total α-T	Animal feeds, human foods (unfortified)	Saponification, diethyl ether extraction, evaporation	LiChrosorb Si-60	Hexane + 0.1% Pr-2-OH	Fluorescence: excitation 293 nm emission 326 nm	Manz & Philipp (1981) (Fig. 94)
a-, β-, γ-, δ-T α-, γ-T3	Animal feeds	EtOH extraction in Soxhlet apparatus, saponification, petroleum spirit extraction, evaporation	Chromegasphere Si-60	Isooctane:THF (97.5:2.5)	Fluorescence: excitation 294 nm emission 325 nm	Cort et al. (1983)
α-, β-, γ-, δ-T α, γ-T3	Corn grain (maize)	Saponification, hexane extraction, evaporation	Ultrasphere-Si	Hexane + 1.2–1.3% Pr-2-OH	Fluorescence: excitation 205 nm emission 330 nm	Weber (1984)

Contd.

Table 27—*Cont.*

Analyte	Sample type	Sample preparation	Stationary phase	Mobile phase	Detection	Reference/Fig. no.
				Quantitative HPLC		
α-, β-, γ-, δ-T	Fats and oils	Alkaline digestion (ambient), diethyl ether extraction, evaporation	LiChrosorb Si-60 (column temperature 44°C)	Hexane + 0·4% Pr-2-OH	UV 295 nm	Zonta & Stancher (1983)
α-, β-, γ-, δ-T β-T3	Meat and meat products	Alkaline digestion (ambient), hexane extraction, evaporation	LiChrosorb Si-60	Hexane: diisopropyl ether (93:7)	Fluorescence: excitation 292 nm emission 324 nm	Piironen et al. (1985)
α-, β-, γ-, δ-T α-, β-T3	Fish and fish products	Alkaline digestion (ambient), hexane extraction, evaporation	LiChrosorb Si-60	Hexane: diisopropyl ether (93:7)	Fluorescence: excitation 292 nm emission 324 nm	Syväoja et al. (1985)
Total α-T	Animal feeds	Solvent extraction, saponification, CH_2Cl_2 extraction, evaporation, Sep-Pak (silica) clean-up, evaporation of eluate	Partisil PAC	Hexane:CH_2Cl_2 (70:30) + 0·2% Pr-2-OH	UV 292 nm	Cohen & Lapointe (1980a) (Fig. 95)
α-T	Fish liver	Solvent extraction, evaporation, extraction with MeCN then partition into isooctane, evaporation	μBondapak C_{18}	MeOH:H_2O (90:10)	UV 280 nm	Hung et al. (1980)

Vitamin E acetate	Gelatin-coated supplemental vitamin E in animal feeds	Gelatin coating dissolved in water at 60°C, extraction with perchloroethylene, evaporation	μBondapak C_{18}	MeOH:H_2O (95:5)	UV 280 nm	Eriksen (1980) (Fig. 96)
Vitamin E acetate	Animal feeds	MeOH extraction	μBondapak C_{18}	MeOH:H_2O (98:2)	UV 280 nm	Shaikh et al. (1977)
α-, β-, γ-, δ-T	Condensed milk, milk substitutes	Saponification, diethyl ether extraction, evaporation, precipitation of sterols from a methanolic solution at $-20°C$	μBondapak C_{18}	MeOH:H_2O (90:10)	UV 280 nm	Pickston (1978)
α-, β + γ-, δ-T	Breakfast cereals, margarine, chocolate bars	Saponification, precipitation of soaps with acetic acid in MeCN	LiChrosorb RP-8	MeOH:H_2O (95:5), pH 4·0 with acetic acid	UV 308 nm or fluorescence: excitation 295 nm emission 330 nm	DeVries et al. (1979)
Total α-T	Animal feeds	Saponification, hexane extraction, evaporation	μBondapak C_{18}	MeOH:H_2O (95:5)	Fluorescence: excitation 296 nm emission 330 nm	McMurray et al. (1980) (Fig. 97)
α-T	Liver	Saponification, hexane extraction	Partisil ODS	Hexane:Pr-2-OH (99:1)	Fluorescence: excitation 210 nm emission 325 nm	Rammell et al. (1983) (Fig. 98)

Abbreviations: see foot of Table 24.

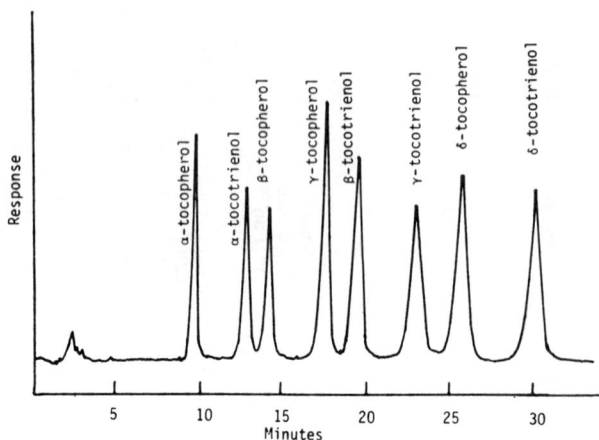

Fig. 88. Adsorption HPLC of E vitamers in standard solution. Column, 5 µm Chromegasphere Si-60; mobile phase, isooctane:tetrahydrofuran (97·5:2·5); fluorescence detection, 294 nm (excitation) and 325 nm (emission) (Reprinted with permission from Cort, W. M., Vincente, T. S., Waysek, E. H. & Williams, B. D. (1983). Vitamin E content of feedstuffs determined by high-performance liquid chromatographic fluorescence. *J. agric. Fd Chem.*, **31**, 1330–3). Copyright (1983) American Chemical Society.

used (Woollard *et al.*, 1987). Glycerides and sterols do not fluoresce, hence do not interfere in the analysis. The only substances found in crude lipid extracts of unfortified foods, which produced peaks near to those of the E vitamers, were plastochromanol-8 and BHA.

Alpha-tocopheryl acetate possesses only 9% of the fluorescence activity of the free tocopherol under normal-phase conditions at specific wavelengths (290 nm excitation; 330 nm emission) (Barnes & Taylor, 1980; Håkansson *et al.*, 1987). The latter authors obtained a detection limit of 0·02 µg for the acetate ester, which was equivalent to a supplementation level of only 0·5 µg/g of food. The levels of the ester in fortified foods range from 5–500 µg/g (Thompson, 1982), hence there is sufficient fluorescence emission to permit its measurement. Woollard *et al.* (1987) employed wavelengths of 280 nm (excitation) and 335 nm (emission) for the simultaneous fluorometric determination of α-tocopheryl acetate and endogenous α-tocopherol in infant formulae. They observed that changing the excitation wavelength to 220 nm enhanced the fluorescence signal of the acetate ester by a factor of three.

The distribution of naturally occurring tocopherols and tocotrienols in oils and fats may be determined by simply dissolving the sample in hexane

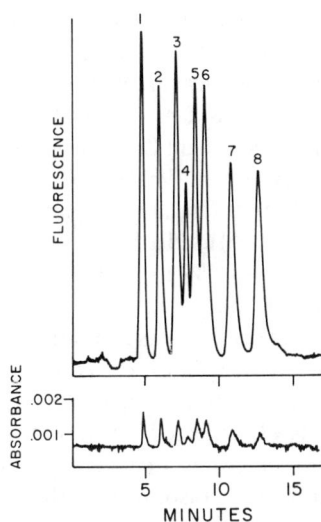

Fig. 89. Adsorption HPLC of E vitamers and BHA comparing fluorescence activity (upper trace) with UV absorbance activity (lower trace). Amount of sample injected: 100 ng of each E vitamer and 20 ng BHA. Peaks: (1) α-T; (2) α-T3; (3) β-T; (4) BHA; (5) γ-T; (6) β-T3; (7) γ-T3; (8) δ-T. (T = tocopherol; T3 = tocotrienol). Column, LiChrosorb Si-60; mobile phase, hexane:diethyl ether (95:5); fluorescence detection, 290 nm (excitation) and 330 nm (emission); UV detection, 295 nm (Reprinted from Thompson & Hatina, 1979, p. 333, by courtesy of Marcel Dekker, Inc.).

(typically 0·5 g in 50 ml), and analysing an aliquot of the hexane extract by normal-phase HPLC. The relatively high concentrations of vitamin E that occur naturally in vegetable oils and certain other fats allow this technique to be performed without the need to concentrate the hexane fraction. Fluorescence detection is obligatory, as UV absorption detection is insufficiently selective, and reveals peaks that interfere with the peaks of the E vitamers. Silica columns can tolerate heavy loads of triglyceride and other non-polar material, which can be easily washed from the column with 25% diethyl ether in hexane after the analyses. External calibration is usually employed with pure standards of those tocopherols and tocotrienols that are available, or can be prepared (Coors & Montag, 1982).

Taylor & Barnes (1981) injected hexane solutions of vegetable oils onto a 250 mm × 4·6 mm i.d. Partisil 5 Silica column eluted with 50% water-saturated hexane:dibutyl ether (90:10) containing 0·05% isopropanol. Fluorescence detection was employed at wavelengths of 290 nm (excitation) and 330 nm (emission). Chromatograms of maize germ oil (corn oil) and cottonseed oil obtained by absorbance detection at 292 nm showed a broad peak which interfered with the measurement of β-tocopherol and γ-tocopherol; fluorescence detection did not show this interference (Fig. 90). Gertz & Herrmann (1982) used a 7 μm LiChrosorb Si-60 column eluted with isooctane:*tert*-butyl methyl ether (98:2), and fluorescence detection at 295 nm (excitation) and 330 nm (emission) to analyse hexane solutions of fats and oils. Syväoja *et al.* (1986) used a 5 μm LiChrosorb Si-60 column and a diisopropyl ether gradient of 8% to 17·6% in hexane to determine the tocopherols and tocotrienols in hexane extracts of vegetable oils, cod liver oil, margarine and butter. Detection was by fluorescence using wavelengths of 290 nm (excitation) and 325 nm (emission). The HPLC column temperature was 30°C (45°C for the separation of γ-tocopherol and β-tocotrienol). Speek *et al.* (1985) injected hexane extracts of seed oils directly onto a 250 mm × 4·6 mm i.d. column packed with 5 μm Polygosil 60 and eluted with hexane:stabilized diisopropyl ether (90:10). Fluorescence detection was used at wavelengths of 296 nm (excitation) and 320 nm (emission). BHT was added as an antioxidant to the diisopropyl ether at 10 mg/litre to prevent the E vitamers from oxidative decomposition. The BHT also improved the chromatography by adsorbing to the silica stationary phase, reducing its polarity, and thus speeding up the analysis. The fluorescence response was reported to be linear for concentrations corresponding to approximately 0·5 μg/g up to 2 mg/g of maize germ oil for each vitamer. The detection limit for each vitamer corresponded to a concentration of 0·5 μg/g. Rammell & Hoogenboom (1985) used a Partisil PAC column with amino–cyano functionality, and a mobile phase of hexane:tetrahydrofuran (94:6) to separate the eight E vitamers, together with plastochromanol-8, in hexane solutions of seed oils. Fluorescence detection was employed using a 210 nm interference filter for excitation and a 325 nm band filter for emission.

Brubacher *et al.* (1985) purified palm oil by freezing the oil at -80°C in a solid CO_2/acetone mixture, and filtering. The HPLC of the E vitamers was performed on a 5 μm LiChrosorb Si-60 column using a mobile phase of hexane:dioxan (96:4) and fluorometric detection at 296 nm (excitation) and 326 nm (emission).

Electrochemical detection has been utilized in the determination of α-, β-, γ- and δ-tocopherols in wheat germ oil using adsorption HPLC, with the electrolyte added postcolumn (Hiroshima *et al.*, 1981). Oil samples were dissolved in hexane and injected onto a 250 mm × 2·1 mm i.d. Zorbax SIL column eluted with hexane:diisopropyl ether (87·5:12·5). The electrolyte

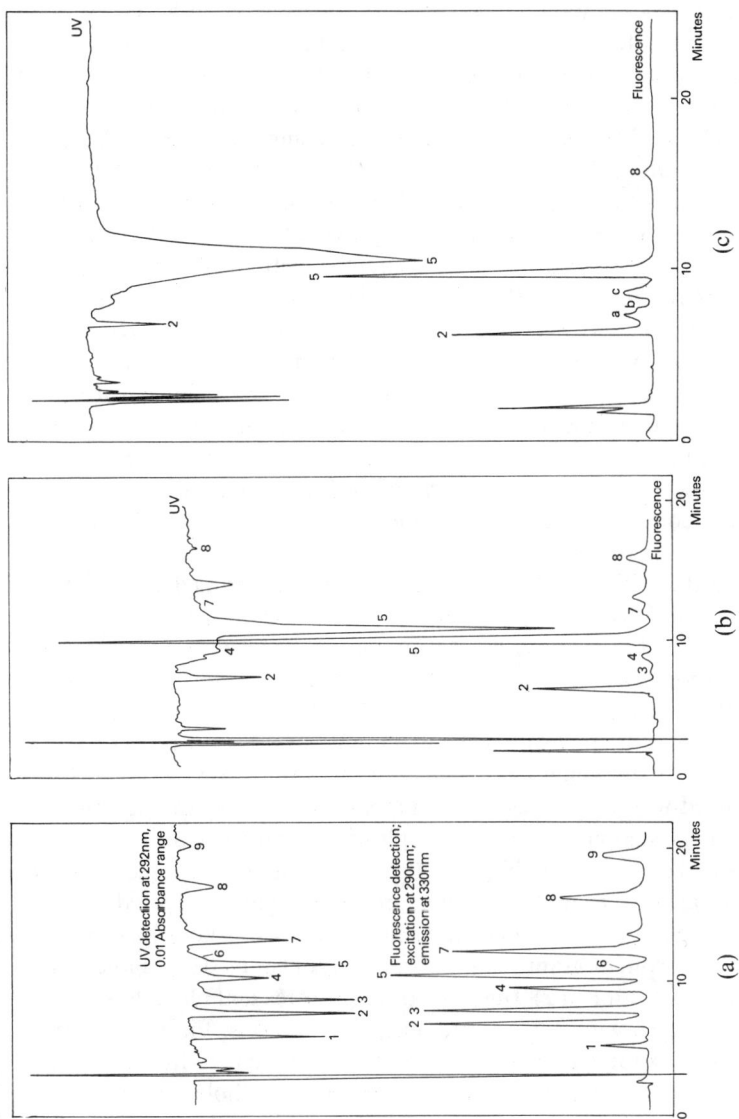

Fig. 90. Adsorption HPLC of E vitamers in hexane solutions of (a) standards, (b) corn oil, and (c) cottonseed oil. Peaks: (1) α-T acetate; (2) α-T; (3) α-T3; (4) β-T; (5) γ-T; (6) β-T3; (7) γ-T3; (8) δ-T; (9) δ-T3; a, b, c unknown, possibly hydrotocopherols or tocodienols. (T = tocopherol; T3 = tocotrienol). Column, Partisil Silica; mobile phase, 50% water-saturated hexane:dibutyl ether (90:10) containing 0·05% isopropanol; dual detection, UV (292 nm) and fluorescence (290 nm, excitation; 330 nm, emission) (from Taylor & Barnes, 1981).

solution was methanol:ethanol (9:1) containing 0·1 M sodium perchlorate, and the applied potential was +0·7 V versus a silver/silver chloride reference electrode. The detection limit of the method was estimated at 1 ng.

Food samples demand a more rigorous method of solvent extraction than simple dissolution in hexane. Wheat products were extracted with hexane in a Soxhlet extractor and analysed using fluorescence detection (290 nm excitation; 330 nm emission) on a 250 mm × 4·6 mm i.d. LiChrosorb Si-60 column eluted with 50% water-saturated hexane:diethyl ether (95:5) (Barnes & Taylor, 1980) or hexane:diisopropyl ether (97:3) (Håkansson *et al.*, 1987). Food composites were extracted with boiling isopropanol, followed by re-extraction with acetone and partitioning of the lipid fraction into hexane (Thompson & Hatina, 1979). The hexane extract was concentrated by evaporation under vacuum before analysis on a 250 mm × 3·2 mm i.d. 5 μm LiChrosorb Si-60 column eluted with 50% water-saturated hexane containing 0·2% isopropanol or 5% diethyl ether. This system, with fluorescence detection (290 nm excitation; 330 nm emission), facilitated the measurement of the four tocopherols (α-, β-, γ- and δ-), three tocotrienols (α-, β- and γ-), and BHA. The efficiency of extraction was reported to be better than 97%.

Woollard & Blott (1986) extracted vitamin E-fortified milk powder formulations with a ternary non-aqueous solvent, followed by partitioning of the total lipid into hexane. An aliquot of the hexane extract, after centrifugation, was analysed on a 10 cm × 8 mm i.d. radially compressed Radial-PAK cartridge containing 5 μm RESOLVE spherical silica, using a mobile phase consisting of hexane containing 0·08% isopropanol. The α-tocopheryl acetate, which was eluted after 7 to 8 min, was visualized using a 280 nm fixed-wavelength detector. Lipid material was rapidly cleared from the column by stepping up the mobile phase flow-rate. The use of a radially compressed cartridge enabled a high flow-rate to be used, without operating at an elevated back-pressure. This significantly reduced the analysis time compared to flow limitations of narrower-bore stainless steel columns. A chromatogram of a fortified whole milk powder obtained using absorbance detection at 280 nm, together with a reagent blank to show the effect of the step-wise flow programme, is depicted in Fig. 91. Complete separation of α-tocopheryl acetate from accompanying vitamin A esters was achieved. A chromatogram of an unfortified whole milk powder is included to confirm the absence of interfering peaks in the area of interest. Figure 92 shows a chromatogram of a typical infant formula containing 4% corn oil, also obtained using absorbance detection at 280 nm. A chromatogram of a fully-filled infant formula containing corn, soya and

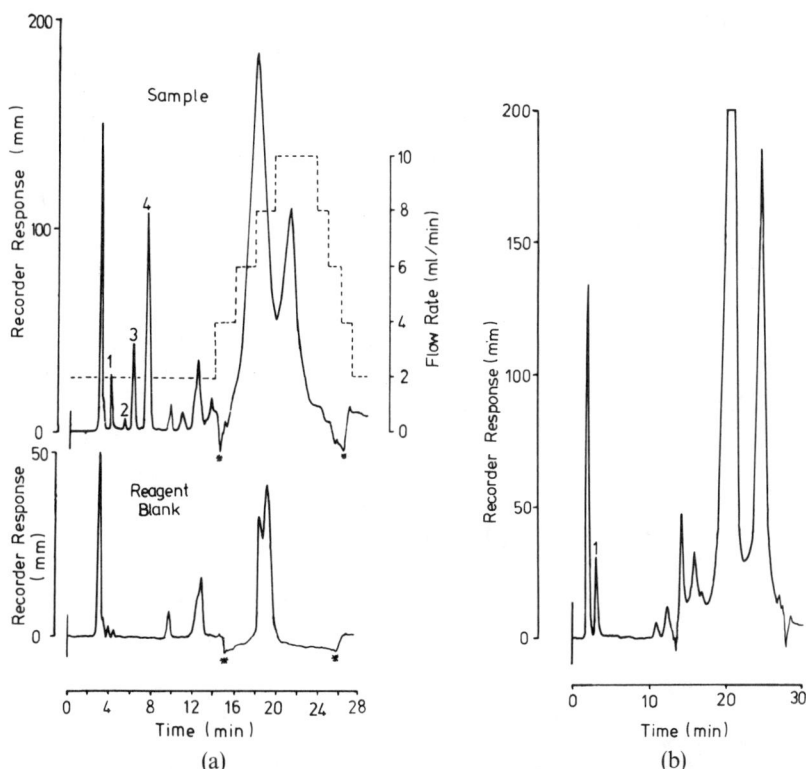

Fig. 91. Adsorption HPLC of vitamin E acetate in lipid extract of (a) vitamin E-fortified infant formula and (b) unfortified infant formula. Dotted lines indicate solvent flow programme. Peaks: (1) retinyl palmitate; (2) 13-*cis*-retinyl acetate; (3) all-*trans*-retinyl acetate; (4) α-tocopheryl acetate.
*Baseline disturbances are due to flow changes. Column, Radial-PAK silica cartridge (5 μm, 8 mm i.d.); mobile phase, 0·08% isopropanol in hexane; UV detection, 280 nm (from Woollard & Blott, 1986).

coconut oils (Fig. 93) demonstrates the benefit of dual absorbance and fluorescence detection. The fluorescence was measured using an excitation wavelength of 295 nm and a 335 nm cut-off emission filter. The fluorescence trace allows the native vitamin E (α-tocopherol) concentration of milk powder to be conveniently estimated, whereas the UV trace is used to quantify the supplemental α-tocopheryl acetate. Retinyl acetate could be assayed simultaneously with α-tocopheryl acetate using absorbance detection or with endogenous α-tocopherol using fluorometric detection. The authors pointed out that a non-programmable

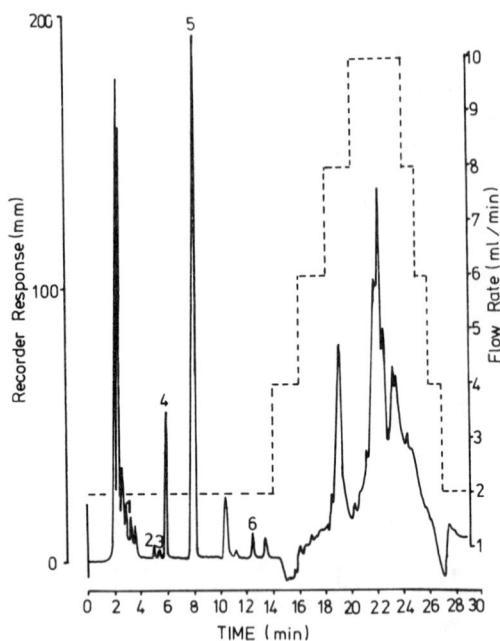

Fig. 92. Adsorption HPLC of vitamin E acetate in lipid extract of vitamin E-fortified infant formula containing 4% corn oil. Peaks: (1) retinyl palmitate; (2) 13-*cis*-retinyl acetate; (3) 9-*cis*-retinyl acetate; (4) all-*trans*-retinyl acetate; (5) α-tocopheryl acetate; (6) α-tocopherol. Chromatographic conditions as for Fig. 91 (from Woollard & Blott, 1986).

dual monochromator fluorescence detector cannot be used to obtain simultaneous detection of vitamins A and E as the increased emission selectivity removes all retinyl fluorescence. The techniques described have also been applied to the determination of α-tocopheryl acetate in animal feeds (Blott & Woollard, 1986).

With the aid of a programmable dual monochromator fluorescence detector, i.e. an instrument which automatically changes the excitation and emission wavelengths with respect to time, the selectivity and sensitivity of the analysis can be optimized. Such an instrument has been utilized in the analysis of serum by adsorption HPLC using the excitation maxima of 295 nm and 325 nm for vitamin E and vitamin A, respectively. The emission maximum (480 nm) was selected for vitamin A, whilst 390 nm was selected as the emission wavelength for vitamin E. Use of the maximum emission wavelength for vitamin E (330 nm) would have resulted in the α-tocopherol peak being 25-fold larger than that of retinol (Rhys Williams, 1985).

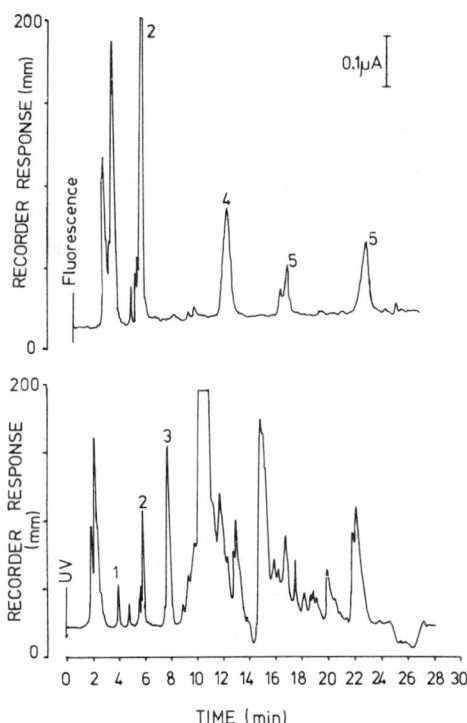

Fig. 93. Adsorption HPLC of vitamin E in lipid extract of vitamin E-fortified fully filled infant formula containing corn, soya and coconut oils. Dual detection: fluorescence, 295 nm excitation with a 335 nm cut-off emission filter (upper trace); UV, 280 nm (lower trace). Peaks: (1) retinyl palmitate; (2) retinyl acetate; (3) α-tocopheryl acetate; (4) α-tocopherol; (5) unidentified E vitamers. Chromatographic conditions as for Fig. 91 (from Woollard & Blott, 1986).

In the analysis of animal feeds, saponification is carried out to hydrolyse the supplemental α-tocopheryl acetate to the free tocopherol, thus providing a measure of the total α-tocopherol content (Cohen & Lapointe, 1980a; McMurray et al., 1980; Manz & Philipp, 1981).

Normal-phase HPLC methods that employ saponification can utilize absorbance detection as well as fluorescence detection, since the unsaponifiable matter is usually free from the interfering material that is present in direct hexane solutions of oils and fats. The lower sensitivity of absorbance detection compared with fluorescence detection is compensated by the concentration step, whereby the ether or hexane solution containing the unsaponifiable matter is evaporated to dryness and redissolved in a small volume of solvent. If fluorescence detection is employed, the hydrolysis step increases the sensitivity as the alcohol exhibits a much stronger fluorescence signal than does the ester.

Manz & Philipp (1981) used saponification in a routine assay for total α-tocopherol of animal feeds. The HPLC system comprised a column of 125 mm length packed with 5 μm LiChrosorb Si-60, a mobile phase of hexane containing 0·1% isopropanol, and a fluorescence detector set at 293 nm (excitation) and 326 nm (emission). Fluorescence detection was essential in the method employed; absorbance detection at 280 nm yielded interfering peaks as well as a lower response (see Fig. 94). Feedstuffs and premixes contain considerable amounts of vitamin A in addition to α-tocopherol. Manz & Philipp (1981) pointed out the importance of awaiting the elution of retinol, which has a longer retention time on a silica column than the tocopherols, before injecting the next sample. Although retinol does not fluoresce at the wavelength set for tocopherols, it quenches their fluorescence because its absorption maximum (325 nm) is in the range of the emission wavelength of the tocopherols.

Cort et al. (1983) separated and identified the naturally occurring tocopherols and tocotrienols in animal feeds, such as soy bean meal, corn, fish meal, cottonseed meal and alfalfa. Samples were extracted with alcohol for 90 min in a Soxhlet apparatus prior to saponification. Analysis was performed using a 5 μm Chromegasphere Si-60 column eluted with isooctane:tetrahydrofuran (97·5:2·5), and detected by fluorescence at wavelengths of 294 nm (excitation) and 325 nm (emission). The average recovery of α-tocopherol added to feed (soy bean oil) was 99·4%; the RSD of the method was 2·7%.

Weber (1984) determined the tocopherols and tocotrienols in corn grain (maize) following direct saponification and extraction. The HPLC system comprised a 250 mm × 4·6 mm i.d. Ultrasphere-Si column eluted with hexane containing 1·2–1·3% isopropanol. Fluorescence was measured using an excitation wavelength of 205 nm and a 330 nm cut-off emission filter. The maize was found to contain only the α- and β-forms of the tocopherols and tocotrienols.

Thompson & Hatina (1979) analysed infant formula foods fortified with α-tocopheryl acetate using a 250 mm × 3·2 mm i.d. 5 μm LiChrosorb Si-60 column, a mobile phase of 50% water-saturated hexane containing 0·2% isopropanol, and a fluorescence detector set at 290 nm (excitation) and 330 nm (emission). The HPLC system was capable of measuring seven out of the eight possible E vitamers (δ-tocotrienol was not detected), but only the four tocopherols were found in the infant formulations tested.

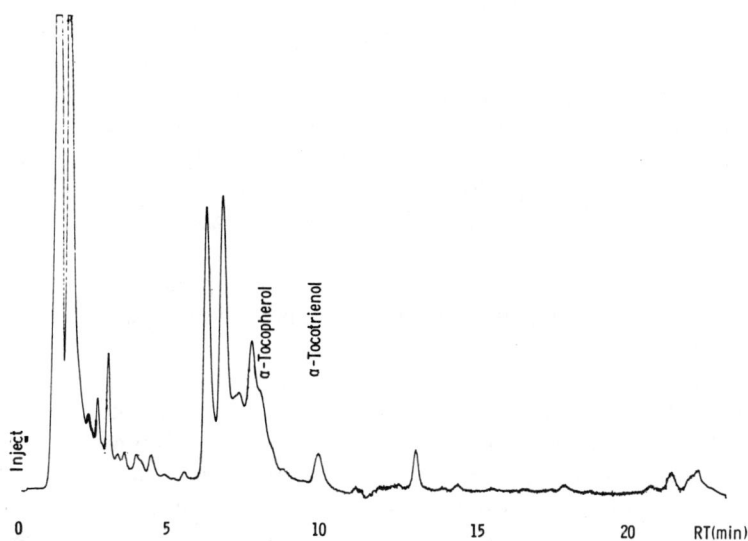

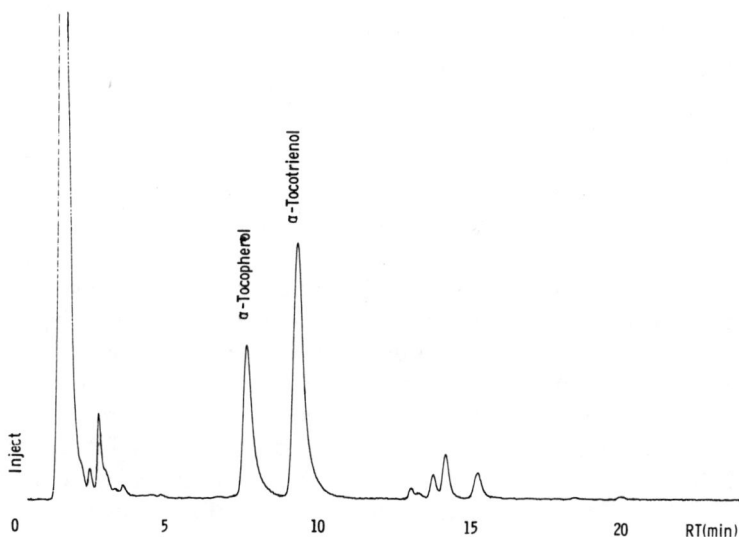

Fig. 94. Adsorption HPLC of vitamin E in the unsaponifiable matter from barley. Upper trace, UV detection at 280 nm; lower trace, fluorescence detection at 293 nm (excitation) and 326 nm (emission). Column, LiChrosorb Si-60; mobile phase, hexane containing 0·1% isopropanol (from Manz & Philipp, 1981).

Zonta & Stancher (1983) hydrolysed oils and fats by alkaline digestion at room temperature. The unsaponifiable matter was analysed on a 250 mm × 2·6 mm i.d. 5 μm LiChrosorb Si-60 column and a guard column dry-packed with 40 μm pellicular silica. The mobile phase was hexane containing 0·4% isopropanol, and the column temperature was 44°C. The four tocopherols were detected spectrophotometrically at 295 nm, and the peaks were characterized by stop-flow analysis; the tocotrienols were not investigated.

Piironen *et al.* (1985) subjected meat and meat products to alkaline digestion at room temperature. The unsaponifiable matter was analysed on a 250 mm × 4 mm i.d. column of 5 μm LiChrosorb Si-60, preceded by a guard column containing pellicular silica, and maintained at 37°C. The mobile phase of hexane:diisopropyl ether (93:7) was monitored by a fluorescence detector set at 292 nm (excitation) and 324 nm (emission). α-Tocopherol was the predominant E vitamer, but small amounts of α-tocotrienol and γ-tocopherol were found in almost every sample. Recoveries of added α-, β-, and γ-tocopherols from meat samples were within the range of 94–100%. The recovery of δ-tocopherol was low, but this vitamer was not detected in any sample. The RSDs for α-, β- and γ-tocopherols were 3·7%, 6·7% and 6·7%, respectively. A similar procedure was employed for the analysis of fish and fish products (Syväoja *et al.*, 1985).

Cohen & Lapointe (1980*a*) employed a polar bonded stationary phase for the determination of total α-tocopherol in animal feeds. Samples were extracted by shaking with a mixture of isooctane:dioxan (80:20) containing ascorbic acid, then filtered and evaporated to dryness under vacuum at 50°C. The residue was saponified and the unsaponifiable components were extracted with dichloromethane, then evaporated to dryness. The residue was dissolved in isooctane and passed into a Sep-Pak (Waters Associates) silica cartridge. The Sep-Pak was eluted with isooctane:dioxan (98:2) and the eluate was evaporated to dryness. The residue was dissolved in a small volume of the HPLC mobile phase, and an aliquot was injected onto a 250 mm × 4 mm i.d. 10 μm Partisil PAC polar bonded-phase column with both nitrile and amino functional groups. The mobile phase of hexane:dichloromethane (70:30) containing 0·2% isopropanol was monitored spectrophotometrically at 292 nm. Chromatograms of extracts from poultry feeds are illustrated in Fig. 95. The average recovery of vitamin E was 96·6% with an RSD of 5·4% in four different animal feeds; the minimum detectable amount of vitamin E in an animal feed was 10 μg/g.

In reversed-phase HPLC, the E vitamers are eluted in the order:

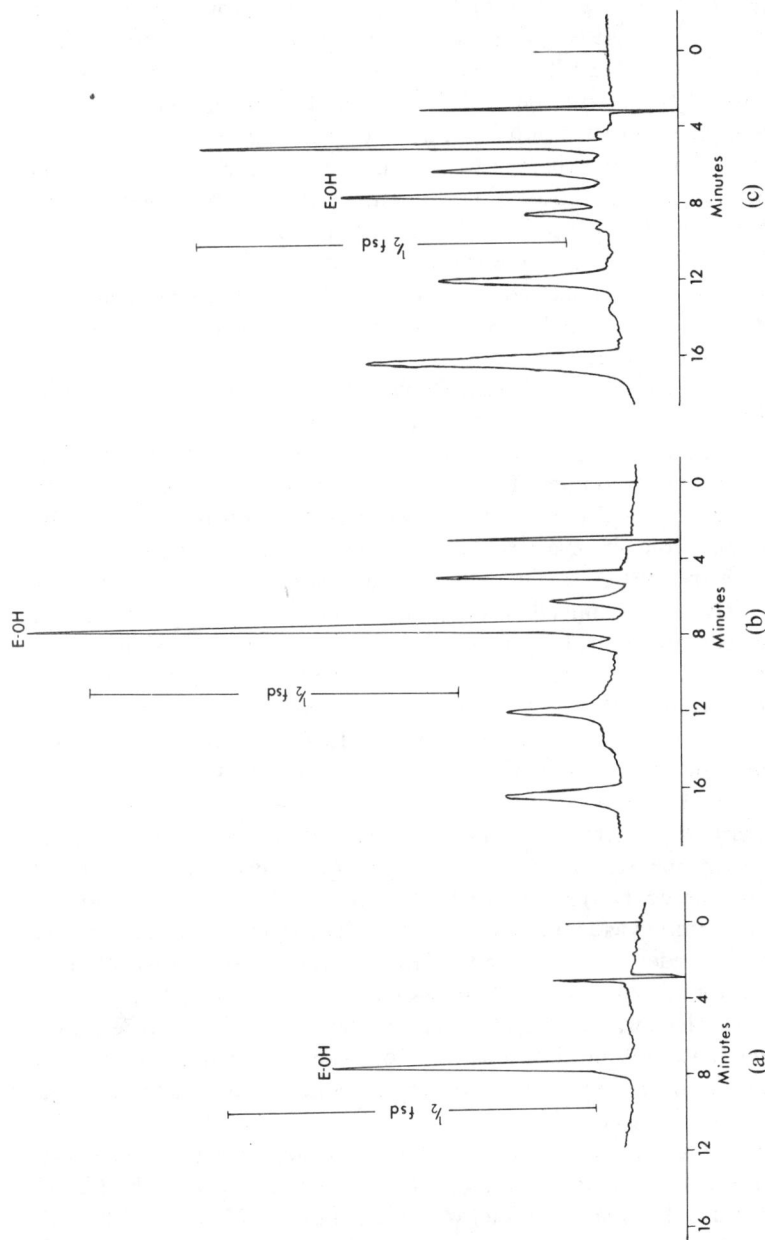

Fig. 95. Normal-phase HPLC of α-tocopherol (E·OH) in (a) α-tocopherol standard (206 ng injected) and the unsaponifiable matter of animal feeds after Sep-Pak filtration: (b) chicken grower containing 72·5 IU added vitamin E/kg, (c) broiler finisher containing 18·2 IU added vitamin E/kg. Column, Partisil PAC; mobile phase, hexane:dichloromethane (70:30) containing 0·2% isopropanol; UV detection, 292 nm (from Cohen & Lapointe, 1980a).

δ-T_3, ($\gamma + \beta$)-T_3, α-T_3, δ-T, ($\gamma + \beta$)-T, α-T. This elution profile contrasts with that of normal-phase HPLC, in which α-tocopherol is eluted first and δ-tocotrienol is eluted last. The positional β- and γ-vitamin E isomers cannot be separated by reversed-phase HPLC, even if gradient elution is used. Reversed-phase columns with isocratic elution are capable of separating α-tocopherol from α-tocopheryl acetate and, because of their easier operation compared with silica adsorption columns, are often preferred for the determination of α-tocopherol or supplemental α-tocopheryl acetate in foods and animal feeds. If the reversed-phase system is operated with a semi-aqueous mobile phase, direct solvent extracts of the sample must be evaporated to dryness, and redissolved in a polar solvent that is compatible with the mobile phase.

The above technique has been employed for the determination of α-tocopherol in fish liver (Hung et al., 1980). The liver sample was homogenized with isooctane:dioxan (80:20), and the combined extracts were dried under vacuum. The residue was extracted three times with acetonitrile, from which α-tocopherol was then partitioned into isooctane. The residue from the evaporated isooctane solution was dissolved in a portion of the HPLC mobile phase, and an aliquot was injected directly onto a 300 mm $\times$ 3·9 mm i.d. μBondapak C_{18} column preceded by a guard column containing pellicular Bondapak C_{18}/Corasil (37–50 μm). The mobile phase of methanol:water (90:10) was monitored spectrophotometrically at 280 nm. Recovery of α-tocopherol added to the sample was 80–92%, with a mean of 86·2%, and an RSD of 4·9%. The minimum concentration of α-tocopherol that could be accurately determined by the method was 1 μg/g of liver.

Eriksen (1980) described a rapid method for the determination of gelatin-coated supplemental vitamin E in feeds. Samples were mixed with water and left on a water bath at 60°C to dissolve the coating. Ethanol was added, and the mixture was extracted with perchloroethylene. The solvent was evaporated under vacuum at 60°C, and the residue was redissolved in methanol for injection onto a 300 mm $\times$ 4 mm i.d. μBondapak C_{18} column. The mobile phase was methanol:water (95:5) and the absorbance detection wavelength was 280 nm. The separation of α-tocopherol and α-tocopheryl acetate is illustrated in Fig. 96, which also depicts chromatograms obtained from two animal feeds.

Shaikh et al. (1977) avoided the evaporation step by extracting animal feedstuffs with methanol, which was directly compatible with the HPLC mobile phase. The filtered extract was injected onto a 300 mm $\times$ 4 mm i.d. μBondapak C_{18} column with a guard column containing pellicular

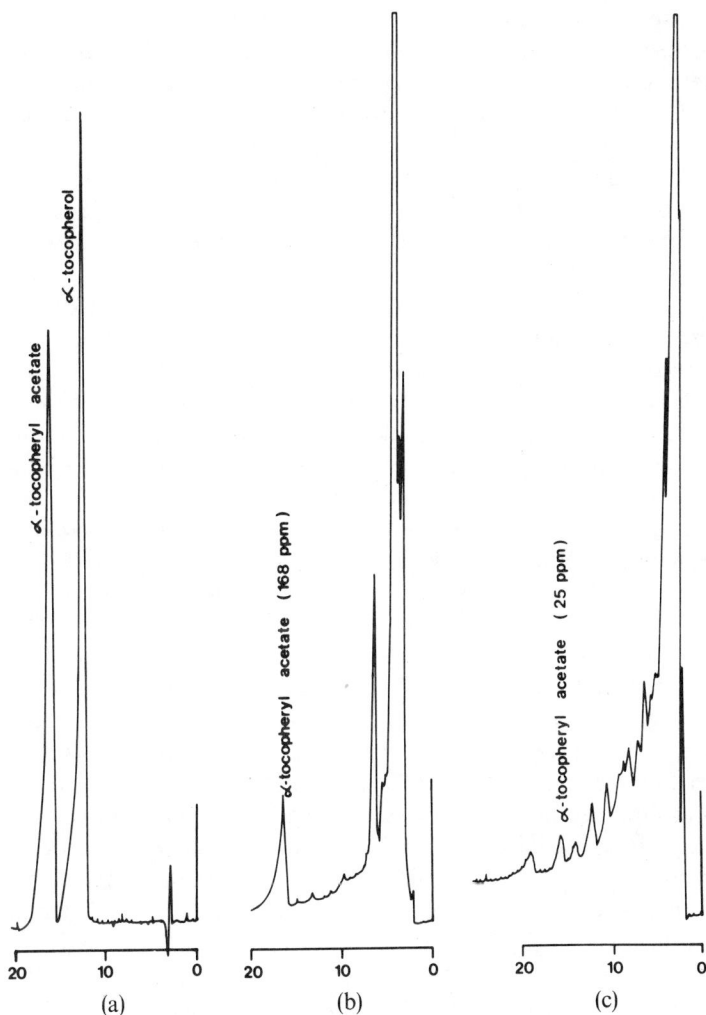

Fig. 96.   Reversed-phase HPLC of α-tocopheryl acetate. (a) Standard solution of α-tocopherol (14·9 μg injected) and α-tocopheryl acetate (17·2 μg injected); and extracts from (b) feed concentrate, (c) pig feed mixture. Column, μBondapak C$_{18}$; mobile phase, methanol:water (95:5); UV detection, 280 nm (from Eriksen, 1980).

Bondapak C_{18}/Corasil. The mobile phase of methanol:water (98:2) was monitored photometrically at 280 nm.

Pickston (1978) determined the tocopherols (α-, $\beta + \gamma$- and δ-) in saponified condensed milks and milk substitutes. The dried unsaponifiable matter was dissolved in methanol and further purified by storing at $-20°C$ for 16 h to precipitate out interfering compounds (presumably sterols). The solution was filtered, and an aliquot of the filtrate was injected onto a 300 mm × 4 mm i.d. μBondapak C_{18} column. The mobile phase of methanol:water (90:10) was monitored photometrically at 280 nm.

DeVries et al. (1979) saponified foods (breakfast cereals, margarine and chocolate bars) in the presence of pyrogallol, and precipitated the fatty acid salts (soaps) with acetic acid in acetonitrile. An aliquot of the filtered material was analysed on a LiChrosorb RP-8 column eluted with methanol:water (95:5) adjusted to pH 4·0 with acetic acid. Detection of the tocopherol (α-, $\beta + \gamma$- and δ-) was performed either by absorbance measurement at 308 nm or by fluorescence at 295 nm (excitation) and 330 nm (emission). The average recovery of added α-tocopheryl acetate was 98·4%, and the RSD of the α-tocopherol content was 4·2%.

McMurray et al. (1980) found that saponification, followed by extraction of the unsaponifiable matter with hexane, more efficiently released natural α-tocopherol from feedstuffs than extraction before saponification. The former method yielded higher recoveries of α-tocopherol (92–95%) compared with recoveries of 85–89% obtained with the latter method, and gave less trouble with emulsions. Aliquots of the concentrated hexane extracts containing the unsaponifiable components were analysed on a 300 mm × 3·9 mm i.d. μBondapak C_{18} column eluted with methanol:water (95:5). Fluorescence detection (296 nm excitation; 330 nm emission) rather than absorbance detection was used, since absorbance measurement at 280 nm revealed peaks with similar retention times to the α-tocopherol peak. Figure 97 shows the peaks of $\gamma + \beta$-tocotrienols, α-tocotrienol and $\gamma + \beta$-tocopherols, as well as α-tocopherol, in the unsaponifiable matter of animal feeds.

Ueda & Igarashi (1985) employed electrochemical detection to determine α-, $\beta + \gamma$-, and δ-tocopherols in saponified animal feeds. The reversed-phase HPLC system comprised a 250 mm × 4·0 mm i.d. Yanapak ODS-T column eluted with methanol containing 0·05 M sodium perchlorate as the conducting electrolyte. An amperometric detector was operated with an applied potential of $+0·8$ V versus a silver/silver chloride reference electrode. The detector could measure α-tocopherol down to 0·1 ng, and was twenty times more sensitive than fluorescence detection.

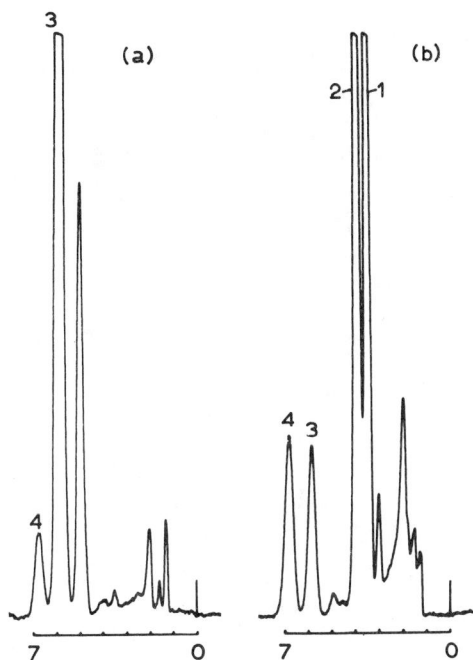

Fig. 97. Reversed-phase HPLC of α-tocopherol in the unsaponifiable matter from two animal feeds (a) and (b). Peaks: (1) $\gamma + \beta$-T3; (2) α-T3; (3) $\gamma + \beta$-T; (4) α-T. (T = tocopherol; T3 = tocotrienol). Column, μBondapak C_{18}; mobile phase, methanol: water (95:5); fluorescence detection, 296 nm (excitation) and 330 nm (emission) (from McMurray *et al.*, 1980).

Non-aqueous mobile phases permit hexane extracts of the unsaponifiable matter to be injected directly onto the reversed-phase HPLC column, thus avoiding the evaporation step necessary to dissolve the unsaponifiable matter in a polar solvent. Rammell *et al.* (1983) injected acid-washed hexane extracts of saponified liver onto a 10 μm Partisil ODS column eluted with hexane:isopropanol (99:1). The isopropanol acted as a polar modifier to resolve the α-tocopherol in a short time. Fluorescence detection was employed using a 210 nm interference filter for excitation, whilst the emission wavelength was provided by a 295 nm cut-off filter and a 325 nm band filter. Although the method was devised primarily for α-tocopherol, it was also capable of separating and measuring $(\beta + \gamma)$-tocopherol and δ-tocopherol (see Fig. 98).

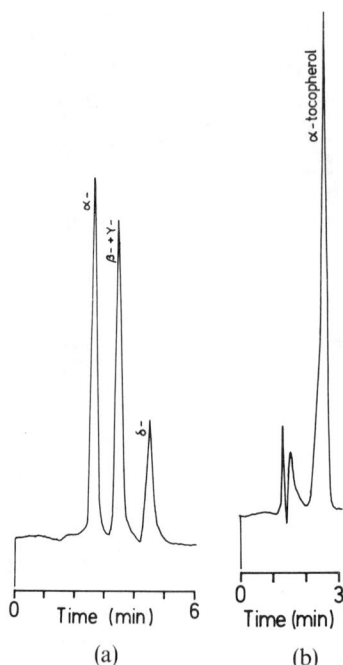

Fig. 98.   NARP of α-tocopherol and other tocopherols. (a) Standard solution of α-, β-, γ- and δ-tocopherols, (b) unsaponifiable matter from liver. Column, Partisil ODS; mobile phase, hexane containing 1% isopropanol; fluorescence detection, 210 nm (excitation) and 325 nm (emission) (Reprinted from Rammell *et al.*, 1983, pp. 1127–8, by courtesy of Marcel Dekker, Inc.).

8.3.5 Vitamin K

Adsorption HPLC facilitates the separation of *cis*- and *trans*-vitamin K_1 from one another, and from the menaquinones, MK-4 to MK-10. A mobile phase of hexane:50% water-saturated dichloromethane (75:25), used with a 5 μm spherical (Spherisorb) or an irregular (Partisil) silica column packing separated, in order of elution: *cis*-K_1, *trans*-K_1, MK-10 and MK-4 (see Fig. 99). The menaquinones of intermediate side chain length could not be resolved from each other, and vitamin K_1 could not be separated from its epoxide metabolite. The elution order of the menaquinones was related to their polarity, MK-10 being more lipophilic than MK-4. Polar-bonded stationary phases with nitrile or amino-nitrile functionality (Spherisorb-5 CN and Partisil 10 PAC) produced similar separations to those produced by the underivatized silica (Haroon *et al.*, 1981).

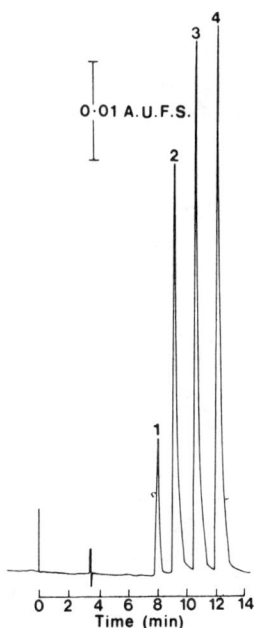

Fig. 99. Adsorption HPLC of vitamin K compounds. Peaks: (1) *cis*-K$_1$; (2) *trans*-K$_1$; (3) MK-10; (4) MK-4. (MK = menaquinone). Column, 5 µm Spherisorb; mobile phase, hexane:50% water-saturated dichloromethane (75:25); UV detection, 250 nm (from Haroon *et al.*, 1981).

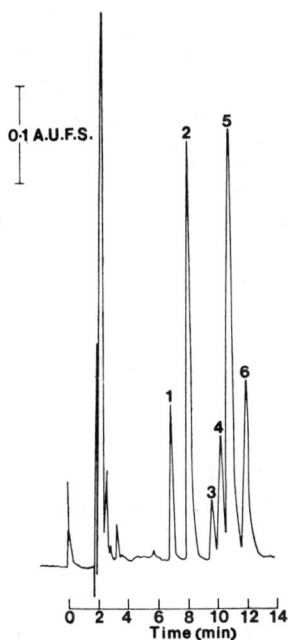

Fig. 100. Adsorption HPLC of *cis* and *trans* isomers of vitamin K compounds. Peaks: (1) *cis*-chloro-K$_1$; (2) *trans*-chloro-K$_1$; (3) *cis*-K$_1$; (4) *cis*-K$_1$ epoxide; (5) *trans*-K$_1$ epoxide; (6) *trans*-K$_1$. Column, 5 µm Spherisorb; mobile phase, hexane:dry dichloromethane (75:25); UV detection, 250 nm (from Haroon *et al.*, 1980).

The use of dry dichloromethane as a polar modifier in hexane, and a column packed with spherical microparticulate silica, facilitated the separation of *cis*- and *trans*-vitamin K$_1$ from their corresponding epoxide metabolites (Haroon *et al.*, 1980). A mobile phase of hexane:dry dichloromethane (75:25), used with a 5 µm Spherisorb column separated, in order of elution, *cis*-K$_1$, *cis*-K$_1$ epoxide, *trans*-K$_1$ epoxide and *trans*-K$_1$. Chloro-K$_1$ (*cis* and *trans* isomers), which is a synthetic antagonist of vitamin K$_1$, was eluted before *cis*-K$_1$ (see Fig. 100). However, the use of dry dichloromethane resulted in considerable peak tailing and low column efficiency with the spherical (Spherisorb) silica column packing, whilst irregular silica microparticles (Partisil 5) failed to separate *trans*-K$_1$ and the K$_1$ epoxide (*cis* and *trans* isomers unresolved).

In contrast to the results obtained by Haroon *et al.* (1980, 1981), Lefevere *et al.* (1985) encountered difficulties in equilibrating the columns, and eliminating strong peak tailing, when they used dichloromethane (either dry or partially saturated with water) as a modifier in hexane. The latter authors suggested that these conflicting observations might be attributable to the presence of different stabilizers in the dichloromethane from different suppliers. They preferred the use of diisopropyl ether or isopropanol as modifiers for the separation of *cis*- and *trans*-vitamin K_1.

HPLC methods for estimating vitamin K in foods and feeds are summarized in Table 28.

Hwang (1985) employed adsorption column chromatography as a clean-up step and adsorption HPLC to determine *cis* and *trans* isomers of vitamin K_1 in infant formula foods. Samples (20 ml) of ready-to-feed liquid products, diluted concentrates or reconstituted powders, were mixed with concentrated ammonium hydroxide and methanol by swirling in a separating funnel. The mixture was then extracted twice with dichloro-methane:isooctane (2:1), and the organic extracts were combined and evaporated under vacuum at 70°C. The oil residue was further dried by co-evaporating three times with acetone, and flushed with nitrogen to produce a clear dry oil. The dried oil residue was dissolved in 10 ml of isooctane containing 0·01% isopropanol and loaded onto a glass column containing dry-packed silica. The vitamin K_1 was eluted from the column with isooctane:dichloromethane:isopropanol (85:15:0·02), and the eluate was evaporated to near dryness under vacuum at 70°C. The oil residue was then dissolved in isooctane and analysed on a 250 mm × 4·5 mm i.d. 5 μm Apex Silica column eluted with isooctane:dichloromethane:isopropanol (70:30:0·02) using photometric detection at 254 nm. Typical chromato-grams of milk-based and soy-based infant formula powders and of vitamin K_1 standard are shown in Fig. 101. The method precision for *trans*-vitamin K_1 was 3·3% RSD, and the recovery was 98 ± 4%. The detection limit was 0·3 ng for both *cis* and *trans* isomers of vitamin K_1.

Manz & Maurer (1982) devised a simple method for determining water-soluble derivatives of menadione in premixes and animal feedstuffs using adsorption HPLC. The active compound was extracted and converted to the free menadione by agitating a sample weighing between 1 and 10 g sequentially with chloroform, dilute ammonia solution, and a Celite/sodium sulphate mixture in a 100 ml centrifuge tube, and then centrifuging. The chloroform extract was diluted or concentrated so that the final solution contained about 0·5–5 μg of menadione per ml. An aliquot of this solution containing carbazole as an internal standard was injected onto a

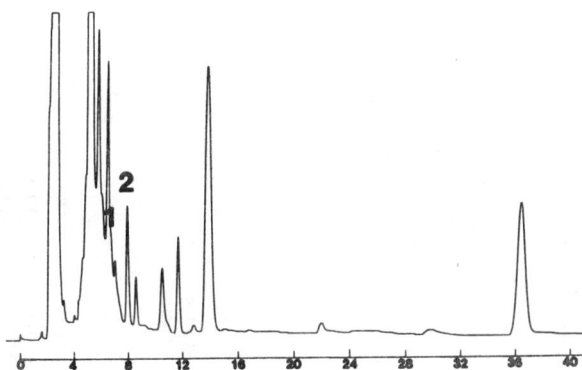

(a)

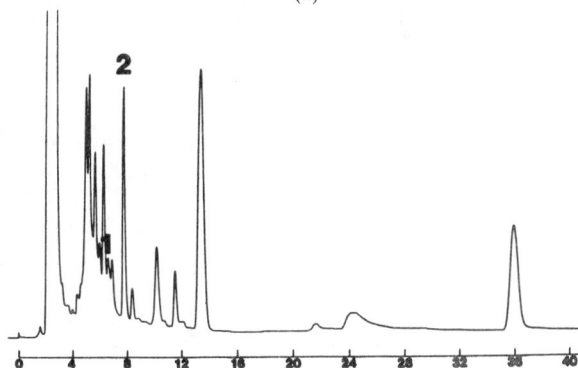

(b)

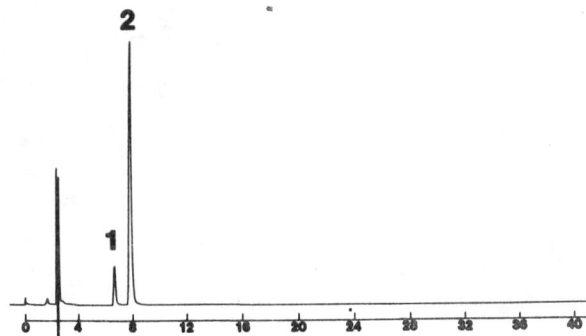

TIME (MIN)

(c)

Fig. 101. Adsorption HPLC of vitamin K_1 *cis* and *trans* isomers. Purified lipid extracts of (a) milk-based, and (b) soy protein-based infant formula powders; (c) vitamin K_1 standard. Peaks: (1) *cis*-K_1; (2) *trans*-K_1. Column, 5 μm Apex Silica; mobile phase, isooctane:dichloromethane:isopropanol (70:30:0·02); UV detection, 254 nm (from Hwang, 1985).

Table 28

HPLC methods used for vitamin K compounds

Analyte	Sample type	Sample preparation	Semi-preparative HPLC	Quantitative HPLC	Reference/ Fig. no.
Cis- and trans-vitamin K_1	Infant formulae			Apex Silica (5 μm) Isooctane:CH_2Cl_2:Pr-2-OH (70:30:0·02) UV 254 nm	Hwang (1985) (Fig. 101)
Water-soluble derivatives of menadione	Animal feeds	Conversion to free menadione by sequential treatment with $CHCl_3$, dilute NH_4OH and Celite/Na_2SO_4; $CHCl_3$ extract analysed by HPLC		LiChrosorb Si-60 5% THF (or 4% $CHCl_3$) in hexane UV 251 or 254 nm	Manz & Maurer (1982)
Vitamin K_1	Fruit, vegetables, milk (unfortified)	Successive extraction with Pr-2-OH and acetone, partition into hexane, evaporation, hydroxyalkoxypropyl Sephadex column chromatography	LiChrosorb Si-60 (10 mm i.d. preparative column) Hexane + 0·03% Pr-2-OH UV 262 nm	LiChrosorb RP-18 Methanol gradient of 85% to 100% in water UV 262 nm	Thompson et al. (1979) (Figs 102–104)

Vitamin K_1	Infant formulae	Enzymatic hydrolysis, pentane extraction, evaporation	μBondapak C_{18} MeOH:MeCN:THF: H_2O (39:39:16:6) UV 254 nm	Bueno & Villalobos (1983) (Fig. 105)
Vitamin K_1	Soy bean oil	Enzymatic hydrolysis, pentane extraction, evaporation, alumina column chromatography, evaporation of eluate	Supelcosil LC-18 MeOH:MeCN:H_2O (88:10:2) UV 270 nm	Zonta & Stancher (1985) (Fig. 106)
Vitamin K_1	Whole fluid milk, infant formulae (unfortified and fortified)	$CHCl_3$/MeOH extraction, vitamin K_1 epoxide added as internal standard, filtration, evaporation of $CHCl_3$ phase, Kieselgel 60 column chromatography, evaporation of eluate, semi-preparative HPLC, evaporation of eluate	Partisil Silica or Partisil PAC Hexane:50% H_2O-saturated CH_2Cl_2 (8:2) UV 254 nm	Haroon et al. (1982) (Figs 110, 111)

Zorbax ODS MeOH:CH_2Cl_2 (8:2) UV 270 nm

Abbreviations: see foot of Table 24.

250 mm × 3·2 mm i.d. 5 μm LiChrosorb Si-60 column eluted with 5% tetrahydrofuran in hexane (or 4% chloroform in hexane). The mobile phase was monitored using a variable wavelength spectrophotometric detector set at 251 nm or a 254 nm fixed-wavelength detector. In the case of low concentrations (< 2 ppm) of menadione the extraction solvent (chloroform) was replaced by the elution solvent used for the HPLC. The procedure had a detection limit of 0·5 ppm menadione, and the RSD determined with an 8 ppm feed sample was ±6% ($n = 9$).

Reversed-phase HPLC can resolve individual menaquinones and phylloquinones, but the technique cannot separate the inactive *cis* isomer of vitamin K_1 from the active *trans* isomer. Thompson *et al.* (1979) described a procedure for determining vitamin K_1 in fruit, vegetables and milk, in which the lipid fraction was purified by open-column chromatography on hydroxyalkoxypropyl Sephadex (HAPS), followed by preparative HPLC on a wide-bore silica column. Analysis of the vitamin K_1 fraction was performed by reversed-phase HPLC using gradient elution. The procedure was as follows.

Food samples (10 g) were extracted with hot isopropanol, followed by acetone extraction, and partitioning of the vitamin K and accompanying lipids into hexane. The pooled hexane extracts were washed with water, and evaporated to dryness under vacuum. The residue was redissolved in hexane and applied to a short (3 cm×1 cm) HAPS column, using hexane elution to remove polar lipids and chlorophylls from the lipid fraction. Extracts from milk were applied to a longer (120 cm × 1 cm) HAPS column, also eluted with hexane, and monitored photometrically at 254 nm. This column separated vitamin K_1 and the lower menaquinones from the triglycerides. The vitamin K fraction from the HAPS column was then subjected to preparative HPLC, using a system which comprised a 250 mm × 10 mm i.d. LiChrosorb Si-60 column, a mobile phase of hexane containing 0·03% isopropanol, and an absorbance detector set at 262 nm. The preparative HPLC separated a phylloquinone peak from a menaquinone peak (Fig. 102). A fraction was collected to include the phylloquinone peak, and the fraction was analysed on a 250 mm × 3·2 mm i.d. LiChrosorb RP-18 column, using a 30 min linear gradient of 85% methanol in water to 100% methanol, and absorbance detection at 262 nm. The quantitative reversed-phase system was capable of separating individual menaquinones and phylloquinones (Fig. 103). A chromatogram showing the vitamin K_1 peak in a purified extract of lettuce is depicted in Fig. 104.

Bueno & Villalobos (1983) determined vitamin K_1 in infant formula

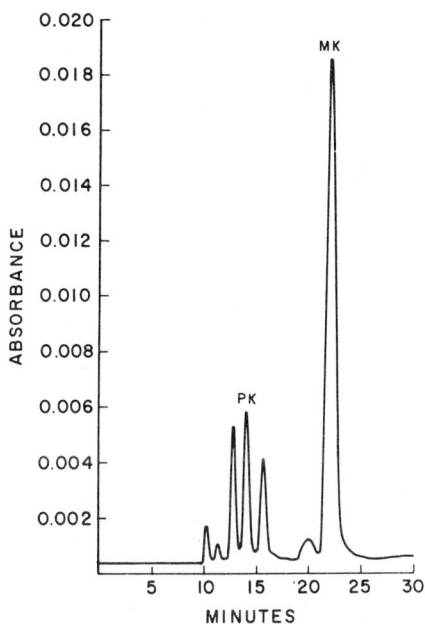

Fig. 102. Preparative adsorption HPLC of purified lipid extract from food showing the separation of phylloquinones (PK) from menaquinones (MK). Column, wide-bore LiChrosorb Si-60; mobile phase, hexane containing 0·03% isopropanol; UV detection, 262 nm (from Thompson *et al.*, 1979).

foods by reversed-phase HPLC after enzymatic hydrolysis and extraction with pentane. Samples of ready-to-feed formulations, diluted concentrates, and reconstituted powders containing 0·01–0·02 mg of vitamin K_1 and <4 g fat were digested with lipase for 1·5 h at 37°C at a pH of 7·7. The hydrolysate was transferred to a separating funnel containing ethanolic sodium hydroxide solution, then immediately extracted three times with pentane. The combined pentane extracts were washed with water to neutral pH, then dried over anhydrous sodium sulphate, and evaporated to dryness under vacuum at 40°C. The residue was dissolved in 10 ml of hexane, then quantitatively transferred to a 15 ml conical centrifuge tube, and evaporated to 1 ml. Aliquots (10 μl) of the concentrated hexane solution were analysed on a 250 mm × 4 mm i.d. column of μBondapak C_{18} using a mobile phase of methanol:acetonitrile:tetrahydrofuran:water (39:39:16:6) and a 254 nm photometric detector. Chromatograms of vitamin K_1 standard, sample, and sample spiked with vitamin K_1 are

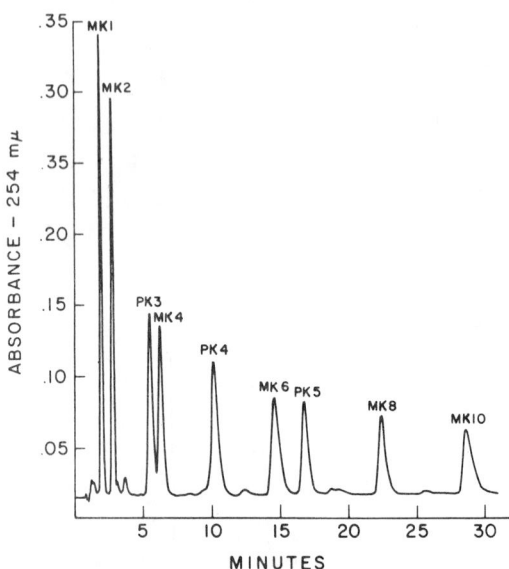

Fig. 103. Reversed-phase HPLC showing the separation of individual mena-quinones and phylloquinones. (PK4 = vitamin K_1). Column, LiChrosorb RP-18; gradient elution programme, 30 min linear gradient of 85% to 100% methanol (in water); UV detection, 262 nm (from Thompson *et al.*, 1979).

shown in Fig. 105. The recovery of vitamin K_1 added to five infant formula foods ranged from 84 to 103%. RSD values of duplicate assays on six samples ranged from 1·33 to 6·71%.

Zonta & Stancher (1985) determined vitamin K_1 in soy bean oil by reversed-phase HPLC after removal of the triglycerides by enzymatic hydrolysis and extraction with pentane, and further purification on a gravity-flow alumina column. Quantification was performed using the standard addition method. The sample/standard mixtures were digested with lipase for 15 h at 37°C at a pH of 5·5, then extracted with pentane. Before separating the organic and aqueous layers, ethanolic KOH was added in order to obtain the fatty acid soaps. Separation of the layers was then performed rapidly. The aqueous layer was re-extracted with pentane, and the pooled organic extract was washed with phosphate buffer (pH 7·7), followed by distilled water. The organic extract was dried over anhydrous sodium sulphate, then evaporated to dryness under vacuum. The dried extract was redissolved in hexane and loaded onto an alumina column. The column was eluted with 7% diethyl ether in hexane, discarding the first

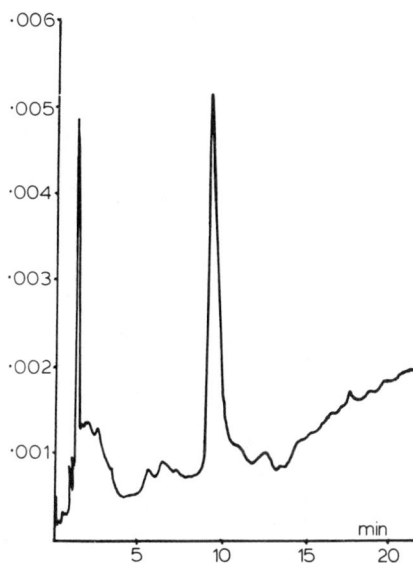

Fig. 104. Reversed-phase HPLC of the phylloquinone fraction isolated by preparative HPLC (Fig. 102) from purified extract of lettuce. The major peak is PK4 (vitamin K_1). Chromatographic conditions as for Fig. 103 (from Thompson *et al.*, 1979).

45 ml of eluate. The next 50 ml was collected, evaporated, and redissolved in hexane. A 25 μl aliquot of the hexane solution was analysed on a 150 mm × 4·6 mm i.d. column of 5 μm Supelcosil LC-18 using a mobile phase of methanol:acetonitrile:water (88:10:2) and absorbance detection at 270 nm (Fig. 106). The mean recovery of the whole procedure was 88·2%.

Speek *et al.* (1984) described a method for determining menadione sodium bisulphite in animal feeds and premixes at concentrations as low as 0·02 μg/g. After aqueous extraction, the vitamin derivative was converted into menadione, which was extracted and separated on a 250 mm × 4·6 mm i.d. 5 μm Hypersil ODS column eluted with ethanol:water (60:40). The menadione was reduced to 2-methyl-1,4-dihydroxynaphthalene by sodium borohydride reagent in a post-column reaction coil, then detected spectrofluorometrically at wavelengths of 325 nm (excitation) and 425 nm (emission).

Langenberg *et al.* (1986) employed an electrochemical detector as a post column reactor in the analysis of vegetables to reduce vitamin K_1 to its hydroquinone form, which was then detected fluorometrically. The selectivity of the method eliminated the need for clean-up or fractionation

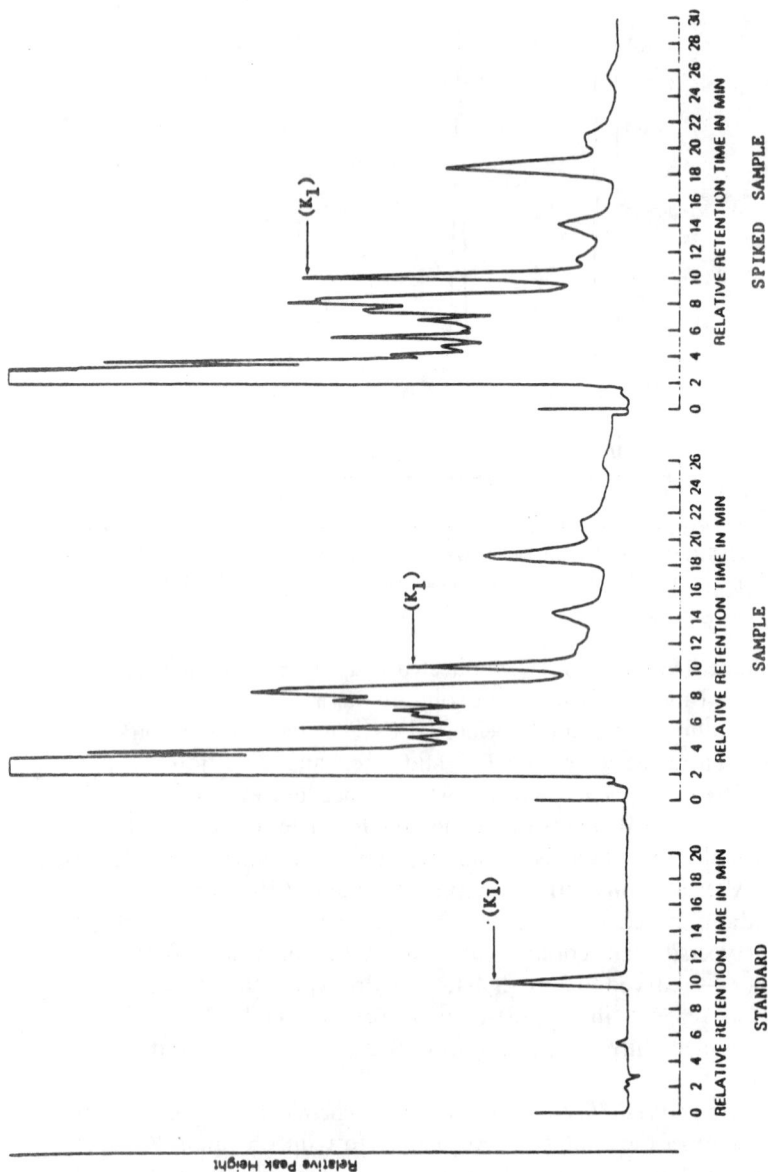

Fig. 105. Reversed-phase HPLC of vitamin K_1. (a) Vitamin K_1 standard, (b) enzymatic hydrolysate of an infant formula, and (c) the same hydrolysate spiked with vitamin K_1. Column, μBondapak C_{18}; mobile phase, methanol:acetonitrile:tetrahydrofuran:water (39:39:16:6); UV detection, 254 nm (from Bueno & Villalobos, 1983).

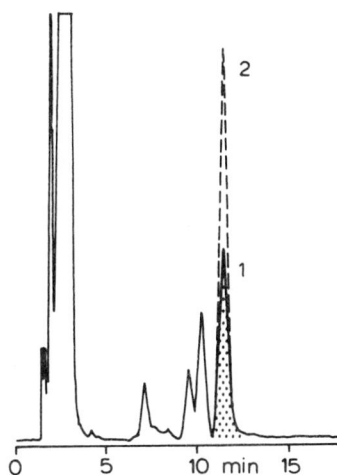

Fig. 106. Reversed-phase HPLC of soy bean oil after enzymatic hydrolysis and alumina column clean-up. Peaks: (1) vitamin K_1 endogenous to the oil; (2) endogenous vitamin K_1 plus vitamin K_1 added for determining recovery. Column, $5\,\mu m$ Supelcosil LC-18; mobile phase, methanol:acetonitrile:water (88:10:2); UV detection, 270 nm (from Zonta & Stancher, 1985).

of the crude lipid extracts. The vegetable material was homogenized with isopropanol in the presence of MK-6 as an internal standard. The vitamin K and accompanying lipids were then partitioned into hexane, an aliquot of which was evaporated to dryness under vacuum at ambient temperature. The residue was redissolved in methanol for reversed-phase HPLC on a 100 mm × 3·0 mm i.d. 5 μm Hypersil-MOS column eluted with methanol: water (92·5:7·5) containing a 0·03 molar concentration of sodium perchlorate as the supporting electrolyte. The spectrofluorometric detector was operated at an excitation wavelength of 320 nm and an emission wavelength of 430 nm. A chromatogram of an extract of raw kale is depicted in Fig. 107. The recovery of the extraction procedure was about 92·5% and the limit of detection was 50 pg of vitamin K_1 injected.

Haroon et al. (1987) reported that 95% of the injected K vitamins could be reduced to their corresponding hydroquinones by postcolumn reaction with zinc metal compared to 60% reduction using an electrochemical detector. Furthermore, the zinc/vitamin K reaction method permits the use of highly efficient NARP systems, which are precluded during electrochemical reduction as the mobile phase cannot dissolve the supporting electrolyte.

Indyk (1988) reported that a commercial fluorescence detector equipped with a high intensity xenon lamp source facilitated the photochemical reduction and simultaneous fluorescence detection of vitamin K_1 during normal passage of the column effluent through the flow cell. The technique, which was applied to vitamin premixes, allowed both normal-phase and

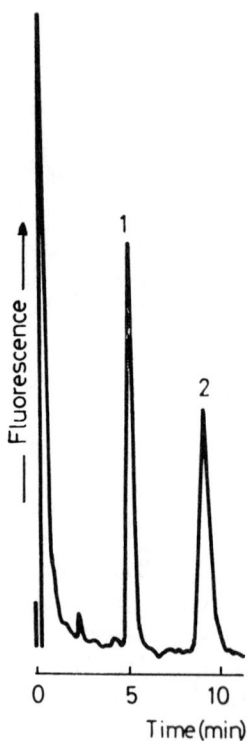

Fig. 107. Reversed-phase HPLC of an extract of raw kale after electrochemical reduction of vitamin K_1 and menaquinone-6 (internal standard) to their respective hydroquinones. Peaks: (1) vitamin K_1; (2) MK-6. Column, 5 μm Hypersil MOS; mobile phase, methanol: water (92·5:7·5) containing 0·03 mol sodium perchlorate; potential applied to the coulometric cell, -500 mV; fluorescence detection, 320 nm (excitation) and 430 nm (emission) (from Langenberg *et al.*, 1986).

reversed-phase HPLC to be employed at detection wavelengths of 325 nm (excitation) and 420 nm (emission).

NARP facilitates the separation of the various analogues of the K_1 and MK-$_n$ series; the technique is well-suited for the long chain menaquinones, which are so lipophilic that they are insoluble in pure methanol. Geometric isomers are not separated by NARP. Shearer *et al.* (1980) obtained baseline separation of eight different K vitamins in a single run within 20 min using NARP with gradient elution. The resolution of K_1 and menaquinones (MK-4 to MK-10) was obtained on a 250 mm × 4·6 mm i.d. 6 μm Zorbax ODS column using a solvent gradient in which the concentration of dichloromethane in methanol was increased linearly at a rate of 5% per min from an initial concentration of 20% to a final concentration of 50% (see Fig. 108). Haroon *et al.* (1981) reported that, with isocratic elution, it was possible to resolve completely K_1, K_1 epoxide and menaquinones (MK-4 to MK-10) using a mobile phase of methanol:dichloromethane (70:30). A linear relationship between the logarithm of the capacity factor (k) and the

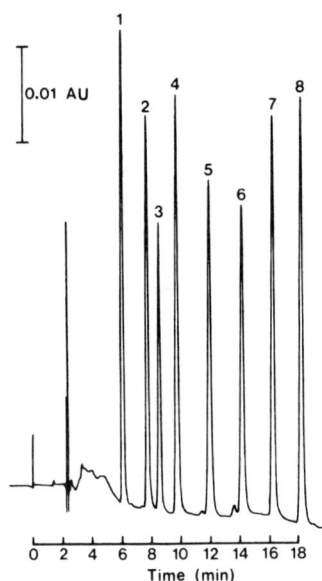

Fig. 108. Separation of vitamin K compounds by NARP. Peaks: (1) MK-4; (2) MK-5; (3) vitamin K_1; (4) to (8) MK-6 to MK-10. (MK = menaquinone). Column, Zorbax ODS; mobile phase, linear gradient in which the concentration of dichloromethane in methanol was increased from an initial concentration of 20% to a final concentration of 50% at a rate of 5%/min; UV detection, 270 nm (from Shearer *et al.*, 1980).

carbon number of the menaquinone side chain was observed under isocratic conditions. Haroon *et al.* (1980) achieved the separation, in elution order, of K_1 epoxide, chloro-K_1 and K_1 on Zorbax ODS with a mobile phase of acetonitrile:dichloromethane (70:30) (see Fig. 109). The resolution of K_1 and its epoxide metabolite was better than that obtained by adsorption HPLC.

Haroon *et al.* (1982) determined vitamin K_1 in milk and unsupplemented infant formula foods using a fractionation scheme which involved lipid extraction, gravity-flow adsorption chromatography, semi-preparative normal-phase HPLC, and quantitative NARP. The procedure was as follows.

Samples of milk (5–10 ml) and dry powder forms of infant formula foods (1–10 g) were extracted directly with chloroform: methanol (2:1) according to the method of Folch *et al.* (1957). A known amount of vitamin K_1 epoxide was added to the mixture as an internal standard and, after mixing, flocculated proteins were removed by centrifugation or by filtration through a glass microfibre filter. The mixture was washed with the appropriate volumes of water to achieve the separation of two phases. The upper methanol–water phase was discarded, and the lower chloroform phase containing K vitamins, the internal standard and other lipids was

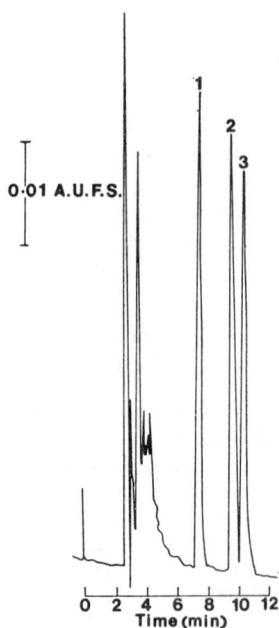

Fig. 109. Separation of vitamin K compounds by NARP. Peaks: (1) K_1 epoxide; (2) chloro-K_1; (3) K_1. Column, Zorbax ODS; mobile phase, acetonitrile:dichloromethane (70:30); UV detection, 270 nm (from Haroon *et al.*, 1980).

evaporated to dryness under vacuum at 60°C. The lipid extract was chromatographed on a slurry-packed column of Kieselgel 60, and the non-polar lipids were removed by elution with petroleum spirit. A fraction containing vitamin K_1, the internal standard, and other lipids of similar polarity was obtained by elution with petroleum spirit:diethyl ether (97:3). After removal of solvents by rotary evaporation, the vitamin K fraction was dissolved in 50–100 μl of the mobile phase, and subjected to semi-preparative HPLC on a column containing either underivatized silica (Partisil 5 Silica) or an amino-nitrile bonded phase (Partisil 10 PAC). The mobile phase used for the elution of either column was hexane:50% water-saturated dichloromethane (8:2) and the detector was a 254 nm photometer. Typical chromatograms obtained from cows' milk and infant formula food are shown in Fig. 110. The fraction of the eluate that corresponded to the retention times of vitamin K_1 and the internal standard was collected and evaporated to dryness under nitrogen. The residue was dissolved in 50–100 μl of the mobile phase and injected onto a reversed-phase column of Zorbax ODS. The mobile phase was methanol:dichloromethane (8:2) and the spectrophotometric detection wavelength was 270 nm. Typical chromatograms are shown in Fig. 111. The recovery of

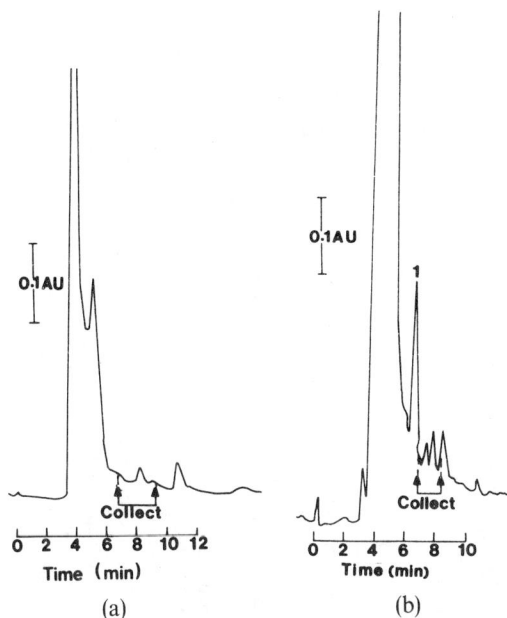

Fig. 110. Semi-preparative normal-phase HPLC of vitamin K_1 in the lipid fraction of (a) cows' milk, and (b) unsupplemented infant formula food, after clean-up on a column of Kieselgel 60. Peak (1) is *cis*-chloro-K_1, which acts as a marker to facilitate the collection of the vitamin K_1 fraction. Column, Partisil PAC; mobile phase, hexane:50% water-saturated dichloromethane (8:2); UV detection, 254 nm (from Haroon *et al.*, 1982 © *J. Nutr.*, **112**, 1105–17, American Institute of Nutrition).

vitamin K_1 added at different levels to a formula food ranged from 90–100%; RSDs were 5·4% and 10·6%.

8.3.6 Concurrent or Simultaneous Determination of Two or More Vitamins

Applications for determining two or more vitamins concurrently or simultaneously are summarised in Tables 29 and 30, respectively.

Reynolds & Judd (1984) determined vitamins A and D concurrently in fortified skimmed milk powder using reversed-phase HPLC with a semi-aqueous mobile phase. The unsaponifiable fraction of the milk powder, after concentration by evaporation, was assayed without preliminary clean-up for vitamin A. For the determination of vitamin D, the unsaponifiable concentrate was purified by Sep-Pak filtration. Vitamin D_3 was added as an internal standard to the milk powder before saponification to compensate for any losses of vitamin D_2 in the sample, including

Table 29

HPLC methods used for the concurrent determination of vitamins A and D

Analyte	Sample type	Sample preparation		Quantitative HPLC	Reference/ Fig. no.
		Vitamin A	Vitamin D		
Total retinol, vitamin D_2 or D_3	Fortified skimmed milk powder	Saponification, ether extraction, evaporation, residue dissolved in 25 ml MeOH, 5 ml aliquot removed for HPLC	Remaining 20 ml MeOH solution evaporated, Sep-Pak (reversed-phase) clean-up. (Vitamin D_2 or D_3 added before saponification as internal standard)	Spherisorb ODS MeOH:H_2O (97.5:2.5) UV 325 nm (vitamin A) UV 265 nm (vitamin D)	Reynolds & Judd (1984) (Fig. 112)
Total retinol, vitamin D_2 or D_3	Fortified fluid milk (whole, semi-skimmed, skimmed)	Alkaline digestion (ambient), hexane extraction, evaporation, residue redissolved in 6 ml hexane, 1 ml aliquot removed for HPLC	Remaining 5 ml hexane solution evaporated, alumina column chromatography, evaporation of eluate	Vydac TP 201 C_{18} Vitamin A MeOH:H_2O (90:10) UV 325 nm Vitamin D MeCN:MeOH (90:10) UV 265 nm	Wickroski & McLean (1984) (Fig. 113)

Abbreviations: see foot of Table 24.

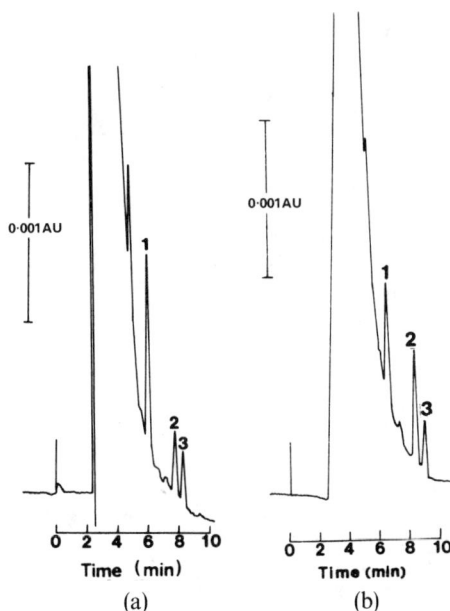

Fig. 111. NARP of vitamin K_1 fraction isolated by semi-preparative HPLC (Fig. 110) from (a) cows' milk, and (b) unsupplemented infant formula food. Peaks: (1) vitamin K_1 epoxide (internal standard); (2) cis-chloro-K_1 (marker compound); (3) vitamin K_1. Column, Zorbax ODS; mobile phase, methanol:dichloromethane (8:2); UV detection, 270 nm (from Haroon et al., 1982 © J. Nutr., **112**, 1105–17, American Institute of Nutrition).

conversion to previtamin D_2 by thermal isomerization. The procedure was as follows.

Samples (10 g) of skimmed milk powder were saponified by refluxing in the presence of the vitamin D internal standard and ascorbic acid, and in an atmosphere of nitrogen. The unsaponifiable matter was extracted with diethyl ether:petroleum spirit (1:1) and the organic layer was washed free from alkali with water. The extract was evaporated to dryness under vacuum at 50°C, using a gentle stream of nitrogen to complete the evaporation, and the residue was dissolved in 25 ml of methanol. A 5 ml aliquot of the methanolic solution was diluted to 15 ml with methanol, and used for the quantification of vitamin A on a 250 mm × 4·6 mm i.d. column of 5 µm Spherisorb ODS with a 75 mm × 2·1 mm i.d. guard column of pellicular reversed-phase material. The mobile phase was methanol:water (97·5:2·5) and the absorbance detection wavelength was 325 nm. The retention time of vitamin A was about 6 min (see Fig. 112(a)).

Table 30

HPLC methods used for the simultaneous determination of two or more vitamins

Analyte	Sample type	Sample preparation	Quantitative HPLC		Detection	Reference/ Fig. no.
			Stationary phase	Mobile phase		
Total retinol, vitamin D_2 or D_3	Fortified chocolate milk, skimmed milk	Saponification, hexane extraction, evaporation, residue dissolved in 0·1 ml MeOH for vitamin A and D assay by HPLC	Vydac TP 201 C_{18}	MeCN:MeOH (90:10)	UV 325 nm (vitamin A) UV 265 nm (vitamin D)	Henderson & McLean (1979) (Fig. 114)
Vitamin A palmitate, vitamin E acetate	Breakfast cereals	Extraction with $CHCl_3$/EtOH/H_2O at 50°C, $CHCl_3$ extract evaporated	μPorasil	Hexane:$CHCl_3$ + 1% EtOH (85:15)	Vitamin A palmitate: UV 280 and 313 nm Fluorescence: excitation 360 nm emission 415 nm Vitamin E acetate: UV 280 nm	Widicus & Kirk (1979) (Fig. 115)
Total retinol, total α-tocopherol	Animal feeds	Saponification, hexane extraction, evaporation	Spherisorb ODS	MeOH:H_2O (90:10)	UV 280 nm	Söderhjelm & Andersson (1978) (Fig. 116)

Analyte	Sample matrix	Extraction/clean-up procedure	Column	Mobile phase	Detection	Reference
Vitamin A palmitate, vitamin E acetate	Infant formulae	Solvent extraction, evaporation, removal of lipid by GP–HPLC on three μStyragel 100 Å columns eluted with CH_2Cl_2 (UV 340 nm), evaporation of eluate	Zorbax ODS (6 μm)	$MeCN:CH_2Cl_2$:MeOH (70:30:0·2)	Vitamin A palmitate: UV 313 nm Vitamin E acetate: UV 280 nm	Landen (1982) (Figs 117, 118)
Vitamin A (alcohol, acetate, palmitate), vitamin D_3, vitamin E (alcohol, acetate)	Animal feeds	Solvent extraction, evaporation, extraction with MeCN then partition into isooctane, evaporation	μBondapak C_{18}	$MeOH:H_2O$ (95:5)	UV 280 nm	Cohen & Lapointe (1978) (Figs 119, 120)
Vitamin A (alcohol, palmitate); vitamin D_2 or D_3; vitamin E (α-, $\beta+\gamma$-, δ-T, acetate); vitamin K_1	Dairy products, infant formulae	Enzymatic hydrolysis, pentane extraction, evaporation	Zorbax ODS (two columns)	Gradient elution: MeOH:EtOAc (86:14)/MeCN	UV 325 nm (retinol) UV 365 nm (vitamin A palmitate) UV 265 nm (vitamins D_2, D_3, E, K_1)	Barnett et al. (1980) (Fig. 122)

Abbreviations: see foot of Table 24.

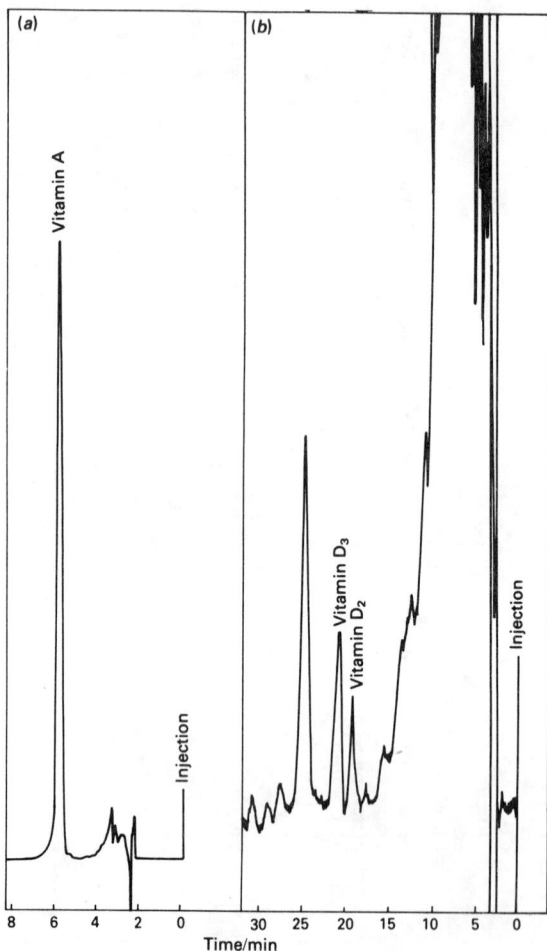

Fig. 112. Concurrent determination of vitamins A and D in fortified skimmed milk powder by reversed-phase HPLC. (a) Chromatogram of vitamin A in the unsaponifiable matter; (b) vitamin D in the unsaponifiable matter after clean-up on a reversed-phase Sep-Pak cartridge. Column, Spherisorb ODS; mobile phase, methanol:water (97·5:2·5); UV detection, 325 nm (vitamin A); 265 nm (vitamin D) (from Reynolds & Judd, 1984).

The remaining 20 ml of methanolic solution was evaporated to dryness under vacuum and the residue was dissolved in 2 ml of ethanol for vitamin D determination. The ethanolic solution was diluted with 1 ml of water, and pumped by means of a glass syringe through a reversed-phase Sep-Pak cartridge packed with C_{18}-bonded silica (Waters Associates). The cartridge was flushed with a polar solvent (methanol:tetrahydrofuran:water; 1:1:2) to elute the material that was more polar than vitamin D. The vitamin D was eluted with a solvent of intermediate polarity (methanol), leaving the more strongly retained material adsorbed on the cartridge, which was then discarded. The methanol eluate was retained for HPLC analysis. Vitamins D_2 and D_3 were separated on the same HPLC column and with the same mobile phase as employed for vitamin A, but using a detection wavelength of 265 nm. Vitamins D_2 and D_3 were completely separated from one another at retention times of approximately 20 min (see Fig. 112(b)). The mean recovery (9 determinations) of retinyl acetate added at different levels to unfortified skimmed milk powder was 96·8% (range 90·3–101·2%) and the RSD was 2·0%. Recoveries of vitamin D_3 relative to D_2 after complete analysis of spiked samples of skimmed milk powder were 100·4%, 101·0% and 100·5%; the RSD was 3·5%. The authors commented that more extensive clean-up techniques, involving sterol precipitation and preparative HPLC, were necessary before vitamin D could be quantified precisely.

Wickroski & McLean (1984) reduced the amount of interfering cholesterol to a minimum in the analysis of skimmed and homogenized whole milk fortified with vitamins A and D by using a sample size of only 6 ml; cf. 100 ml sample size of whole milk (Muniz et al., 1982). The unsaponifiable fraction, after concentration by evaporation, was analysed directly for vitamin A using a reversed-phase column with a semi-aqueous mobile phase. For the determination of vitamin D, the cholesterol was removed from the concentrated unsaponifiable fraction by gravity-flow chromatography on dry-packed alumina, before analysis by NARP. The procedure was as follows.

Samples (6 ml) of fortified fluid milk were subjected to overnight alkaline digestion at ambient temperature with slow, constant stirring in the presence of pyrogallol, and the unsaponifiable matter was extracted with hexane. The hexane extract was washed with aqueous KOH solution; washed with water until free from alkali; evaporated to dryness under vacuum; and the residue was redissolved in 6 ml of hexane. A 1 ml aliquot of the hexane solution was transferred to a 2 ml vial and evaporated to dryness at 30°C in a stream of nitrogen. The residue was dissolved in 100 μl of methanol for vitamin A determination. The HPLC column

(250 mm × 3·2 mm i.d.) contained 10 μm Vydac TP 201 C_{18}; the mobile phase was methanol:water (90:10); and the absorbance detection wavelength was 325 nm. A chromatogram showing the vitamin A peak from a sample of skimmed milk is depicted in Fig. 113(a).

To the remaining 5 ml of hexane solution was added a special indicator (chlorophyll-a) and 1 g of dry, deactivated, neutral alumina. This mixture was evaporated to dryness under vacuum at 30°C, and the alumina was poured on top of a prepared dry alumina column (300 mm × 10 mm i.d.). The column was washed with hexane followed by benzene, and the vitamin

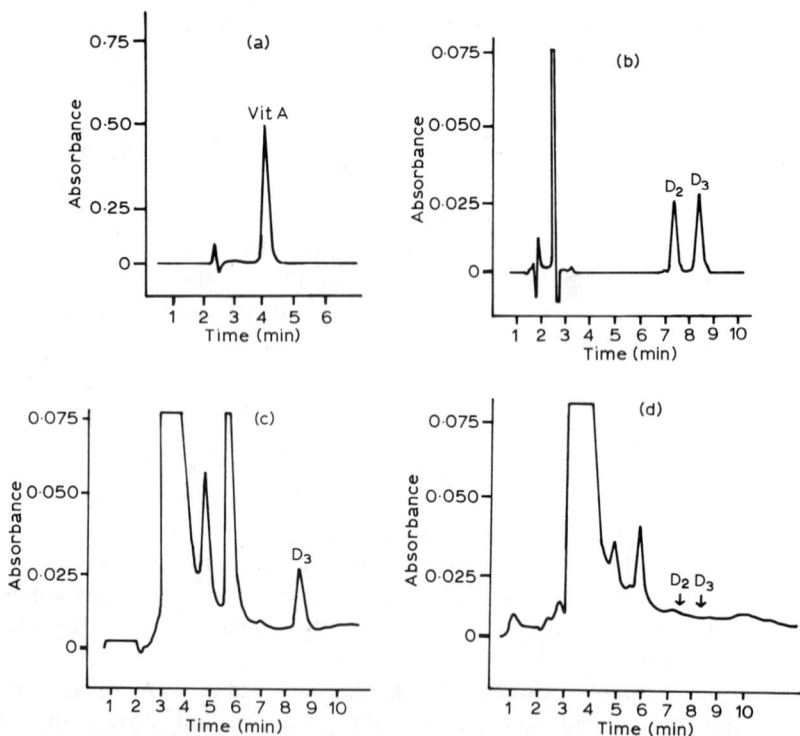

Fig. 113. Concurrent determination of vitamins A and D in fortified milk by reversed-phase HPLC. Chromatograms depict (a) vitamin A in the unsaponifiable matter of skimmed milk, (b) vitamin D_2 and vitamin D_3 standards, (c) vitamin D_3 in the unsaponifiable matter of homogenized whole milk after alumina column clean-up, (d) eluting positions of vitamins D_2 and D_3 in a purified extract of unfortified whole milk. Column, Vydac TP 201 C_{18}. Vitamin A mobile phase, methanol:water (90:10) monitored at 325 nm; vitamin D mobile phase, acetonitrile:methanol (90:10) monitored at 265 nm (from Wickroski & McLean, 1984).

D fraction (6–8 ml), delineated by means of the indicator, was eluted with chloroform. The vitamin D fraction was evaporated to approximately 1 ml under vacuum at 30°C. The contents of the flask were then quantitatively transferred to a 3 ml vial and evaporated to dryness in a stream of nitrogen at 30°C. The residue was dissolved in 100 μl of methanol for vitamin D quantification using the same HPLC column system as employed for vitamin A. The mobile phase was acetonitrile:methanol (90:10), and the detection wavelength was 265 nm. This system completely separated vitamins D_2 and D_3 with elution times between 7 and 9 min. Chromatograms of vitamin D_2 and D_3 standards, and of vitamin D-fortified and unfortified samples of homogenized whole milk are depicted in Fig. 113(b), (c), (d). Percentage recoveries (and standard deviations) of added vitamins A, D_2 and D_3 from non-fat skimmed milk were, respectively, 92·2 (2·6), 94·1 (4·8) and 91·1 (5·2). Corresponding values for vitamins D_2 and D_3 in homogenized whole milk were 86·5 (9·4) and 83·7 (4·9). Minimum detectable amounts were 3·2 μg of vitamin A per 100 ml and 0·13 μg of vitamin D per 100 ml.

Henderson & McLean (1979) devised a rapid screening method for the simultaneous determination of vitamins A and D in fortified skimmed milk and chocolate milk using NARP. Two different wavelengths were used to analyse the concentrated unsaponifiable matter. Milk samples (1 ml) were saponified for 20 min at 80°C in the presence of pyrogallol. The unsaponifiable matter was extracted with hexane, and the combined hexane extracts were washed with water, then evaporated to dryness under nitrogen. The residue was dissolved in 0·1 ml methanol, and 20 μl of this solution was injected onto a 250 mm × 3·5 mm i.d. Vydac TP 201 C_{18} column eluted with acetonitrile:methanol (90:10). Chromatograms of vitamins A and D in fortified chocolate milk measured spectrophotometrically at 325 nm and 265 nm, respectively, are shown in Fig. 114. Vitamins D_2 and D_3 were completely resolved. Recovery studies were performed on samples containing vitamins A and D in ten times the equivalent amounts found in fortified milk. Percentage recoveries (and standard deviations) for vitamin D_3 and vitamin A were, respectively, 98·4 (3·4) and 99·0 (2·9).

Adsorption HPLC has been employed for the simultaneous determination of supplemental retinyl palmitate and α-tocopheryl acetate in breakfast cereals (Widicus & Kirk, 1979). The concentrated lipid extract was injected directly onto a silica HPLC column without prior sample purification. The procedure was as follows.

Samples (2 g) of fortified breakfast cereals were extracted with a chloroform/ethanol/water mixture by refluxing with shaking in a 50°C water bath. The chloroform extract was dried over anhydrous sodium

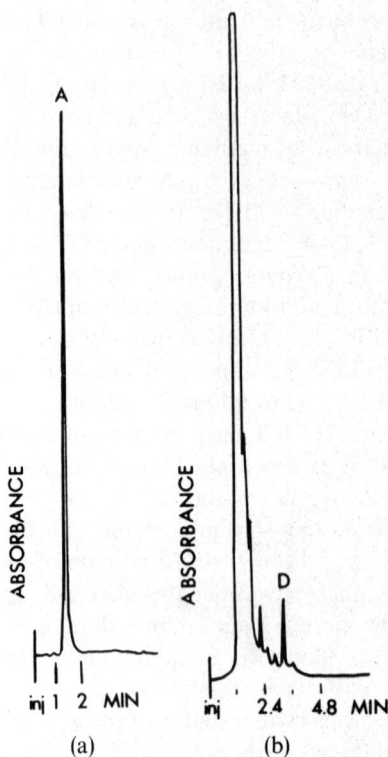

Fig. 114. Simultaneous determination of vitamins A and D by NARP in the unsaponifiable matter of fortified chocolate milk. (a) Chromatogram of vitamin A detected at 325 nm; (b) vitamin D detected at 265 nm. Column, Vydac TP 201 C_{18}; mobile phase, acetonitrile:methanol (90:10) (from Henderson & McLean, 1979).

sulphate, then evaporated to dryness under vacuum at 35°C. The residue was dissolved in 10 ml of the HPLC mobile phase (hexane:chloroform containing 1% ethanol; 85:15), filtered through a 0.45μ syringe filter, and injected ($10 \mu l$ aliquot) onto a 300 mm × 4 mm i.d. μPorasil silica column. Tocopheryl acetate was monitored photometrically at 280 nm, while retinyl palmitate was monitored at 280 nm and 313 nm, and by fluorescence (360 nm excitation; 415 nm emission) (see Fig. 115). Standard curves of retinyl palmitate and α-tocopheryl acetate were prepared each day of analysis. The recoveries of retinyl palmitate and α-tocopheryl acetate added to the cereal products during the extraction procedure were, with standard deviations, 99·2% (4·28%) and 94·9% (4·10%), respectively. Extraction of an unfortified cereal showed no appreciable absorbance or fluorescence.

Reversed-phase HPLC using a 250 mm × 3·2 mm i.d. 10 μm Spherisorb ODS column and a methanol:water (90:10) mobile phase has been used to

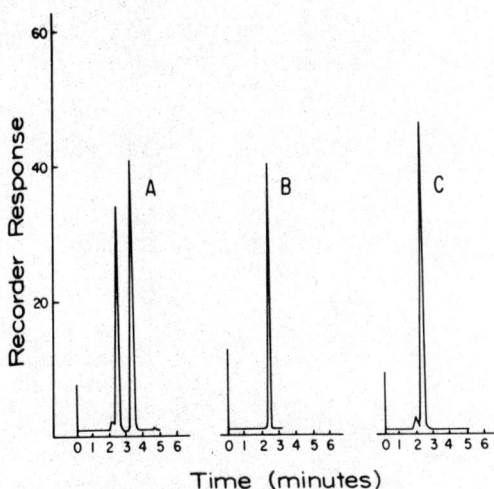

Fig. 115. Simultaneous determination of vitamins A and E by adsorption HPLC in lipid extract of whole wheat-based fortified breakfast cereal. (A) UV absorbance measurement at 280 nm (first peak, retinyl palmitate; second peak, α-tocopheryl acetate); (B) absorbance at 313 nm (retinyl palmitate); (C) fluorescence of retinyl palmitate (excitation, 360 nm; emission, 415 nm). Column, μPorasil; mobile phase, hexane:chloroform containing 1% ethanol (85:15) (from Widicus & Kirk, 1979).

determine retinol and α-tocopherol in the unsaponifiable fraction of animal feeds fortified with vitamins A and E (Söderhjelm & Andersson, 1978). Figure 116 shows a typical chromatogram obtained using a 280 nm fixed-wavelength detector. The molar absorptivity coefficient at 280 nm was about half of its value at the λ_{max} for vitamin A (325 nm) and about one-tenth for vitamin E (λ_{max} 294 nm) in the methanol:water mobile phase.

Landen (1982) employed NARP for the determination of supplemental retinyl palmitate and α-tocopheryl acetate in infant formula foods, following removal of the triglycerides by gel-permeation HPLC. The procedure was as follows.

The lipid-soluble components were extracted from the sample (6·5 g of liquid or reconstituted powdered milk) by homogenizing in a solvent mixture of isopropanol and dichloromethane with magnesium sulphate added to remove water. The extract was evaporated to dryness under vacuum below 30°C; dissolved in dichloromethane; filtered; re-evaporated; and dissolved in 5 ml of dichloromethane. This solution was fractionated on three μStyragel 100 Å columns (300 mm × 7·8 mm i.d.) connected in series, using a mobile phase of dichloromethane containing 0·001%

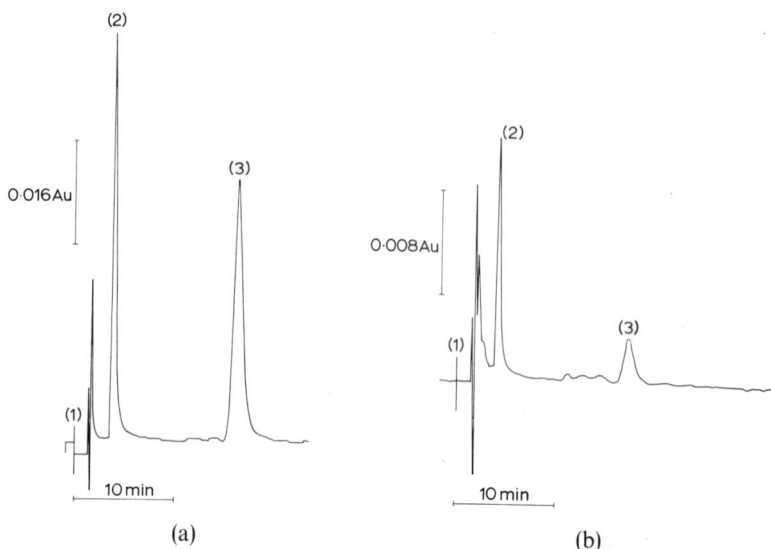

Fig. 116. Simultaneous determination of vitamins A and E in fortified animal feeds by reversed-phase HPLC. Chromatograms depict (a) standard solution containing vitamins A and E, (b) vitamins A and E in the unsaponifiable matter from a cattle feed. (1) Injection mark; (2) retinol peak; (3) α-tocopherol peak. Column, Spherisorb ODS; mobile phase, methanol:water (90:10); UV detection, 280 nm (from Söderhjelm & Andersson, 1978).

triethylamine. The column effluent was continuously monitored with refractive index and absorbance detectors. After elution of the oil fraction, as monitored by refractive index, the vitamin fraction detected at 340 nm was collected (3·5 ml) (see Fig. 117).

The vitamin fraction was evaporated to dryness under reduced pressure at 20°C in an atmosphere of helium. If the sample was known to contain β-carotene, 10 μl of dichloromethane containing 0·001% triethylamine and 0·01% BHA was added to the vitamin fraction before evaporation. The dried residue was immediately dissolved in 0·5–1·0 ml of the non-aqueous mobile phase (acetonitrile:dichloromethane containing 0·001% triethylamine:methanol; 70:30:0·2) for analysis on a 250 mm × 4·6 mm i.d. column of 6 μm Zorbax ODS. The column effluent was monitored spectrophotometrically for retinyl palmitate and α-tocopheryl acetate at 313 nm and 280 nm, respectively (Fig. 118). If the product was labelled to contain β-carotene, the effluent was continuously monitored for retinyl palmitate and β-carotene at 313 nm and 436 nm, respectively. Recoveries of

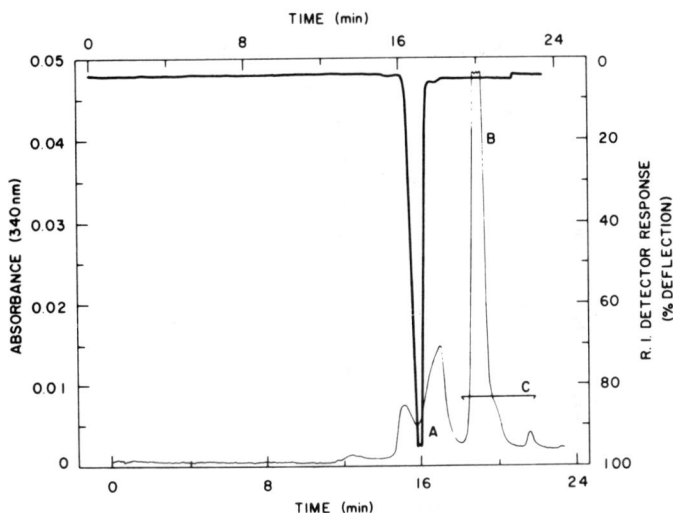

Fig. 117.   Gel-permeation HPLC of the lipid fraction of a vitamin A- and vitamin E-fortified infant formula food showing the separation of the lipid (peak A) from the vitamin A/E fraction (peak B). Position of the vitamin fraction collected is indicated by C. Column, three μStyragel 100 Å columns connected in series; mobile phase, dichloromethane containing 0·001% triethylamine; dual detection, UV (340 nm) and refractive index (from Landen, 1982).

added retinyl palmitate from infant formula foods were 95·0% and 92·1%; recoveries of α-tocopheryl acetate were 95·2% and 97·1%.

Cohen & Lapointe (1978) used reversed-phase HPLC to determine vitamins A, D and E in animal feeds after extraction with a solvent mixture and purification by solvent partitioning. Feed samples (5 g) were ground and shaken with a solution of isooctane:dioxan (80:20). The mixture was filtered, and the filtrate was shaken with 0·3 ml of tetraethylenepentamine to render the chlorophyll partly insoluble before evaporation to near dryness under vacuum. The residue was extracted three times with acetonitrile and the filtered extracts were evaporated to 60–80 ml. The acetonitrile solution was extracted three times with isooctane, and the isooctane solution was shaken with sodium phosphate tribasic to precipitate inorganic salts and to remove any traces of amine. After filtration and evaporation to dryness, the residue was dissolved in methanol for injection onto a 250 mm × 4·2 mm i.d. column packed with μBondapak C_{18}. The mobile phase of methanol:water (95:5) was monitored photometrically at 280 nm. Separation of retinol, retinyl acetate, vitamin

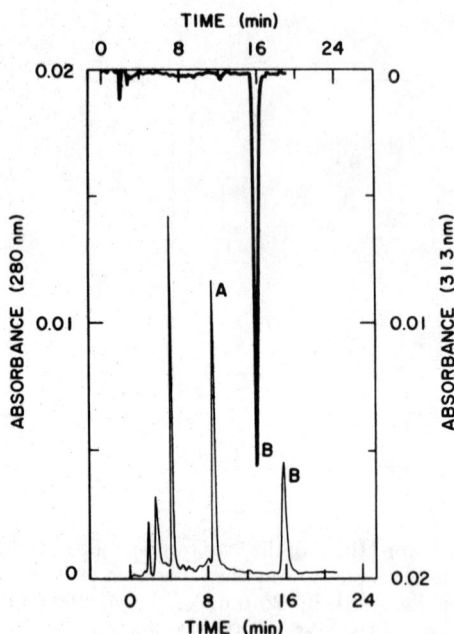

Fig. 118. NARP of the vitamin A/E fraction isolated by gel-permeation HPLC (Fig. 117) from a fortified infant formula food. Peaks: (A) α-tocopheryl acetate; (B) retinyl palmitate. Column, 6 μm Zorbax ODS; mobile phase, acetonitrile: dichloromethane containing 0·001 % triethylamine: methanol (70:30:0·2); dual UV detection, 280 nm (α-tocopheryl acetate); 313 nm (retinyl palmitate) (from Landen, 1982).

D_3, tocopherol and α-tocopheryl acetate was achieved within 18 min (Fig. 119(a)); retinyl palmitate was eluted at 39 min (Fig. 119(b)). Chromatograms of the vitamins extracted from a feed sample and from a poultry vitamin premix are shown in Fig. 120. The average recovery percentages were: retinyl acetate 96·4% ± 2·4; vitamin D_3 91·25% ± 5·9; α-tocopheryl acetate 92·6% ± 2·9.

Zonta *et al.* (1982) used reversed-phase HPLC with gradient elution to separate vitamins A, D, E, K_1 and carotene in the unsaponifiable fraction of foods. Samples such as olive oil and butter, were subjected to overnight alkaline digestion at ambient temperature in a sealed, nitrogen-flushed flask with the inclusion of ascorbic acid as antioxidant. The unsaponifiable matter was extracted with hexane; evaporated to dryness under vacuum at <40°C; and the residue was dissolved in methanol for direct analysis by

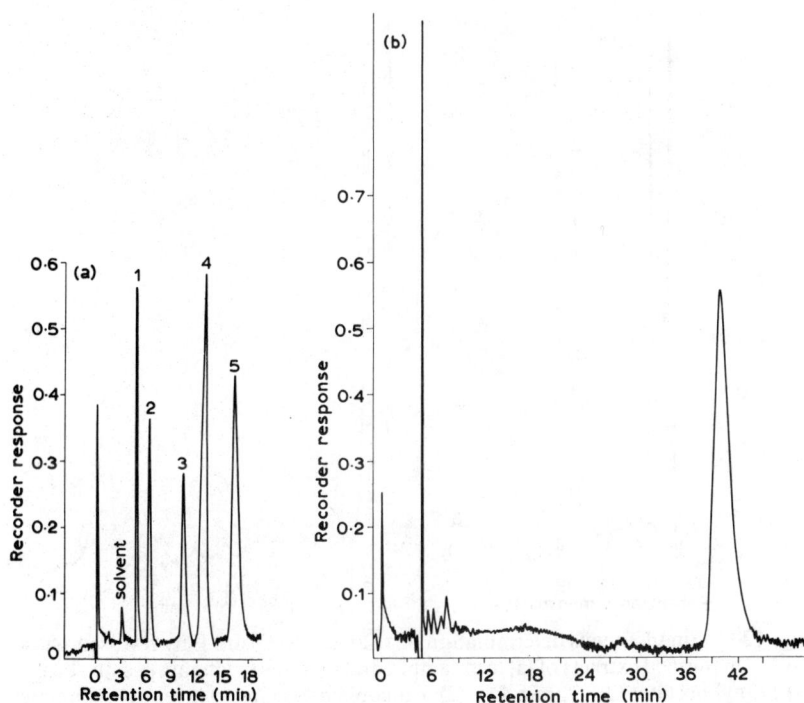

Fig. 119. Reversed-phase HPLC of fat-soluble vitamin standards, A, D and E. (a) Mixture of 33 ng retinol (peak 1), 13·1 ng retinyl acetate (peak 2), 25 ng vitamin D_3 (peak 3), 474 ng α-tocopherol (peak 4), 500 ng α-tocopheryl acetate (peak 5); (b) 325·5 ng retinyl palmitate. Column, μBondapak C_{18}; mobile phase, methanol: water (95:5); UV detection, 280 nm (Reprinted with permission from Cohen, H. & Lapointe, M. (1978). Method for the extraction and cleanup of animal feed for the determination of liposoluble vitamins D, A and E by high-pressure liquid chromatography. *J. agric. Fd Chem.*, **26**, 1210–13). Copyright (1978) American Chemical Society.

HPLC. Two reversed-phase columns connected in series were used: 250 mm × 2·6 mm i.d. ODS-HC-Sil-X-1 (Perkin-Elmer) and 150 mm × 4·6 mm i.d. Supelcosil LC-18. A Supelco guard column dry-packed with 40 μm pellicular packing was also employed. A gradient elution programme was adopted where the mobile phase at pump A was acetonitrile:methanol (80:20), whilst pump B delivered distilled water. The column operating temperature was 44°C; the reduced viscosity obtained with this gentle heating permitted the use of higher flow rates with not too great a pressure drop. Wavelength programming was adopted so that each

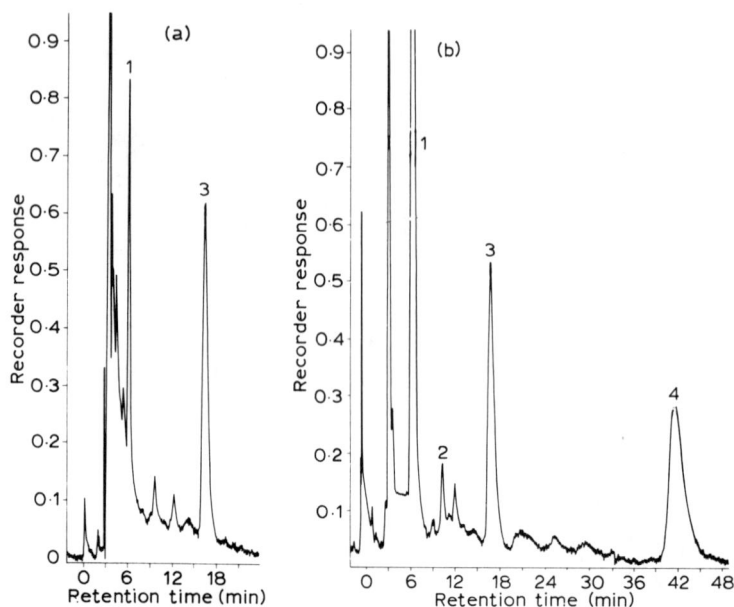

Fig. 120. Simultaneous determination of vitamins A, D and E by reversed-phase HPLC in purified extracts of (a) feed sample, and (b) poultry vitamin premix. Peaks: (1) retinyl acetate; (2) vitamin D_3; (3) α-tocopheryl acetate; (4) retinyl palmitate. Chromatographic conditions as for Fig. 119 (Reprinted with permission from Cohen, H. & Lapointe, M. (1978). Method for the extraction and cleanup of animal feed for the determination of liposoluble vitamins D, A, and E by high-pressure liquid chromatography. *J. agric. Fd Chem.*, **26**, 1210–13). Copyright (1978) American Chemical Society.

vitamin was detected as its λ_{max}. Figure 121 shows the separation of vitamins A, D_2, D_3, E, K_1 and carotene in standard solution, and in extracts from cod liver oil and butter. The HPLC system was also capable of resolving vitamins D_2 and D_3, together with their corresponding previtamins and provitamins. No quantitative data were reported.

Barnett *et al.* (1980) employed NARP with gradient elution to determine vitamins A, D, E and K_1 in fortified milk- and soy-based infant formula foods, and dairy products. Sample preparation entailed enzymatic hydrolysis of the fats and solvent extraction of the hydrolysate. The lipase enzyme effectively hydrolyses the triglycerides into their component fatty acids and glycerol, but only partially converts retinyl palmitate and α-tocopheryl acetate to their alcohol forms; vitamins D_2 and K_1 are unaffected. The procedure was as follows.

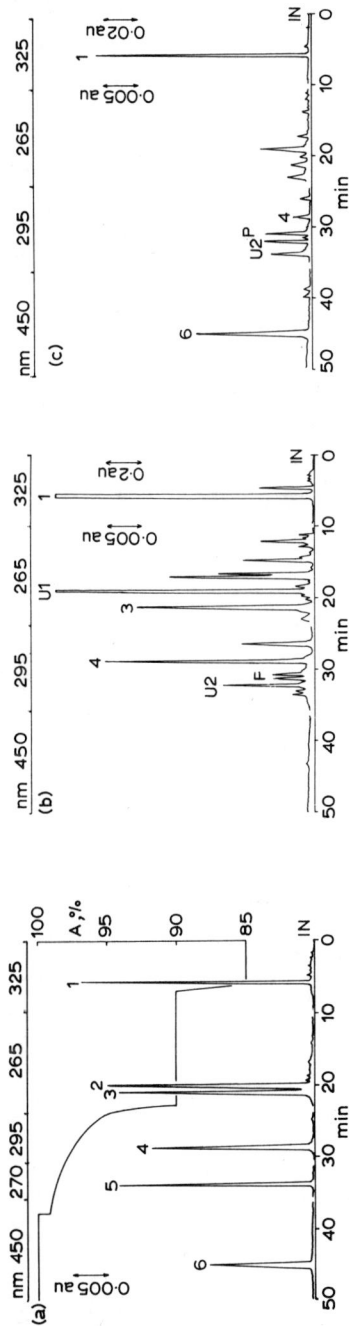

Fig. 121. Simultaneous determination of vitamins A, D₂, D₃, E, K₁, and carotene by reversed-phase HPLC in (a) standard solution, and in the unsaponifiable material from (b) cod liver oil, (c) butter. Peaks: (1) retinol; (2) vitamin D₂; (3) vitamin D₃; (4) α-tocopherol; (5) vitamin K₁; (6) carotene; P = provitamin D₃; U1 and U2 are unidentified peaks. Two-column system, ODS-HC-Sil-X-1 and Supelcosil LC-18 connected in series; gradient elution programme, percentage of mixture A (acetonitrile:methanol, 80:20) referred to the total volume of A + B (B is water) is superimposed in (a); UV wavelength programme (see top of figures); column temp., 44°C (from Zonta *et al.*, 1982).

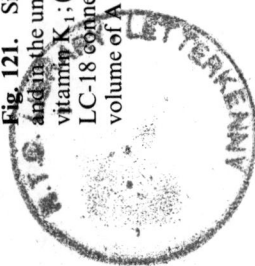

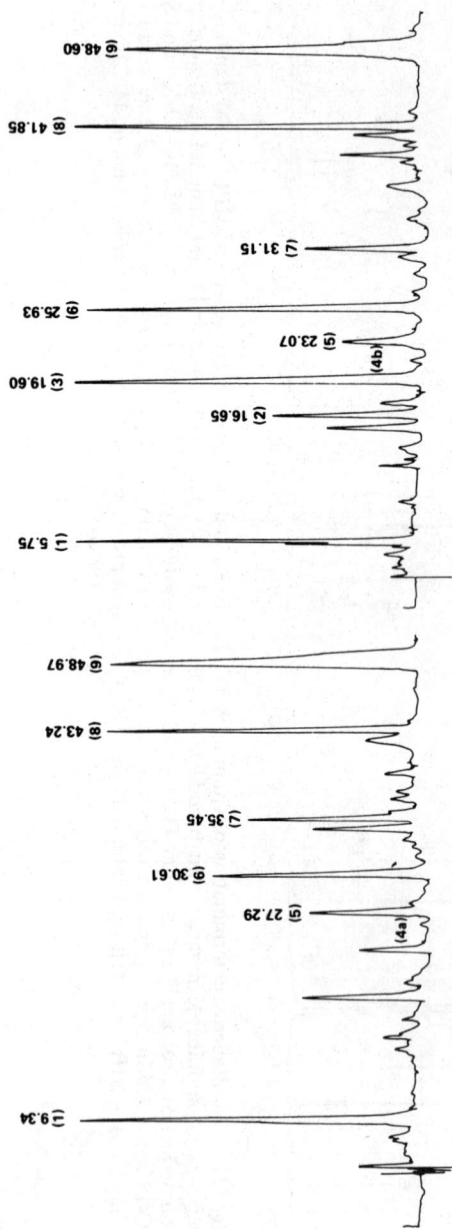

Fig. 122. Simultaneous determination of vitamins A, D₂ or D₃, E and K₁ using NARP with gradient elution. Chromatograms show soy-based infant formula products after enzymatic hydrolysis. Peaks: (1) retinol; (2) δ-tocopherol; (3) β + γ-tocopherol; (4a) vitamin D₂; (4b) vitamin D₃; (5) α-tocopherol; (6) α-tocopheryl acetate; (7) vitamin K₁; (8) cholesteryl phenylacetate (internal standard); (9) retinyl palmitate. Column, Zorbax ODS; gradient elution programme, methanol: ethyl acetate (86:14) against 100% acetonitrile; UV wavelength programming: peak (1) 325 nm; peaks (2) to (8) 265 nm; peak (9) 365 nm (Reprinted with permission from Barnett, S. A., Frick, L. W. & Baine, H. M. (1980). Simultaneous determination of vitamins A, D₂ or D₃, E and K₁ in infant formulas and dairy products by reversed-phase liquid chromatography. *Analyt. Chem.*, **52**, 610–14). Copyright (1980) American Chemical Society.

An amount of sample containing approximately 3·5–4·0 g of fat was taken, and the lipid component was subjected to enzymatic hydrolysis by incubation with lipase for 1 h at 37°C. The hydrolysate was made alkaline, then diluted with ethanol and extracted with pentane. The combined pentane extracts were washed to neutral pH with water, filtered through sodium sulphate, then evaporated to dryness under vacuum at 40°C. The residue was dissolved in diethyl ether (approximately 2 ml) and re-evaporated to dryness in a stream of nitrogen. A solution of cholesteryl phenylacetate in ethyl acetate:acetonitrile (1:1) was added as an internal standard, and an aliquot of the diluted sample was injected onto two 250 mm × 4·6 mm i.d. Zorbax ODS reversed-phase columns connected in series and eluted with a gradient programme of methanol:ethyl acetate (86:14) against 100% acetonitrile. The following vitamins, with their elution times in min, were identified after enzymatic hydrolysis of soy-based infant formula foods: retinol (5·75), δ-tocopherol (16·65), $\beta + \gamma$-tocopherol (19·60), vitamin D_2 or D_3 (minor peaks), α-tocopherol (23·07), α-tocopheryl acetate (25·93), vitamin K_1 (31·15), cholesteryl phenylacetate (internal standard) (41·85) and retinyl palmitate (48·60) (Fig. 122). Detection of the vitamins was accomplished using a wavelength-programmable spectrophotometric detector. The first component of interest, retinol, was detected at 325 nm; the following components, up to and including the internal standard, were detected at 265 nm; and the final component of interest, retinyl palmitate, was detected at 365 nm. The recoveries of vitamins A, D, E and K_1 added to milk-based or soy-based infant formula foods were greater than 93%.

References

Aaron, J. J. (1980). Photochemical-fluorometric determination of the K vitamins. *Meth. Enzym.*, **67F**, 140–8.

Aitzetmüller, K., Pilz, J. & Tasche, R. (1979). Fast determination of vitamin A palmitate in margarines by HPLC. *Fette Seifen Anstrichmittel*, **81**, 40–3.

Albers, N., Behm, G., Dressler, D., Klaus, W., Küther, K. & Lindner, H. (1984). *Vitamins in Animal Nutrition*, Arbeitsgemeinschaft für Wirkstoffe in der Tierernährung eV (AWT), Bonn.

Ames, S. R. (1966). Methods for evaluating vitamin A isomers. *J. Ass. off. analyt. Chem.*, **49**, 1071–8.

Ames, S. R. (1972a). Tocopherols. 5. Occurrence in foods. In *The Vitamins*, 2nd edn, Vol. V (W. H. Sebrell, Jr & R. S. Harris, eds), Academic Press, New York, pp. 233–48.

Ames, S. R. (1972b). Tocopherols. 4. Estimation in foods and food supplements. *Ibid.*, pp. 225–33.

Ames, S. R. & Tinkler, F. H. (1962). Determination of supplemental alpha-tocopheryl acetate in premixes, feeds and pet foods. *J. Ass. off. analyt. Chem.*, **45**, 425–33.

Analytical Methods Committee (1959). The determination of tocopherols in oils, foods and feeding stuffs. *Analyst, Lond.*, **84**, 356–72.

Analytical Methods Committee (1985). Determination of vitamin A in animal feedingstuffs by high-performance liquid chromatography. *Analyst, Lond.*, **110**, 1019–26.

Anon. (1976). *Vitamin Compendium. The Properties of the Vitamins and their Importance in Human and Animal Nutrition*, F. Hoffmann–La Roche & Co. Ltd, Basle, Switzerland.

Anon. (1985). Why vitamin fortification? *Fd Engng*, Feb., 1985, pp. 96–7.

AOAC (1984a). Nomenclature for vitamin E. Final action. In *Official Methods of Analysis*, 14th edn (S. Williams, ed.), Association of Official Analytical Chemists, Inc., Arlington, Va., 43.128.

AOAC (1984b). Carotenes and xanthophylls in dried plant materials and mixed feeds. Spectrophotometric method. Final action. *Ibid.*, 43.018–43.023.

AOAC (1984c). Carotenes in fresh plant materials and silages. Spectrophotometric method. Final action. *Ibid.*, 43.014–43.017.

AOAC (1984*d*). Alpha-tocopherol and alpha-tocopheryl acetate in foods and feeds. Colorimetric method. Final action. *Ibid.*, 43.129–43.137.

AOAC (1984*e*). Alpha-tocopheryl acetate (supplemental) in foods and feeds. Colorimetric method. Final action. *Ibid.*, 43.147–43.151.

AOAC (1984*f*). Vitamin A in margarine. Spectrophotometric method. First action. *Ibid.*, 43.001–43.007.

AOAC (1984*g*). Vitamin A in mixed feeds, premixes and foods. Colorimetric method. First action. *Ibid.*, 43.008–43.013.

AOAC (1984*h*). Menadione sodium bisulfite (water-soluble vitamin K_3) in feed premixes. Gas chromatographic method. Final action. *Ibid.*, 43.161–43.166.

AOAC (1984*i*). Vitamin D in fortified milk and milk powder. Liquid chromatographic method. Final action. *Ibid.*, 43.110–43.117.

AOAC (1984*j*). Vitamin D in mixed feeds, premixes, and pet foods. Liquid chromatographic method. Final action. *Ibid.*, 43.118–43.127.

Association of Vitamin Chemists, Inc. (1966). *Methods of Vitamin Assay*, 3rd edn, Interscience Publishers, New York.

Atuma, S. S. (1975). Electrochemical determination of vitamin E in margarine, butter and palm oil. *J. Sci. Fd Agric.*, **26**, 393–9.

Atuma, S. S. & Lindquist, J. (1973). Voltammetric determination of tocopherols by use of a newly developed carbon paste electrode. *Analyst, Lond.*, **98**, 886–94.

Avioli, L. V. & Lee, S. W. (1966). Detection of nanogram quantities of vitamin D by gas–liquid chromatography. *Analyt. Biochem.*, **16**, 193–9.

Ball, G. F. M. & Ratcliff, P. W. (1978). The analysis of tocopherols in corn oil and bacon fat. *J. Fd Technol.*, **13**, 433–43.

Barnes, P. J. & Taylor, P. W. (1980). The composition of acyl lipids and tocopherols in wheat germ oils from various sources. *J. Sci. Fd Agric.*, **31**, 997–1006.

Barnett, S. A., Frick, L. W. & Baine, H. M. (1980). Simultaneous determination of vitamins A, D_2 or D_3, E and K_1 in infant formulas and dairy products by reversed-phase liquid chromatography. *Analyt. Chem.*, **52**, 610–14.

Bauernfeind, J. C. (1977). The tocopherol content of food and influencing factors. *CRC crit. Rev. Fd Sci. Nutr.*, **8**, 337–82.

Bauernfeind, J. C. (1980). Tocopherols in foods. In *Vitamin E. A Comprehensive Treatise* (L. J. Machlin, ed.), Marcel Dekker, Inc., New York, pp. 99–167.

Bayfield, R. F. & Cole, E. R. (1980). Colorimetric estimation of vitamin A with trichloroacetic acid. *Meth. Enzym.*, **67**F., 189–95.

Bechthold, H. & Jähnchen, E. (1979). Quantitative analysis of vitamin K_1 and vitamin K_1 2,3-epoxide in plasma by electron-capture gas–liquid chromatography. *J. Chromat. Biomed. Appl.*, **164**, 85–90.

Behrens, W. A. & Madère, R. (1983). Interrelationship and competition of α- and γ-tocopherol at the level of intestinal absorption, plasma transport and liver uptake. *Nutr. Res.*, **3**, 891–7.

Bell, J. G. (1971). Separation of oil-soluble vitamins by partition chromatography on Sephadex LH 20. *Chemy Ind.*, **7**, 201–2.

Bell, J. G. & Christie, A. A. (1973). Gas–liquid chromatographic determination of vitamin D in cod-liver oil. *Analyst, Lond.*, **98**, 268–73.

Bell, J. G. & Christie, A. A. (1974). Gas–liquid chromatographic determination of vitamin D_2 in fortified full-cream dried milk. *Analyst, Lond.*, **99**, 385–96.

Bender, A. E. (1979). The effects of processing on the stability of vitamins in foods. In *Proceedings of the Kellogg Nutrition Symposium*, London, 14th–15th Dec., 1978 (T. G. Taylor, ed.), MTP Press, Lancaster, pp. 111–25.

Berridge, J. C. (1985). *Techniques for the Automated Optimization of HPLC Separations*, John Wiley & Sons, Inc., Chichester.

Bieri, J. G. & McKenna, M. C. (1981). Expressing dietary values for fat-soluble vitamins: changes in concepts and terminology. *Am. J. clin. Nutr.*, **34**, 289–95.

Blott, A. D. & Woollard, D. C. (1986). Rapid determination of α-tocopheryl acetate in animal feeds by high-performance liquid chromatography. *J. Micronutr. Anal.*, **2**, 259–74.

Bolliger, H. R. & König, A. (1969*a*). Vitamin D group. In *Thin-Layer Chromatography* (E. Stahl, ed.), Allen & Unwin Ltd, London, pp. 275–83.

Bolliger, H. R. & König, A. (1969*b*). Vitamin E group. *Ibid.*, pp. 283–8.

Booth, V. H. (1961). Spurious recovery tests in tocopherol determinations. *Analyt. Chem.*, **33**, 1224–6.

Borsje, B., de Vries, E. J., Zeeman, J. & Mulder, F. J. (1982). Analysis of fat-soluble vitamins. 26. High performance liquid chromatographic determination of vitamin D in fortified milk and milk powder. *J. Ass. off. analyt. Chem.*, **65**, 1225–7.

Bristow, P. A. (1976). *Liquid Chromatography in Practice*, hetp, Wilmslow, Cheshire.

Bro-Rasmussen, F. & Hjarde, W. (1957*a*). Determination of α-tocopherol by chromatography on secondary magnesium phosphate. *Acta chem. scand.*, **11**, 34–43.

Bro-Rasmussen, F. & Hjarde, W. (1957*b*). Quantitative determination of the individual tocopherols by chromatography on secondary magnesium phosphate. *Ibid.*, **11**, 44–52.

Brown, F. (1952). The estimation of vitamin E. *Biochem. J.*, **51**, 237–9.

Brubacher, G. (1968). The determination of vitamins and carotenoids in fats. In *Analysis and Characterization of Oils, Fats and Fat Products*, Vol. II (H. A. Boekenoogen, ed.), Interscience Publishers, New York, pp. 607–54.

Brubacher, G., Müller-Mulot, W. & Southgate, D. A. T. (1985). *Methods for the Determination of Vitamins in Food*, Elsevier Applied Science Publishers, London.

Budowski, P. & Bondi, A. (1957). Determination of vitamin A by conversion to anhydrovitamin A. *Analyst, Lond.*, **82**, 751–60.

Bueno, M. P. & Villalobos, M. C. (1983). Reverse phase high pressure liquid chromatographic determination of vitamin K_1 in infant formulas. *J. Ass. off. analyt. Chem.*, **66**, 1063–6.

Bui, M. H. (1987). Sample preparation and liquid chromatographic determination of vitamin D in food products. *J. Ass. off. analyt. Chem.*, **70**, 802–5.

Bui-Nguyên, M. & Blanc, B. (1980). Measurement of vitamin A in milk and cheese by means of high pressure liquid chromatography (HPLC). *Experimentia*, **36**, 374–5.

Bunnell, R. H. (1967). Vitamin E assay by chemical methods. In *The Vitamins*, 2nd edn, Vol. VI (P. György & W. N. Pearson, eds), Academic Press, New York, pp. 261–304.

Bunnell, R. H., Keating, J., Quaresimo, A. & Parman, G. K. (1965). Alpha-tocopherol content of foods. *Am. J. clin. Nutr.*, **17**, 1–10.

Burton, G. W. & Ingold, K. U. (1981). Autoxidation of biological molecules. 1. The antioxidant activity of vitamin E and related chain-breaking phenolic antioxidants *in vitro*. *J. Am. Chem. Soc.*, **103**, 6472–7.

Bushway, R. J. (1985). Separation of carotenoids in fruits and vegetables by high performance liquid chromatography. *J. Liquid Chromat.*, **8**, 1527–47.

Bushway, R. J. & Wilson, A. M. (1982). Determination of α- and β-carotene in fruit and vegetables by high performance liquid chromatography. *Can. Inst. Fd Sci. Technol. J.*, **15**, 165–9.

Buttriss, J. L. & Diplock, A. T. (1984). High-performance liquid chromatography methods for vitamin E in tissues. *Meth. Enzym.*, **105**, 131–8.

Cain, R. F. (1975). Factors influencing the nutritional quality and fortification of fruits and vegetables. In *Technology of Fortification of Foods*, Food and Nutrition Board, NRC, Nat. Acad. Sci., Washington, DC.

Carpenter, A. P., Jr (1979). Determination of tocopherols in vegetable oils. *J. Am. Oil Chem. Soc.*, **56**, 668–71.

Chen, P. S., Jr, Terepka, R. & Lane, K. (1964). Sensitive fluorescence reaction for vitamins D and dihydrotachysterol. *Analyt. Biochem.*, **8**, 34–42.

Chen, P. S., Jr, Terepka, R., Lane, K. & Marsh, A. (1965). Studies of the stability and extractability of vitamin D. *Analyt. Biochem.*, **10**, 421–34.

Chow, C. K., Draper, H. H. & Saari Csallany, A. (1969). Method for the assay of free and esterified tocopherols. *Analyt. Biochem.*, **32**, 81–90.

Christie, A. A. (1971). Chemical methods for the determination of vitamins A, C, D and E in food. In *The University of Nottingham Seminar on Vitamins* (M. Stein, ed.), Churchill Livingstone, Edinburgh and London, pp. 146–64.

Christie, A. A. (1975). Analysis for selected vitamins in a nutritional labelling programme. *Inst. Fd Sci. Technol. Proc.*, **8**, 163–8.

Christie, A. A. & Wiggins, R. A. (1978). Developments in vitamin analysis. In *Developments in Food Analysis Techniques*, Vol. I (R. D. King, ed.), Applied Science Publishers, London, pp. 1–42.

Christie, A. A., Dean, A. C. & Millburn, B. A. (1973). The determination of vitamin E in food by colorimetry and gas–liquid chromatography. *Analyst, Lond.*, **98**, 161–7.

Cohen, H. & Lapointe, M. (1978). Method for the extraction and cleanup of animal feed for the determination of liposoluble vitamins D, A, and E by high-pressure liquid chromatography. *J. agric. Fd Chem.*, **26**, 1210–13.

Cohen, H. & Lapointe, M. (1979). Quantitative analysis of vitamin D_3 in a feed using normal phase high pressure liquid chromatography. *J. chromatogr. Sci.*, **17**, 510–13.

Cohen, H. & Lapointe, M. R. (1980*a*). Determination of vitamin E in animal feeds by normal phase high pressure liquid chromatography. *J. Ass. off. analyt. Chem.*, **63**, 1254–7.

Cohen, H. & Lapointe, M. (1980*b*). Determination of low levels of vitamin D_3 in animal feeds, using Sephadex LH-20 and normal phase high pressure liquid chromatography. *J. Ass. off. analyt. Chem.*, **63**, 1158–62.

Cohen, H. & Wakeford, B. (1980). High pressure liquid chromatographic determination of vitamin D_3 in instant nonfat dried milk. *J. Ass. off. analyt. Chem.*, **63**, 1163–7.

Cooke, N. H. C., Archer, B. G., Olsen, K. & Berick, A. (1982). Comparison of three- and five-micrometer column packings for reversed-phase liquid chromatography. *Analyt. Chem.*, **54**, 2277–83.

Coors, U. & Montag, A. (1982). Separation of tocopherols and tocotrienols besides α-tocopherol acetate by high pressure liquid chromatography. *Fd Sci. Technol. Abstr.*, **14**, 1A61.

Cort, W. M., Mergens, W. & Greene, A. (1978). Stability of alpha-and gamma-tocopherol: Fe^{3+} and Cu^{2+} interactions. *J. Fd Sci.*, **43**, 797–8.

Cort, W. M., Vicente, T. S., Waysek, E. H. & Williams, B. D. (1983). Vitamin E content of feedstuffs determined by high-performance liquid chromatographic fluorescence. *J. agric. Fd Chem.*, **31**, 1330–3.

Coulter, S. T. & Thomas, E. L. (1968). Enrichment and fortification of dairy products and margarine. *J. agric. Fd Chem.*, **16**, 158–62.

Cox, G. B. (1977). Practical aspects of bonded phase chromatography. *J. chromatogr. Sci.*, **15**, 385–92.

Cremin, F. M. & Power, P. (1985). Vitamins in bovine and human milks. In *Developments in Dairy Chemistry*, Vol. III (P. F. Fox, ed.), Elsevier Applied Science Publishers, London and New York, pp. 337–98.

Dam, H. & Søndergaard, E. (1967). The determination of vitamin K. In *The Vitamins*, 2nd edn, Vol. VI (P. György & W. N. Pearson, eds), Academic Press, New York, pp. 245–60.

Dean, A. C. (1971). The separation of dimeric tocopherol products from vitamin E in food by dry-column chromatography. *Chemy Ind.*, 12th June, 677–8.

Deldime, P., Jacobsberg, B. & Belhassine, M. (1978). Contribution to the assessment of tocopherols in plant oils and fats by differential pulse voltammetry. *Analyt. Lett.*, **AII**(1), 63–72.

De Leenheer, A. P. & Cruyl, A. A. M. (1980). Gas–liquid chromatography of vitamin D and analogs. *Meth. Enzym.*, **67**F, 335–43.

DeLuca, H. F. (1975). Function of the fat-soluble vitamins. *Am. J. clin. Nutr.*, **28**, 339–45.

DeLuca, H. F. (1978). Vitamin D. In *Handbook of Lipid Research*, Vol. II (H. F. DeLuca, ed.), Plenum Press, New York, pp. 69–132.

DeLuca, H. F. & Blunt, J. W. (1971). Vitamin D. *Meth. Enzym.*, **18**C, 709–33.

DeLuca, H. F., Zile, M. H. & Neville, P. F. (1969). Chromatography of vitamins A and D. In *Lipid Chromatographic Analysis*, Vol. 2 (G. V. Marinetti, ed.), Marcel Dekker, Inc., New York, pp. 345–457.

de Man, J. M. (1981). Light-induced destruction of vitamin A in milk. *J. Dairy Sci.*, **64**, 2031–2.

Dennison, D. B. & Kirk, J. R. (1977). Quantitative analysis of vitamin A in cereal products by high speed liquid chromatography. *J. Fd Sci.*, **42**, 1376–9.

Department of Health & Social Security (1969). *Recommended intakes of nutrients for the United Kingdom*. Reports on Public Health and Medical Subjects. No. 120, HM Stationery Office, London.

Department of Health & Social Security (1979). *Recommended daily amounts of food energy and nutrients for groups of people in the United Kingdom.* Report on Health and Social Subjects, No. 15, HM Stationery Office, London.

De Ritter, E. (1977). *Stability Characteristics of Vitamins in Processed Foods*, F. Hoffmann–La Roche & Co. Ltd, Basle, Switzerland.

De Ritter, E. & Purcell, A. E. (1981). Carotenoid analytical methods. In *Carotenoids as Colorants and Vitamin A Precursors* (J. C. Bauernfeind, ed.), Academic Press, New York, pp. 815–82.

Desai, I. D. (1980). Assay methods. In *Vitamin E. A Comprehensive Treatise* (L. J. Machlin, ed.), Marcel Dekker, Inc., New York, pp. 67–98.

Desai, I. D. & Machlin, L. J. (1985). Vitamin E. In *Methods of Vitamin Assay*, 4th edn (J. Augustin, B. P. Klein, D. Becker & P. B. Venugopal, eds), John Wiley, New York, pp. 255–83.

de Vries, E. J. & Borsje, B. (1982). Analysis of fat-soluble vitamins. 27. High performance liquid chromatographic and gas–liquid chromatographic determination of vitamin D in fortified milk and milk powder: collaborative study. *J. Ass. off. analyt. Chem.*, **65**, 1228–34.

de Vries, E. J., Mulder, F. J. & Keuning, K. J. (1969). Determination of vitamin D in blood. *J. Vitam.*, **15**, 189–97.

de Vries, E. J., Zeeman, J., Esser, R. J. E., Borsje, B. & Mulder, F. J. (1979). Analysis of fat-soluble vitamins. XXI. High pressure liquid chromatographic assay methods for vitamin D in vitamin D concentrates. *J. Ass. off. analyt. Chem.*, **62**, 129–35.

de Vries, E. J., van Bemmel, P. & Borsje, B. (1983). Analysis of fat-soluble vitamins. XXVIII. High performance liquid chromatographic determination of vitamin D in pet foods and feeds: collaborative study. *J. Ass. off. analyt. Chem.*, **66**, 751–8.

DeVries, J. W. (1985). Chromatographic assay of vitamins. In *Methods of Vitamin Assay*, 4th edn (J. Augustin, B. P. Klein, D. Becker & P. B. Venugopal, eds), John Wiley, New York, pp. 65–94.

DeVries, J. W., Egberg, D. C. & Heroff, J. C. (1979). Concurrent analysis of vitamin A and vitamin E by reversed phase high performance liquid chromatography. In *Liquid Chromatographic Analysis of Food and Beverages*, Vol. II (G. Charalambous, ed.), Academic Press, New York, pp. 477–97.

Dialameh, G. H. & Olson, R. E. (1969). Gas–liquid chromatography of phytyl ubiquinone, vitamin E, vitamin K_1, and homologs of vitamin K_2. *Analyt. Biochem.*, **32**, 263–72.

DiCesare, J. L., Dong, M. W. & Atwood, J. G. (1981). Very-high-speed liquid chromatography. II. Some instrumental factors influencing performance. *J. Chromat.*, **217**, 369–86.

Dicks-Bushnell, M. W. (1967). Column chromatography in the determination of tocopherol: Florisil, silicic acid, and secondary magnesium phosphate. *J. Chromat.*, **27**, 96–103.

Draper, H. H. (1970). The tocopherols. In *Fat-soluble Vitamins* (R. A. Morton, ed.), Pergamon Press, New York, pp. 333–93.

Dugan, R. E., Frigerio, N. A. & Siebert, J. M. (1964). Colorimetric determination of vitamin A and its derivatives with trifluoroacetic acid. *Analyt. Chem.*, **36**, 114–17.

Duggan, D. E., Bowman, R. L., Brodie, B. B. & Udenfriend, S. (1957). A spectrophotofluorometric study of compounds of biological interest. *Archs Biochem. Biophys.*, **68**, 1–14.

Dunphy, P. J. & Brodie, A. F. (1971). The structure and function of quinones in respiratory metabolism. *Meth. Enzym.*, **18C**, 407–61.

Egan, H., Kirk, R. S. & Sawyer, R. (1981). *Pearson's Chemical Analysis of Foods*, 8th edn, Churchill Livingstone, London.

Egberg, D. C., Heroff, J. C. & Potter, R. H. (1977). Determination of all-*trans* and 13-*cis* vitamin A in food products by high-pressure liquid chromatography. *J. agric. Fd Chem.*, **25**, 1127–32.

Eisner, J., Iverson, J. L. & Firestone, D. (1966). Gas chromatography of unsaponifiable matter. 4. Aliphatic alcohols, tocopherols and triterpenoid alcohols in butter and vegetable oils. *J. Ass. off. analyt. Chem.*, **49**, 580–90.

Eisses, J. & de Vries, H. (1969). Chemical method for the determination of vitamin D in evaporated milk with the elimination of cholesterol by digitonin precipitation. *J. Ass. off. analyt. Chem.*, **52**, 1189–95.

Elkins, E. R. & Dudek, J. A. (1985). Sampling for vitamin analyses. In *Methods of Vitamin Assay*, 4th edn (J. Augustin, B. P. Klein, D. Becker & P. B. Venugopal, eds), John Wiley, New York, pp. 135–51.

Engelhardt, H. (1977). The role of moderators in liquid–solid chromatography. *J. chromatogr. Sci.*, **15**, 380–4.

Engelhardt, H. (ed.) (1986). *Practice of High Performance Liquid Chromatography. Applications, Equipment and Quantitative Analysis*, Springer-Verlag, Berlin, Heidelberg, New York, Tokyo.

Erdman, J. W., Jr, Hou, S. F. & Lachance, P. A. (1973). Fluorometric determination of vitamin A in foods. *J. Fd Sci.*, **38**, 447–9.

Erickson, D. R. & Dunkley, W. L. (1964). Spectrophotometric determination of tocopherol in milk and milk lipides. *Analyt. Chem.*, **36**, 1055–8.

Erickson, J. A., Weissberger, W. & Keeney, P. G. (1973). Tocopherols in the unsaponifiable fraction of cocoa lipids. *J. Fd Sci.*, **38**, 1158–61.

Eriksen, S. (1980). Rapid high performance liquid chromatographic method for determination of gelatin-coated supplemental vitamin E in feeds. *J. Ass. off. analyt. Chem.*, **63**, 1154–7.

Ettre, L. S. (1981). The nomenclature of chromatography. II. Liquid chromatography. *J. Chromat. chromatogr. Rev.*, **220**, 29–63.

Fallick, G. J. & Rausch, C. W. (1979). Radial compression separation system. *Am. Lab.*, **11**, 87–97.

Fenton, T. W., Vogtmann, H. & Clandinin, D. R. (1973). Gas–liquid chromatography of vitamin A_1 alcohol and vitamin A_1 acetate. *J. Chromat.*, **77**, 410–12.

Fisher, A. L., Parfitt, A. M. & Lloyd, H. M. (1972). Gas–liquid chromatography of vitamin D as trimethylsilyl derivatives. *J. Chromat.*, **65**, 493–9.

Fisher, J. F. & Rouseff, R. L. (1986). Solid–phase extraction and HPLC determination of β-cryptoxanthin and α- and β-carotene in orange juice. *J. agric. Fd Chem.*, **34**, 985–9.

Folch, J., Lees, M. & Sloane Stanley, G. H. (1957). A simple method for the isolation and purification of total lipides from animal tissues. *J. biol. Chem.*, **226**, 497–509.

Fong, G. W. K., Johnson, R. N. & Kho, B. T. (1983). Non-aqueous reverse phase liquid chromatographic determination of vitamin D_2 in multi-vitamin tablets, using vitamin D_3 as internal standard. *J. Ass. off. analyt. Chem.*, **66**, 939–45.

Ford, J. E., Porter, J. W. G., Thompson, S. Y., Toothill, J. & Edwards-Webb, J. (1969). Effects of ultra-high-temperature (UHT) processing and of subsequent storage on the vitamin content of milk. *J. Dairy Res.*, **36**, 447–54.

Fukuzawa, K., Tokumura, A., Ouchi, S. & Tsukatani, H. (1982). Antioxidant activities of tocopherols on Fe^{2+}-ascorbate-induced lipid peroxidation in lecithin liposomes. *Lipids*, **17**, 511–13.

Ganguly, J. & Murthy, S. K. (1967). Biogenesis of vitamin A and carotene. In *The Vitamins*, 2nd edn, Vol. I (W. H. Sebrell, Jr & R. S. Harris, eds), Academic Press, New York, pp. 125–53.

Gertz, C. & Herrmann, K. (1982). Analysis of tocopherols and tocotrienols in foods. *Z. Lebensmittelunters. u.-Forsch.*, **174**, 390–4. (German text).

Gharbo, S. A. & Gosser, L. A. (1974). A stable and sensitive colorimetric method for the determination of ergocalciferol (vitamin D_2) by using trifluoroacetic acid. *Analyst, Lond.*, **99**, 222–4.

Gharbo, S. A. & Gosser, L. A. (1975). Differential spectrophotometric method for the determination of vitamin A (retinol) by using trifluoroacetic acid, and its application to related compounds. *Analyst, Lond.*, **100**, 703–7.

Gillan, F. T. & Johns, R. B. (1983). Normal-phase HPLC analysis of microbial carotenoids and neutral lipids. *J. chromatogr. Sci.*, **21**, 34–8.

Govind Rao, M. K. & Perkins, E. G. (1972). Identification and estimation of tocopherols and tocotrienols in vegetable oils using gas chromatography–mass spectrometry. *J. agric. Fd Chem.*, **20**, 240–5.

Grace, M. L. & Bernhard, R. A. (1984). Measuring vitamins A and D in milk. *J. Dairy Sci.*, **67**, 1646–54.

Grady, L. T. & Thakker, K. D. (1980). Stability of solid drugs: degradation of ergocalciferol (vitamin D_2) and cholecalciferol (vitamin D_3) at high humidities and elevated temperatures. *J. Pharm. Sci.*, **69**, 1099–102.

Green, J. (1951). Studies on the analysis of vitamins D. 2. The analytical purification of vitamin D by differential solubility, precipitation reactions, and chromatography. *Biochem. J.*, **49**, 45–54.

Green, J. (1970). Distribution of fat-soluble vitamins and their standardization and assay by biological methods. In *Fat-soluble Vitamins* (R. A. Morton, ed.), Pergamon Press, New York, pp. 71–97.

Grys, S. (1975). An improved and accurate procedure for the determination of vitamin A. *Analyst, Lond.*, **100**, 637–9.

Grys, S. (1980). Indirect spectrophotometry on vitamin A products: peak signal readout. *Meth. Enzym.*, **67F**, 195–9.

Guilbault, G. G. (1973). *Practical Fluorescence. Theory, Methods and Techniques*, Marcel Dekker, Inc., New York.

Gunstone, F. D. & Norris, F. A. (1983). *Lipids in Foods. Chemistry, Biochemistry and Technology*, Pergamon Press, Oxford.

Håkansson, B., Jägerstad, M. & Öste, R. (1987). Determination of vitamin E in wheat products by HPLC. *J. Micronutr. Anal.*, **3**, 307–18.

Hall, G. S. & Laidman, D. L. (1968). The determination of tocopherols and isoprenoid quinones in the grain and seedlings of wheat (*Triticum vulgare*). *Biochem. J.*, **108**, 465–73.

Hamilton, R. J. & Sewell, P. A. (1982). *Introduction to High Performance Liquid Chromatography*, 2nd edn, Chapman & Hall, London & New York.

Hanewald, K. H., Mulder, F. J. & Keuning, K. J. (1968). Thin-layer chromatographic assay of vitamin D in high-potency preparations. *J. pharm. Sci.*, **57**, 1308–12.

Haroon, Y., Shearer, M. J. & Barkhan, P. (1980). Resolution of phylloquinone (vitamin K_1), phylloquinone 2, 3-epoxide, 2-chloro-phylloquinone and their geometric isomers by high-performance liquid chromatography. *J. Chromat.*, **200**, 293–9.

Haroon, Y., Shearer, M. J. & Barkhan, P. (1981). Resolution of menaquinones (vitamins K_2) by high-performance liquid chromatography. *J. Chromat.*, **206**, 333–42.

Haroon, Y., Shearer, M. J., Rahim, S., Gunn, W. G., McEnery, G. & Barkhan, P. (1982). The content of phylloquinone (vitamin K_1) in human milk, cow's milk and infant formula foods determined by high-performance liquid chromatography. *J. Nutr.*, **112**, 1105–17.

Haroon, Y., Bacon, D. S. & Sadowski, J. A. (1987). Chemical reduction system for the detection of phylloquinone (vitamin K_1) and menaquinones (vitamin K_2). *J. Chromat.*, **384**, 383–9.

Harris, P. L. & Embree, N. D. (1963). Quantitative consideration of the effect of polyunsaturated fatty acid content of the diet upon the requirements for vitamin E. *Am. J. clin. Nutr.*, **13**, 385–92.

Hartman, K. T. (1977). A simplified gas liquid chromatographic determination for vitamin E in vegetable oils. *J. Am. Oil Chem. Soc.*, **54**, 421–3.

Hasegawa, K. (1980). Separation of carotenoids on lipophilic Sephadex. *Meth. Enzym.*, **67F**, 261–4.

Hashmi, M. (1973). *Assay of Vitamins in Pharmaceutical Preparations*, John Wiley & Sons, London and New York.

Henderson, S. K. & McLean, L. A. (1979). Screening method for vitamins A and D in fortified skim milk, chocolate milk, and vitamin D liquid concentrates. *J. Ass. off. analyt. Chem.*, **62**, 1358–60.

Hicks, R. M. (1983). The scientific basis for regarding vitamin A and its analogues as anti-carcinogenic agents. *Proc. Nutr. Soc.*, **42**, 83–93.

Hiroshima, O., Ikenoya, S., Ohmae, M. & Kawabe, K. (1981). Electrochemical detector for high-performance liquid chromatography. V. Application to adsorption chromatography. *Chem. Pharm. Bull.*, **29**, 451–5.

Hjarde, W., Leerbeck, E. & Leth, T. (1973). The chemistry of vitamin E (including its chemical determination). *Acta Agric. scand.*, Suppl. 19, 87–96.

HMSO (1982). *The Feeding Stuffs (Sampling and Analysis) Regulations 1982*, Statutory Instruments No. 1144, HM Stationery Office, London.

Holasová, M. & Blattná, J. (1976). Gel chromatographic separation of retinol, retinyl esters and other fat-soluble vitamins. *J. Chromat.*, **123**, 225–30.

Holmes, R. P. & Kummerow, F. A. (1983). The relationship of adequate and excessive intake of vitamin D to health and disease. *J. Am. Coll. Nutr.*, **2**, 173–99.

Horváth, C. (1982). Bonded phase chromatography. In *Techniques in Liquid Chromatography* (C. F. Simpson, ed.), John Wiley & Sons, Chichester, pp. 229–301.

Horwitt, M. K. (1960). Vitamin E and lipid metabolism in man. *Am. J. clin. Nutr.*, **8**, 451–61.

Hsieh, Y-P. C. & Karel, M. (1983). Rapid extraction and determination of α- and β-carotenes in foods. *J. Chromat.*, **259**, 515–18.

Hubbard, R., Brown, P. K. & Bownds, D. (1971). Retinol. *Meth. Enzym.*, **18C**, 644–7.

Hung, S. O., Cho, Y. C. & Slinger, S. J. (1980). High performance liquid chromatographic determination of α-tocopherol in fish liver. *J. Ass. off. analyt. Chem.*, **63**, 889–93.

Hwang, S-M. (1985). Liquid chromatographic determination of vitamin K_1 *trans*- and *cis*-isomers in infant formula. *J. Ass. off. analyt. Chem.*, **68**, 684–9.

Igarashi, O., Hagino, M. & Inagaki, C. (1973). Decomposition of α-tocopheryl spirodimer by alkaline saponification. *J. Nutr. Sci. Vitaminol.*, **19**, 469–74.

Indyk, H. (1982). The routine determination of vitamin A in fortified milk powder products. *NZ Jl Dairy Sci. Technol.*, **17**, 257–67.

Indyk, H. (1983). The routine, simultaneous determination of vitamins A and E in fortified whole milk powders. *NZ Jl Dairy Sci. Technol.*, **18**, 197–208.

Indyk, H. (1988). The photoinduced reduction and simultaneous fluorescence detection of vitamin K_1 with HPLC. *J. Micronutr. Anal.*, **4**, 61–70.

Indyk, H. & Woollard, D. C. (1984). The determination of vitamin D in milk powders by high performance liquid chromatography. *NZ Jl Dairy Sci. Technol.*, **19**, 19–30.

Indyk, H. & Woollard, D. C. (1985*a*). The determination of vitamin D in supplemented milk powders by HPLC. II. Incorporation of internal standard. *NZ Jl Dairy Sci. Technol.*, **20**, 19–28.

Indyk, H. & Woollard, D. C. (1985*b*). The determination of vitamin D in fortified milk powders and infant formulas by HPLC. *J. Micronutr. Anal.*, **1**, 121–41.

Itoh, T., Tamura, T. & Matsumoto, T. (1973). Sterol composition of 19 vegetable oils. *J. Am. Oil Chem. Soc.*, **50**, 122–5.

Jackson, P. A., Shelton, C. J. & Frier, P. J. (1982). High performance liquid chromatographic determination of vitamin D_3 in foods with particular reference to eggs. *Analyst, Lond.*, **107**, 1363–9.

Johnson, F. C. (1979). The antioxidant vitamins. *CRC crit. Rev. Fd Sci. Nutr.*, **11**, 217–309.

Johnson, G. W. & Vickers, C. (1973). The identification and semiquantitative assay of some fat-soluble vitamins and antioxidants in pharmaceutical products and animal feeds by thin-layer chromatography. *Analyst, Lond.*, **98**, 257–67.

Jones, G., Seamark, D. A., Trafford, D. J. H. & Makin, H. L. J. (1985). Vitamin D: cholecalciferol, ergocalciferol, and hydroxylated metabolites. In *Modern Chromatographic Analysis of the Vitamins* (A. P. de Leenheer, W. E. Lambert & M. G. M. de Ruyter, eds), Marcel Dekker, Inc., New York, pp. 73–128.

Jones, S. W., Wilkie, J. B. & Libby, D. A. (1965). Modification of the USP chemical method for determining vitamin D in evaporated milk. *J. Ass. off. analyt. Chem.*, **48**, 1212–17.

Kamangar, T. & Fawzi, A. B. (1978). Spectrophotometric determination of vitamin A in oils and fats. *J. Ass. off. analyt. Chem.*, **61**, 753–5.

Karch, K., Sebastian, I., Halász, I. & Engelhardt, H. (1976). Optimization of reversed-phase separations. *J. Chromat.*, **122**, 171–84.

Kasparek, S. (1980). Chemistry of tocopherols and tocotrienols. In *Vitamin E. A*

Comprehensive Treatise (L. J. Machlin, ed.), Marcel Dekker, Inc., New York, pp. 7–65.

Keverling Buisman, J. A., Hanewald, K. H., Mulder, F. J., Roborgh, J. R. & Keuning, K. J. (1968). Evaluation of the effect of isomerization on the chemical and biological assay of vitamin D. *J. pharm. Sci.*, **57**, 1326–9.

Kläui, H. (1971). The functional (technical) uses of vitamins. In *The University of Nottingham Seminar on Vitamins* (M. Stein, ed.), Churchill Livingstone, Edinburgh and London, pp. 110–43.

Kläui, H. M., Hausheer, W. & Huschke, G. (1970). Technological aspects of the use of fat-soluble vitamins and carotenoids and of the development of stabilized marketable forms. In *Fat-soluble Vitamins* (R. A. Morton, ed.), Pergamon Press, New York, pp. 113–59.

Kobayashi, T. (1965). Studies on the chemical isomerization of vitamin D. I. Chemical isomerization of vitamin D_2 to isotachysterol by acetyl chloride. *J. Vitam.*, **11**, 48–53.

Kobayashi, T. (1967). Studies on the chemical isomerization of vitamin D. V. Chemical isomerization course of vitamin D_2 to isotachysterol$_2$ by acetyl chloride. *J. Vitam.*, **13**, 268–73.

Kobayashi, T., Okano, T. & Takeuchi, A. (1986). The determination of vitamin D in foods and feeds using high-performance liquid chromatography. *J. Micronutr. Anal.*, **2**, 1–24.

Kodicek, E. & Lawson, D. E. M. (1967). Vitamin D. In *The Vitamins*, 2nd edn, Vol. VI (P. György & W. N. Pearson, eds), Academic Press, New York, pp. 211–44.

Koshy, K. T. (1982). Chromatography of vitamin D_3 and metabolites. In *Advances in Chromatography*, Vol. XX (J. C. Giddings, E. Grushka, J. Cazes & P. R. Brown, eds), Marcel Dekker, Inc., New York, pp. 83–138.

Krampitz, G. (1980). *Vitamin D in Animal Nutrition*, F. Hoffmann–La Roche & Co. Ltd, Basle, Switzerland.

Krstulovic, A. M. & Brown, P. R. (1982). *Reversed-phase High-Performance Liquid Chromatography*, John Wiley & Sons, Inc., New York.

Krukovsky, V. N. (1964). The protection of milk fat tocopherols during saponification with ascorbic acid. *J. agric. Fd Chem.*, **12**, 289–92.

Kutsky, R. J. (1973). *Handbook of Vitamins and Hormones*, Van Nostrand Reinhold, New York.

Laidman, D. L. & Hall, G. S. (1971). Adsorption column chromatography of tocopherols. *Meth. Enzym.*, **18C**, 349–56.

Lakowicz, J. R. (1983). *Principles of Fluorescence Spectroscopy*, Plenum Press, New York.

Lambert, W. E., Nelis, H. J., de Ruyter, M. G. M. & de Leenheer, A. P. (1985). Vitamin A: retinol, carotenoids, and related compounds. In *Modern Chromatographic Analysis of the Vitamins* (A. P. de Leenheer, W. E. Lambert & M. G. M. de Ruyter, eds), Marcel Dekker, Inc., New York, pp. 1–72.

Lambertsen, G., Myklestad, H. & Braekkan, O. R. (1964). The determination and contents of α- and γ-tocopherols in margarine. *Analyst, Lond.*, **89**, 164–7.

Landen, W. O., Jr (1980). Application of gel permeation chromatography and nonaqueous reverse phase chromatography to high pressure liquid chromatographic determination of retinyl palmitate in fortified breakfast cereals. *J. Ass. off. analyt. Chem.*, **63**, 131–6.

Landen, W. O., Jr (1981). Resolution of fat-soluble vitamins in high-performance liquid chromatography with methanol- containing mobile phases. *J. Chromat.*, **211**, 155–9.

Landen, W. O., Jr (1982). Application of gel permeation chromatography and nonaqueous reversed-phase chromatography to high performance liquid chromatographic determination of retinyl and α-tocopheryl acetate in infant formulas. *J. Ass. off. analyt. Chem.*, **65**, 810–16.

Landen, W. O., Jr (1985). Liquid chromatographic determination of vitamins D_2 and D_3 in fortified milk and infant formulas. *J. Ass. off. analyt. Chem.*, **68**, 183–7.

Landen, W. O., Jr & Eitenmiller, R. R. (1979). Application of gel permeation chromatography and nonaqueous reverse phase chromatography to high pressure liquid chromatographic determination of retinyl palmitate and β-carotene in oil and margarine. *J. Ass. off. analyt. Chem.*, **62**, 283–9.

Landers, G. M. & Olson, J. A. (1986). Absence of isomerization of retinyl palmitate, retinol, and retinal in chlorinated and nonchlorinated solvents under gold light. *J. Ass. off. analyt. Chem.*, **69**, 50–5.

Langenberg, J. P., Tjaden, U. R., de Vogel, E. M. & Langerak, D.Is. (1986). Determination of phylloquinone (vitamin K_1) in raw and processed vegetables using reversed phase HPLC with electrofluorometric detection. *Acta Alimentaria*, **15**, 187–98.

Lauren, D. R., Agnew, M. P. & McNaughton, D. E. (1986). The use of decanol for improving chromatographic stability in isocratic non-aqueous reversed-phase analysis of carotenoids by high-pressure liquid chromatography. *J. Liquid Chromat.*, **9**, 1997–2012.

Lawn, R. E., Harris, J. R. & Johnson, S. F. (1983). Some aspects of the use of high-performance liquid chromatography for the determination of vitamin A in animal feeding stuffs. *J. Sci. Fd Agric.*, **34**, 1039–46.

Lawson, E. (1985). Vitamin D. In *Fat-Soluble Vitamins. Their Biochemistry and Applications* (A. T. Diplock, ed.), Heinemann, London, pp. 76–153.

Lefevere, M. F. L., Claeys, A. E. & de Leenheer, A. P. (1985). Vitamin K: phylloquinone and menaquinones. In *Modern Chromatographic Analysis of the Vitamins* (A. P. de Leenheer, W. E. Lambert & M. G. M. de Ruyter, eds), Marcel Dekker, Inc., New York, pp. 201–66.

Le Maguer, I. & Jackson, H. (1983). Stability of vitamin A in pasteurized and ultra-high temperature processed milks. *J. Dairy Sci.*, **66**, 2452–8.

Lento, H. G. (1984). Sample preparation and its role in nutritional analysis. In *Modern Methods of Food Analysis* (K. K. Stewart & J. R. Whitaker, eds), AVI Publishing Co., Inc., Westport, CT, pp. 71–9.

Lercker, G. & Caboni, M. F. (1985). GLC analysis of unsaponifiable matter. *Riv. ital. sostanze grasse*, **62**, 193–8. (Italian text).

Loev, B. & Goodman, M. M. (1967). Dry-column chromatography: a preparative chromatographic technique with the resolution of thin-layer chromatography. *Chemy Ind.*, 2nd December 2026–32.

Loev, B. & Snader, K. M. (1965). Dry-column chromatography. A preparative chromatographic technique with the resolvability of thin-layer chromatography. *Chemy Ind.*, 2nd January, 15–16.

Losowsky, M. S. (1979). Vitamin E in human nutrition. In *Proceedings of the Kellogg*

Nutrition Symposium, London, 14th–15th Dec., 1978 (T. G. Taylor, ed.) MTP Press, Lancaster, pp. 101–10.

McBride, H. D. & Evans, D. H. (1973). Rapid voltammetric method for the estimation of tocopherols and antioxidants in oils and fats. *Analyt. Chem.*, **45**, 446–9.

McCormick, R. M. & Karger, B. L. (1980). Distribution phenomena of mobile-phase components and determination of dead volume in reversed-phase liquid chromatography. *Analyt. Chem.*, **52**, 2249–57.

McDonald, P., Edwards, R. A. & Greenhalgh, J. F. D. (1972). *Animal Nutrition*, Oliver & Boyd, Edinburgh.

Machlin, L. J. (1984). Vitamin E. In *Handbook of Vitamins. Nutritional, Biochemical and Clinical Aspects* (L. J. Machlin, ed.), Marcel Dekker, Inc., New York, pp. 99–145.

McLaren, D. (1967a). Effects of vitamin A deficiency in man. In *The Vitamins*, 2nd edn, Vol. I (W. H. Sebrell, Jr & R. S. Harris, eds), Academic Press, New York, pp. 267–80.

McLaren, D. (1967b). Requirements of vitamin A in man. In *The Vitamins*, 2nd edn, Vol. I (W. H. Sebrell, Jr & R. S. Harris, eds), Academic Press, New York, pp. 301–3.

McLaughlin, P. J. & Weihrauch, J. C. (1979). Vitamin E content of foods. *J. Am. Diet. Ass.*, **75**, 647–65.

McMurray, C. H., Blanchflower, W. J. & Rice, D. A. (1980). Influence of extraction techniques on determination of α-tocopherol in animal feedstuffs. *J. Ass. off. analyt. Chem.*, **63**, 1258–61.

Majors, R. E. (1976). Liquid–solid (adsorption) chromatography. In *Practical High Performance Liquid Chromatography* (C. F. Simpson, ed.), Heydon & Son Ltd, London, pp. 89–108.

Majors, R. E. (1980). Recent advances in HPLC packings and columns. *J. chromatogr. Sci.*, **18**, 488–511.

Manes, J. D., Fluckiger, H. B. & Schneider, D. L. (1972). Chromatographic analysis of vitamin K_1; application to infant formula products. *J. agric. Fd Chem.*, **20**, 1130–2.

Manz, U. & Maurer, R. (1982). A method for the determination of vitamin K_3 in premixes and animal feedstuffs with the aid of high performance liquid chromatography. *Int. J. Vitam. Nutr. Res.*, **52**, 248–52.

Manz, U. & Philipp, K. (1981). A method for the routine determination of tocopherols in animal feed and human foodstuffs with the aid of high performance liquid chromatography. *Int. J. Vitam. Nutr. Res.*, **51**, 342–8.

Meijboom, P. W. & Jongenotter, G. A. (1979). A quantitative determination of tocotrienols and tocopherols in palm oil by TLC–GLC. *J. Am. Oil Chem. Soc.*, **56**, 33–5.

Meissonnier, E. (1983). *The Supply of Vitamins to Dairy Cattle*, F. Hoffmann–La Roche & Co. Ltd, Basle, Switzerland.

Merck Index (1983). 10th edn (M. Windholz, ed.), Merck & Co., Inc., Rahway, NJ, USA.

Miller, B. E. & Norman, A. W. (1984). Vitamin D. In *Handbook of Vitamins. Nutritional, Biochemical and Clinical Aspects* (L. J. Machlin, ed.), Marcel Dekker, Inc., New York, pp. 45–97.

Miller, D. R. & Hayes, K. C. (1982). Vitamin excess and toxicity. In *Nutritional Toxicology*, Vol I (J. N. Hathcock, ed.), Academic Press, New York, pp. 81–133.

Mills, R. S. (1985). Comparison of Carr–Price analysis and liquid chromatographic analysis for vitamin A in fortified milk. *J. Ass. off. analyt. Chem.*, **68**, 56–8.

Mordret, F. & Laurent, A. M. (1978). Determination of tocopherols by glass capillary column GLC. *Revue fr. Cps gras*, **25**, 245–50. (French text).

Morris, W. W., Jr & Haenni, E. O. (1962). Characterisation of tocopherols in vegetable oils by infrared spectrophotometry. *J. Ass. off. analyt. Chem.*, **45**, 92–8.

Mulder, F. J. & de Vries, E. J. (1974). Analysis of fat-soluble vitamins. 13. Chemical vitamin D assay in vitamin D and multivitamin preparations. *J. Ass. off. analyt. Chem.*, **57**, 1349–56.

Mulder, F. J., de Vries, E. J. & Borsje, B. (1971). Chemical analysis of vitamin D in concentrates and its problems. 12. Analysis of fat-soluble vitamins. *J. Ass. off. analyt. Chem.*, **54**, 1168–74.

Müller-Mulot, W. (1976). Rapid method for the quantitative determination of individual tocopherols in oils and fats. *J. Am. Oil Chem. Soc.*, **53**, 732–6.

Mulry, M. C., Schmidt, R. H. & Kirk, J. R. (1983). Isomerization of retinyl palmitate using conventional lipid extraction solvents. *J. Ass. off. analyt. Chem.*, **66**, 746–50.

Muniz, J. F., Wehr, C. T. & Wehr, H. M. (1982). Reverse phase liquid chromatographic determination of vitamins D_2 and D_3 in milk. *J. Ass. off. analyt. Chem.*, **65**, 791–7.

Murray, T. K. (1962). Purification of vitamin A by partition chromatography in the analysis of pharmaceuticals and margarine. *Analyt. Chem.*, **34**, 1241–4.

Murray, T. K., Day, K. C. & Kodicek, E. (1966). The differentiation and assay of vitamins D_2 and D_3 by gas–liquid chromatography. *Biochem. J.*, **98**, 293–6.

Murray, T. K., Erdody, P. & Panalaks, T. (1968). Determination of vitamins D_2 and D_3 in pharmaceuticals by gas–liquid chromatography. *J. Ass. off. analyt. Chem.*, **51**, 839–42.

Nair, P. P. (1966). Quantitative methods for the study of vitamin D. In *Advances in Lipid Research*, Vol. IV (R. Paoletti & D. Kritchevsky, eds), Academic Press, New York, pp. 227–56.

Nair, P. P. & Machiz, J. (1967). Gas–liquid chromatography of isomeric methyltocols and their derivatives. *Biochim. biophys. Acta*, **144**, 446–51.

Nair, P. P. & Turner, D. A. (1963). The application of gas–liquid chromatography to the determination of vitamins E and K. *J. Am. Oil Chem. Soc.*, **40**, 353–6.

Nair, P. P., Bucana, C., de Leon, S. & Turner, D. A. (1965). Gas chromatographic studies of vitamins D_2 and D_3. *Analyt. Chem.*, **37**, 631–6.

Nair, P. P., Sarlos, I. & Machiz, J. (1966). Microquantitative separation of isomeric dimethyltocols by gas–liquid chromatography. *Archs Biochem. Biophys.*, **114**, 488–93.

Navia, J. M. (1971). Vitamin D group. 2. Chemistry. In *The Vitamins*, 2nd edn, Vol. III (W. H. Sebrell, Jr & R. S. Harris, eds), Academic Press, New York, pp. 158–203.

Nelis, H. J. C. F. & de Leenheer, A. P. (1983). Isocratic nonaqueous reversed-phase liquid chromatography of carotenoids. *Analyt. Chem.*, **55**, 270–5.

Nelis, H. J., de Bevere, V. O. R. C. & de Leenheer, A. P. (1985). Vitamin E:

tocopherols and tocotrienols. In *Modern Chromatographic Analysis of the Vitamins* (A. P. de Leenheer, W. E. Lambert & M. G. M. de Ruyter, eds), Marcel Dekker, Inc., New York, pp. 129–200.

Nelson, J. P. & Milun, A. J. (1968). Gas chromatographic determination of tocopherols and sterols in soya sludges and residues. *J. Am. Oil Chem. Soc.*, **45**, 848–51.

Nelson, J. P., Milun, A. J. & Fisher, H. D. (1970). Gas chromatographic determination of tocopherols and sterols in soya sludges and residues—an improved method. *J. Am. Oil Chem. Soc.*, **47**, 259–61.

Nield, C. H., Russell, W. C. & Zimmerli, A. (1940). The spectrophotometric determination of vitamins D_2 and D_3. *J. biol. Chem.*, **136**, 73–9.

Nilsson, J. L. G., Daves, G. D., Jr & Folkers, K. (1968). New tocopherol dimers. *Acta chem. scand.*, **22**, 200–6.

Okano, T., Takeuchi, A. & Kobayashi, T. (1981). Simplified assay of vitamin D_2 in fortified dried milk by using two steps of high-performance liquid chromatography. *J. Nutr. Sci. Vitaminol.*, **27**, 539–50.

Olson, J. A. (1965). The determination of the fat-soluble vitamins: A, D, E, and K. In *Newer Methods of Nutritional Biochemistry*, Vol. II (A. A. Albanese, ed.), Academic Press, New York, pp. 345–402.

Olson, J. A. (1984). Vitamin A. In *Handbook of Vitamins. Nutritional, Biochemical and Clinical Aspects* (L. J. Machlin, ed.), Marcel Dekker, Inc., New York, pp. 1–43.

Omaye, S. T. (1984). Safety of megavitamin therapy. In *Nutritional and Toxicological Aspects of Food Safety* (M. Friedman, ed.), Plenum Press, New York, pp. 169–203.

Osborne, D. R. & Voogt, P. (1978). Fat-soluble vitamins. In *The Analysis of Nutrients in Foods*, Academic Press, London, pp. 183–200.

Owen, C. A., Jr (1971). Vitamin K group. 10. Deficiency effects in animals and human beings. In *The Vitamins*, 2nd edn, Vol. III (W. H. Sebrell, Jr & R. S. Harris, eds), Academic Press, New York, pp. 470–91.

Panalaks, T. (1970). A gas-chromatographic method for the determination of vitamin D in fortified non-fat dried milk. *Analyst, Lond.*, **95**, 862–7.

Panalaks, T. (1971). Colorimetric method for the determination of vitamin D in fortified whole and partially skim fluid milks. *J. Ass. off. analyt. Chem.*, **54**, 1299–1303.

Parris, N. A. (1978). Non-aqueous reversed-phase liquid chromatography. A neglected approach to the analysis of low polarity samples. *J. Chromat.*, **157**, 161–70.

Parris, N. A. (1984). *Instrumental Liquid Chromatography*, 2nd edn, Journal of Chromatography Library, Vol. 27, Elsevier, Amsterdam, Oxford, New York and Tokyo.

Parrish, D. B. (1977). Determination of vitamin A in foods—a review. *CRC crit. Rev. Fd Sci. Nutr.*, **9**, 375–94.

Parrish, D. B. (1979). Determination of vitamin D in foods: a review, *Ibid.*, **12**, 29–57.

Parrish, D. B. (1980*a*). Determination of vitamin E in foods—a review. *Ibid.*, **13**, 161–87.

Parrish, D. B. (1980*b*). Determination of vitamin K in foods: a review. *Ibid.*, **13**, 337–52.

Parrish, D. B., Moffitt, R. A., Noel, R. J. & Thompson, J. N. (1985). Vitamin A. In *Methods of Vitamin Assay*, 4th edn (J. Augustin, B. P. Klein, D. Becker & P. B. Venugopal, eds), John Wiley, New York, pp. 153–84.

Passmore, R. & Eastwood, M. A. (1986). *Davidson and Passmore Human Nutrition and Dietetics*, 8th edn, Churchill Livingstone, New York.

Paul, A. A. & Southgate, D. A. T. (1978). *McCance and Widdowson's The Composition of Foods*, 4th edn, HM Stationery Office, London.

Peto, R., Doll, R., Buckley, J. D. & Sporn, M. B. (1981). Can dietary beta-carotene materially reduce human cancer rates? *Nature, Lond.*, **290**, 201–8.

Pickston, L. (1978). Determination of α-tocopherol in condensed milks and milk substitutes by high performance liquid chromatography. *NZ Jl Sci.*, **21**, 383–5.

Piironen, V., Syväoja, E-L., Varo, P., Salminen, K. & Koivistoinen, P. (1985). Tocopherols and tocotrienols in Finnish foods: meat and meat products. *J. agric. Fd Chem.*, **33**, 1215–18.

Pitt, G. A. J. (1985). Vitamin A. In *Fat-Soluble Vitamins. Their Biochemistry and Applications* (A. T. Diplock, ed.), Heinemann, London, pp. 1–75.

Podlaha, O., Eriksson, Å., & Toregård, B. (1978). An investigation of the basic conditions for tocopherol determination in vegetable oils and fats by differential pulse polarography. *J. Am. Oil Chem. Soc.*, **55**, 530–2.

Ponchon, G. & Fellers, F. X. (1968). Thin-layer chromatography of vitamin D and related sterols. *J. Chromat.*, **35**, 53–65.

Poole, C. F. & Schuette, S. A. (1984). *Contemporary Practice of Chromatography*, Elsevier, Amsterdam, Oxford, New York and Tokyo.

Quackenbush, F. W. (1973). Use of heat to saponify xanthophyll esters and speed analysis for carotenoids in feed materials: collaborative study, *J. Ass. off. analyt. Chem.*, **56**, 748–53.

Quackenbush, F. W. & Smallidge, R. L. (1986). Nonaqueous reverse phase liquid chromatographic system for separation and quantitation of provitamins A. *J. Ass. off. analyt. Chem.*, **69**, 767–72.

Rammell, C. G. & Hoogenboom, J. J. L. (1985). Separation of tocols by HPLC on an amino–cyano polar phase column. *J. Liquid Chromat.*, **8**, 707–17.

Rammell, C. G., Cunliffe, B. & Kieboom, A. J. (1983). Determination of alpha-tocopherol in biological specimens by high-performance liquid chromatography. *J. Liquid Chromat.*, **6**, 1123–30.

Reynolds, S. L. (1984). The use of HPLC in the determination of fat-soluble vitamins in a variety of milk-based food products. In *Developments in Applications of High Performance Liquid Chromatography to the Analysis of Foods*, Royal Soc. Chem. Symp., September, 1984, pp. 43–50.

Reynolds, S. L. & Judd, H. J. (1984). Rapid procedure for the determination of vitamins A and D in fortified skimmed milk powder using high-performance liquid chromatography. *Analyst, Lond.*, **109**, 489–92.

Rhys Williams, A. T. (1980). *Fluorescence Detection in Liquid Chromatography*, Perkin–Elmer, Beaconsfield.

Rhys Williams, A. T. (1985). Simultaneous determination of serum vitamin A and E by liquid chromatography with fluorescence detection. *J. Chromat. Biomed. Appl.*, **341**, 198–201.

Roels, O. A. (1967). Vitamins A and carotene. 4. Occurrence in foods. In *The*

Vitamins, 2nd edn, Vol. I (W. H. Sebrell, Jr & R. S. Harris, eds), Academic Press, New York, pp. 113–21.

Roels, O. A. & Mahadevan, S. (1967). Vitamin A. In *The Vitamins*, 2nd edn, Vol. VI (P. György & W. N. Pearson, eds), Academic Press, New York, pp. 139–97.

Russell Eggitt, P. W. & Ward, L. D. (1953). The chemical estimation of vitamin-E activity in cereal products. 1. The tocopherol pattern of wheat-germ oil. *J. Sci. Fd Agric.*, **4**, 569–79.

Ryan, T. H. (ed.) (1984). *Electrochemical Detectors. Fundamental Aspects and Analytical Applications*, Plenum Press, New York.

Schudel, P., Mayer, H. & Isler, O. (1972). Tocopherols. 2. Chemistry. In *The Vitamins*, 2nd edn, Vol. V (W. H. Sebrell, Jr & R. S. Harris, eds), Academic Press, New York, pp. 168–217.

Schwieter, U. & Isler, O. (1967). Vitamins A and carotene. 2. Chemistry. In *The Vitamins*, 2nd edn, Vol. I (W. H. Sebrell, Jr & R. S. Harris, eds), Academic Press, New York, pp. 5–99.

Scott, M. L. (1978). Vitamin E. In *Handbook of Lipid Research*, Vol. II (H. F. DeLuca, ed.), Plenum Press, New York, pp. 133–210.

Scott, R. P. W. (1986). *Liquid Chromatography Detectors*, 2nd edn, Journal of Chromatography Library, Vol. 33, Elsevier, Amsterdam, Oxford, New York and Tokyo.

Seifert, R. M. (1979). Analysis of vitamin K_1 in some green leafy vegetables by gas chromatography. *J. agric. Fd Chem.*, **27**, 1301–4.

Senyk, G. F., Gregory, J. F. & Shipe, W. F. (1975). Modified fluorometric determination of vitamin A in milk. *J. Dairy Sci.*, **58**, 558–60.

Sertl, D. C. & Molitor, B. E. (1985). Liquid chromatographic determination of vitamin D in milk and infant formula. *J. Ass. off. analyt. Chem.*, **68**, 177–82.

Shaikh, R., Huang, H. S. & Zielinski, W. L., Jr (1977). High performance liquid chromatographic analysis of supplemental vitamin E in feed. *J. Ass. off. analyt. Chem.*, **60**, 137–9.

Shaw, W. H. C. & Jefferies, J. P. (1957). The determination of vitamin D and related compounds. *Analyst, Lond.*, **82**, 8–18.

Shearer, M. J. (1983). High-performance liquid chromatography of K vitamins and their antagonists. *Adv. Chromat.*, **21**, 243–301.

Shearer, M. J. (1986). Vitamins. In *HPLC of Small Molecules—a Practical Approach* (C. K. Lim, ed.), IRL Press, Oxford, pp. 157–219.

Shearer, M. J., Allan, V., Haroon, Y. & Barkhan, P. (1980). Nutritional aspects of vitamin K in the human. In *Vitamin K Metabolism and Vitamin K-Dependent Proteins* (J. W. Suttie, ed.), University Park Press, Baltimore, pp. 317–27.

Shen, C-S. J. & Sheppard, A. J. (1986). A rapid high-performance liquid chromatographic method for separating tocopherols. *J. Micronutr. Anal.*, **2**, 43–53.

Sheppard, A. J., La Croix, D. E. & Prosser, A. R. (1968). Separation of vitamins D_2 and D_3 as isotachysterols D_2 and D_3 by gas–liquid chromatography. *J. Ass. off. analyt. Chem.*, **51**, 834–8.

Sheppard, A. J., Prosser, A. R. & Hubbard, W. D. (1971). Gas chromatography of vitamin E. *Meth. Enzym.*, **18C**, 356–65.

Sheppard, A. J., Prosser, A. R. & Hubbard, W. D. (1972). Gas chromatography of the fat-soluble vitamins: a review. *J. Am. Oil Chem. Soc.*, **49**, 619–33.

Simpson, C. F. (ed.) (1982). *Techniques in Liquid Chromatography*, John Wiley & Sons, Chichester.

Simpson, K. L. (1983). Relative value of carotenoids as precursors of vitamin A. *Proc. Nutr. Soc.*, **42**, 7–17.

Simpson, K. L., Tsou, S. C. S. & Chichester, C. O. (1985). Carotenes. In *Methods of Vitamin Assay*, 4th edn (J. Augustin, B. P. Klein, D. Becker & P. B. Venugopal, eds), John Wiley, New York, pp. 185–220.

Sivell, L. M., Bull, N. L., Buss, D. H., Wiggins, R. A., Scuffam, D. & Jackson, P. A. (1984). Vitamin A activity in foods of animal origin. *J. Sci. Fd Agric.*, **35**, 931–9.

Sklan, D. & Budowski, P. (1973). Simple separation of vitamins D from sterols and retinol by argentation thin-layer chromatography. *Analyt. Chem.*, **49**, 200–1.

Slover, H. T. (1980). Nutrient analysis by glass capillary gas chromatography. In *Nutrient analysis of foods: the state of the art for routine analysis*, Proc. Nutrient Analysis Symp., 93rd Ann. Meet. Ass. Off. Analyt. Chem., Washington, DC, Oct. 15–18th, pp. 25–42.

Slover, H. T., Lehmann, J. & Valis, R. J. (1969a). Vitamin E in foods: determination of tocols and tocotrienols. *J. Am. Oil Chem. Soc.*, **46**, 417–20.

Slover, H. T., Lehmann, J. & Valis, R. J. (1969b). Nutrient composition of selected wheats and wheat products. III. Tocopherols. *Cereal Chem.*, **46**, 635–41.

Slover, H. T., Thompson, R. H., Jr & Merola, G. V. (1983). Determination of tocopherols and sterols by capillary gas chromatography. *J. Am. Oil Chem. Soc.*, **60**, 1524–8.

Slover, H. T., Thompson, R. H., Jr, Davis, C. S. & Merola, G. V. (1985). Lipids in margarines and margarine-like foods. *J. Am. Oil Chem. Soc.*, **62**, 775–86.

Snyder, L. R. (1974). Classification of the solvent properties of common liquids. *J. Chromat.*, **92**, 223–30.

Snyder, L. R. (1978). Classification of the solvent properties of common liquids. *J. chromatogr. Sci.*, **16**, 223–34.

Snyder, L. R. & Kirkland, J. J. (1979). *Introduction to Modern Liquid Chromatography*, 2nd edn, John Wiley & Sons, Inc., New York.

Söderhjelm, P. & Andersson, B. (1978). Simultaneous determination of vitamins A and E in feeds and foods by reversed phase high-pressure liquid chromatography. *J. Sci. Fd Agric.*, **29**, 697–702.

Speek, A. J., Schrijver, J. & Schreurs, W. H. P. (1984). Fluorimetric determination of menadione sodium bisulphite (vitamin K_3) in animal feed and premixes by high-performance liquid chromatography with post-column derivatization. *J. Chromat.*, **301**, 441–7.

Speek, A. J., Schrijver, J. & Schreurs, W. H. P. (1985). Vitamin E composition of some seed oils as determined by high-performance liquid chromatography with fluorometric detection. *J. Fd Sci.*, **50**, 121–4.

Speek, A. J., Temalilwa, C. R. & Schrijver, J. (1986). Determination of β-carotene content and vitamin A activity of vegetables by high-performance liquid chromatography and spectrophotometry. *Fd Chem.*, **19**, 65–74.

Stancher, B. & Zonta, F. (1982). High performance liquid chromatographic determination of carotene and vitamin A and its geometric isomers in foods. Applications to cheese analysis. *J. Chromat.*, **238**, 217–25.

Stancher, B. & Zonta, F. (1984). High-performance liquid chromatography of the unsaponifiable from samples of marine and freshwater fish: fractionation and identification of retinol (vitamin A_1) and dehydroretinol (vitamin A_2) isomers. *J. Chromat.*, **287**, 353–64.

Stancher, B., Zonta, F. & Bogoni, P. (1987). Determination of olive oil carotenoids by HPLC. *J. Micronutr. Anal.*, **3**, 97–106.

Stewart, I. (1977). Provitamin A and carotenoid content of citrus juices. *J. agric. Fd Chem.*, **25**, 1132–7.

Strohecker, R. & Henning, H. M. (1966). *Vitamin Assay—Tested Methods* (Translated by D. D. Libman), Verlag Chemie, Weinheim.

Subramanyam, G. B. & Parrish, D. B. (1976). Colorimetric reagents for determining vitamin A in feeds and foods. *J. Ass. off. analyt. Chem.*, **59**, 1125–30.

Suttie, J. W. (1984). Vitamin K. In *Handbook of Vitamins. Nutritional, Biochemical and Clinical Aspects* (L. J. Machlin, ed.), Marcel Dekker, Inc., New York, pp. 147–98.

Suttie, J. W. (1985). Vitamin K. In *Fat-Soluble Vitamins. Their Biochemistry and Applications* (A. T. Diplock, ed.), Heinemann, London, pp. 225–311.

Sweeney, J. P. & Marsh, A. C. (1971). Effect of processing on provitamin A in vegetables. *J. Am. diet. Ass.*, **59**, 238–43.

Syväoja, E-L., Salminen, K., Piironen, V., Varo, P., Kerojoki, O. & Koivistoinen, P. (1985). Tocopherols and tocotrienols in Finnish foods: fish and fish products. *J. Am. Oil Chem. Soc.*, **62**, 1245–8.

Syväoja, E. L., Piironen, V., Varo, P., Koivistoinen, P. & Salminen, K. (1986). Tocopherols and tocotrienols in Finnish foods: oil and fats. *J. Am. Oil Chem. Soc.*, **63**, 328–9.

Takeuchi, A., Okano, T., Teraoka, S., Murakami, Y. & Kobayashi, T. (1984). High-performance liquid chromatographic determination of vitamin D in foods, feeds and pharmaceuticals by successive use of reversed-phase and straight-phase columns. *J. Nutr. Sci. Vitaminol.*, **30**, 11–25.

Taylor, P. & Barnes, P. (1981). Analysis for vitamin E in edible oils by high performance liquid chromatography. *Chemy Ind.*, 17th October, 722–6.

Taylor, R. F. & Ikawa, M. (1980). Gas chromatography, gas chromatography–mass spectrometry, and high-pressure liquid chromatography of carotenoids and retinoids. *Meth. Enzym.*, **67**F, 233–61.

Thompson, J. N. (1982). Trace analysis of vitamins by liquid chromatography. In *Trace Analysis*, Vol. II (J. F. Lawrence, ed.), Academic Press, New York, pp. 1–67.

Thompson, J. N. (1986). Problems of official methods and new techniques for analysis of foods and feeds for vitamin A. *J. Ass. off. analyt. Chem.*, **69**, 727–38.

Thompson, J. N. & Hatina, G. (1979). Determination of tocopherols and tocotrienols in foods and tissues by high performance liquid chromatography. *J. Liquid Chromat.*, **2**, 327–44.

Thompson, J. N. & Maxwell, W. B. (1977). Reverse phase high pressure liquid chromatography of vitamin A in margarine, infant formula, and fortified milk. *J. Ass. off. analyt. Chem.*, **60**, 766–71.

Thompson, J. N., Erdody, P., Brien, R. & Murray, T. K. (1971). Fluorometric determination of vitamin A in human blood and liver. *Biochem. Med.*, **5**, 67–89.

Thompson, J. N., Erdody, P. & Maxwell, W. B. (1972a). Chromatographic separation and spectrophotofluorometric determination of tocopherols using hydroxyalkoxypropyl Sephadex. *Analyt. Biochem.*, **50**, 267–80.

Thompson, J. N., Erdody, P., Maxwell, W. B. & Murray, T. K. (1972*b*). Fluorometric determination of vitamin A in dairy products. *J. Dairy Sci.*, **55**, 1077–80.

Thompson, J. N., Maxwell, W. B. & L'Abbe, M. (1977). High pressure liquid chromatographic determination of vitamin D in fortified milk. *J. Ass. off. analyt. Chem.*, **60**, 998–1002.

Thompson, J. N., Hatina, G. & Maxwell, W. B. (1979). Determination of vitamins E and K in foods and tissues using high performance liquid chromatography. In *Trace Organic Analysis: A New Frontier in Analytical Chemistry* (H. S. Hertz & S. N. Chesler, eds), National Bureau of Standards Special Publication 519, Washington, DC.

Thompson, J. N., Hatina, G. & Maxwell, W. B. (1980). High performance liquid chromatographic determination of vitamin A in margarine, milk, partially skimmed milk, and skimmed milk. *J. Ass. off. analyt. Chem.*, **63**, 894–8.

Thompson, J. N., Hatina, G., Maxwell, W. B. & Duval, S. (1982). High performance liquid chromatographic determination of vitamin D in fortified milks, margarine and infant formulas. *J. Ass. off. analyt. Chem.*, **65**, 624–31.

Thompson, S. Y. (1975). *Vitamin A in Animal Nutrition*, F. Hoffmann–La Roche & Co. Ltd, Basle, Switzerland.

Truswell, A. S. (1985). ABC of nutrition. Vitamins 2. *Br. Med. J.*, **291**, 1103–6.

Tsen, C. C. (1961). An improved spectrophotometric method for the determination of tocopherols using 4,7-diphenyl-1, 10-phenanthroline. *Analyt. Chem.*, **33**, 849–51.

Tsukida, K. & Saika, K. (1970). Determination of vitamins D by gas–liquid chromatography. I. Differentiation and assay of vitamins D_2 and D_3. *J. Vitam.*, **16**, 293–6.

Ueda, T. & Igarashi, O. (1985). Evaluation of the electrochemical detector for the determination of tocopherols in feeds by high-performance liquid chromatography. *J. Micronutr. Anal.*, **1**, 31–8.

Ueda, T. & Igarashi, O. (1987). New solvent system for extraction of tocopherols from biological specimens for HPLC determination and the evaluation of 2,2,5,7,8-pentamethyl-6-chromanol as an internal standard. *J. Micronutr. Anal.*, **3**, 185–98.

Usher, C. D., Favell, D. J. & Lavery, H. (1968). A method for the determination of vitamin A, α- and β-carotene in margarine, including the results of a collaborative test. *Analyst, Lond.*, **93**, 107–10.

van Niekerk, P. J. & Smit, S. C. C. (1980). The determination of vitamin D in margarine by high performance liquid chromatography. *J. Am. Oil Chem. Soc.*, **57**, 417–21.

Vecchi, M., Vesely, J. & Oesterhelt, G. (1973). Applications of high-pressure liquid chromatography and gas chromatography to problems in vitamin A analysis. *J. Chromat.*, **83**, 447–53.

Vecchi, M., Schmid, M., Walther, W. & Gerber, F. (1981). Determination of the diastereomers of vitamin K_1. *J. High Resolut. Chromat. Commun.*, **4**, 257–9.

Vetter, W., Vecchi, M., Gutmann, H., Rüegg, R., Walther, W. & Meyer, P. (1967). Gas chromatographic and mass spectrometric investigation of phytylubiquinone, vitamin K_1 and vitamin K_2. *Helv. chim. Acta*, **50**, 1866–79. (German text).

Vickrey, T. M. (ed.) (1983). *Liquid Chromatography Detectors*, Marcel Dekker, Inc., New York.

Vivilecchia, R. V., Lightbody, B. G., Thimot, N. Z. & Quinn, H. M. (1977). The use of microparticulates in gel permeation chromatography. *J. chromatogr. Sci.*, **15**, 424–33.

Waltking, A. E., Kiernan, M. & Bleffert, G. W. (1977). Evaluation of rapid polarographic method for determining tocopherols in vegetable oils and oil-based products. *J. Ass. off. analyt. Chem.*, **60**, 890–4.

Weber, E. J. (1984). High performance liquid chromatography of the tocols in corn grain. *J. Am. Oil Chem. Soc.*, **61**, 1231–4.

Whittle, K. J. & Pennock, J. F. (1967). The examination of tocopherols by two-dimensional thin-layer chromatography and subsequent colorimetric determination. *Analyst, Lond.*, **92**, 423–30.

Wickroski, A. F. & McLean, L. A. (1984). Improved reverse phase liquid chromatographic determination of vitamins A and D in fortified milk. *J. Ass. off. analyt. Chem.*, **67**, 62–5.

Widicus, W. A. & Kirk, J. R. (1979). High performance liquid chromatographic determination of vitamins A and E in cereal products. *J. Ass. off. analyt. Chem.*, **62**, 637–41.

Wiggins, R. A. (1976). Chemical analysis of vitamins A, D and E. *Proc. analyt. Div. chem. Soc.*, **13**, 133–7.

Wiggins, R. A. (1978). The chemical determination of vitamin D in food. *J. Sci. Fd Agric.*, **29**, 991–2.

Wilson, P. W., Kodicek, E. & Booth, V. H. (1962). Separation of tocopherols by gas–liquid chromatography. *Biochem. J.*, **84**, 524–31.

Wilson, P. W., Lawson, D. E. M. & Kodicek, E. (1969). Gas liquid chromatography of ergocalciferol and cholecalciferol in nanogram quantities. *J. Chromat.*, **39**, 75–7.

Winkler, V. W. (1973). Collaborative study of a gas–liquid chromatographic method for the determination of water-soluble menadione (vitamin K_3) in feed premixes. *J. Ass. off. analyt. Chem.*, **56**, 1277–80.

Winkler, V. W. & Yoder, J. M. (1972). Direct gas–liquid chromatographic determination of water-soluble vitamin K_3 in feed premixes. *J. Ass. off. analyt. Chem.*, **55**, 1219–22.

Woollard, D. C. (1987). Quality control of the fat-soluble vitamins in the New Zealand dairy industry. *Fd Technol. Aust.*, **39**, 250–3.

Woollard, D. C. & Blott, A. D. (1986). The routine determination of vitamin E acetate in milk-powder formulations using high-performance liquid chromatography. *J. Micronutr. Anal.*, **2**, 97–115.

Woollard, D. C. & Fairweather, J. P. (1985). The storage stability of vitamin A in fortified ultra-high temperature processed milk. *J. Micronutr. Anal.*, **1**, 13–21.

Woollard, D. C. & Indyk, H. (1986). The HPLC analysis of vitamin A isomers in dairy products and their significance in biopotency estimations. *J. Micronutr. Anal.*, **2**, 125–46.

Woollard, D. C. & Woollard, G. A. (1981). Determination of vitamin A in fortified milk powders using high performance liquid chromatography. *NZ Jl Dairy Sci. Technol.*, **16**, 99–112.

Woollard, D. C., Blott, A. D. & Indyk, H. (1987). Fluorometric detection of tocopheryl acetate and its use in the analysis of infant formulae. *J. Micronutr. Anal.*, **3**, 1–14.

Yamaoka, M., Tanaka, A. & Kato, A. (1985). Antioxidative activity of tocotrienols. *Yukagaku*, **34**, 120–2.

Yeung, E. S. (ed.) (1986). *Detectors for Liquid Chromatography*, John Wiley & Sons, New York.

Zakaria, M., Simpson, K., Brown, P. R. & Krstulovic, A. (1979). Use of reversed-phase high-performance liquid chromatographic analysis for the determination of provitamin A carotenes in tomatoes. *J. Chromat.*, **176**, 109–17.

Zandi, P. & McKay, J. E. (1976). Determination of tocopherols in soybean oil using fractional crystallisation. *J. Sci. Fd Agric.*, **27**, 843–8.

Ziffer, H., Vanden Heuvel, W. J. A., Haahti, E. O. A. & Horning, E. C. (1960). Gas chromatographic behaviour of vitamins D_2 and D_3. *J. Am. Chem. Soc.*, **82**, 6411–12.

Zonta, F. & Stancher, B. (1983). High performance liquid chromatography of tocopherols in oils and fats. *Riv. ital sostanze grasse*, **60**, 195–9.

Zonta, F. & Stancher, B. (1985). Quantitative analysis of phylloquinone (vitamin K_1) in soy bean oils by high-performance liquid chromatography. *J. Chromat.*, **329**, 257–63.

Zonta, F., Stancher, B. & Bielawny, J. (1982). Separation and identification of vitamins D_2 and D_3 and their isomers in food samples in the presence of vitamin A, vitamin E and carotene. *J. Chromat.*, **246**, 105–12.

Glossary of Terms used in High-Performance Liquid Chromatography

k, *the solute capacity factor*: is a measure of a solute's retention, corrected for the void volume. It is defined as the ratio of the quantity of solute in the stationary phase to the quantity in the mobile phase. A permeating but non-sorbed solute has a k value of zero; the k value increases by one for each column volume needed to elute the solute. A k value of 8–10 means that the solute takes a long time to elute. For rapid analyses a low k value is desired, while for complex separations a high k value is needed. The compromise is a k value of 2–6.

α, *the separation factor or selectivity*: is a measure of how well two peaks are separated, and is defined as the relative retention of two solutes by the stationary phase. The actual separation of two peaks in a chromatogram is not adequately described by α alone, since it does not contain any information about peak widths. The higher the value of α, the greater is the separation between two solutes. If α is 1·0 then the separation between two solutes is zero.

$\varepsilon°$, *the solvent strength parameter*: is defined as the adsorption energy per unit area of standard adsorbent, and is a useful means of quantifying polarity in liquid–solid (adsorption) chromatography. The stronger or more polar solvents (high $\varepsilon°$ values) provide low retention times (small k values), whereas weaker or more non-polar solvents give large k values. For a given solute and adsorbent, log k varies linearly with $\varepsilon°$. All values of $\varepsilon°$ are relative to the value for pentane, which is taken to be zero. Hydrocarbons have low values of $\varepsilon°$ (hexane = 0·01), ethers have medium values (diisopropyl ether = 0·28), and alcohols have very high values (methanol = 0·95).

Specific surface area: can be separated into two components; the surface area within the pores and the external surface area of the particle. Irregular packings will have a greater external surface area than spherical particles. The pore surface area is several orders of magnitude larger than the external surface area and, in general, the larger the surface area of the packing material, the smaller will be the pore diameter. Commercial HPLC silica packings used for fat-soluble vitamin assays in foods have surface areas ranging from 170–500 m^2/g; and pore diameters ranging from 60–125 Å.

Specific pore volume: is defined as the amount of liquid that fills the total volume of the pores per gram of adsorbent, and ranges between 0·7–0·9 cm^3/g.

Index